DATE DUE

AP 20 '09			
MR 30 '00			
MY 7 '00			
NO 09 '00			
AP 15 '02			
MY 6 '02			
MY 28 '02			
OC 7 '02			
NO 15 '04			

DEMCO 38-296

OSTEOPOROSIS

CURRENT ◊ CLINICAL ◊ PRACTICE

OSTEOPOROSIS

DIAGNOSTIC AND THERAPEUTIC PRINCIPLES

Edited by

CLIFFORD J. ROSEN, MD

*Maine Center for Osteoporosis Research
and Education, St. Joseph Hospital, Bangor, Maine*

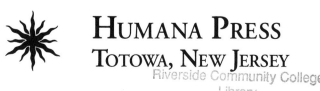

HUMANA PRESS
TOTOWA, NEW JERSEY

© 1996 Humana Press Inc.
999 Riverview Drive, Suite 208
Totowa, New Jersey 07512

For additional copies, pricing for bulk purchases, and/or information about other Humana titles,
contact Humana at the above address or at any of the following numbers: Tel.: 201-256-1699;
Fax: 201-256-8341; E-mail: humana@interramp.com

This publication is printed on acid-free paper. ∞
ANSI Z39.48-1984 (American National Standards Institute) Permanence of Paper for Printed Library Materials.

Printed in the United States of America. 10 9 8 7 6 5 4 3 2 1

ISBN 0-89603-374-0

FOREWORD

Lawrence G. Raisz, MD

Division of Endocrinology and Metabolism,
University of Connecticut Health Center, Farmington, CT

The rapid transfer of new knowledge concerning the pathogenesis, diagnosis, prevention, and treatment of disease into clinical practice has always been a major challenge in medicine. This challenge is particularly difficult to meet in osteoporosis, not only because there has been so much new knowledge generated in recent years, but also because this disorder has not caught the attention of many practicing physicians. The goal of this volume is to help primary care physicians develop a better understanding of osteoporosis and a more effective approach to diagnosis, prevention, and treatment. As primary care physicians become more and more responsible for the maintenance of health and the prevention of disease, osteoporosis must become one of their important concerns.

The magnitude of the problem of osteoporosis has been widely publicized. Within the next 30 years, the cost of hip fractures alone is expected to exceed $40 billion a year in the United States and will be a major cause of increased mortality. In addition, vertebral crush fractures will cripple more and more of our elderly population, both men and women. This enormous toll is not inevitable. Current methods of identifying individuals at risk and applying preventive programs could reduce the incidence of fractures by 50% or more. This should be the minimum goal of clinicians. We must identify and apply the principles and practices that will achieve a substantial reduction in fracture incidence and disability at a manageable cost. This will only occur if there is an effective dialog between health care providers and those who are developing new approaches in osteoporosis.

There are other reasons for the substantial lag between the development of new knowledge and its application in osteoporosis. One important reason is that there are many areas of controversy. For example, there is still no general agreement about the role of screening for osteoporosis or the costs and benefits of hormone replacement therapy. We still are not sure about the relative efficacy of different nonhormonal forms of treatment. This book will neither fully resolve nor avoid these controversies, but try to provide guidance to the practicing physicians so that they can select the best alternatives for their patients. As pointed out by Guyatt, we do not yet have the necessary information from extensive prospective clinical trials that are available for other common disorders, for example, in the treatment of hypertension. This is a common situation in medicine. Physicians make decisions based on limited knowledge, but they can make better decisions if they have ready access to the knowledge that is currently available. The aim of this book is to provide that knowledge as well as the opinions of individuals who have worked extensively in this field. Thus, it will help the reader become acquainted with the fundamental principles of bone biology, as well as the current understanding of pathogenetic mechanisms, clinical features, and therapy of osteoporosis.

One of the most controversial topics is diagnosis. It is easy to diagnose osteoporosis in a patient with fractures. This is accomplished to a great extent by ruling out other disorders that can mimic or aggravate osteoporosis. A more difficult, but potentially more important, approach is to diagnose osteoporosis before fractures occur. Diagnostic criteria have been developed based on bone density, but there is not general agreement about the populations to be screened. Part III on "The Diagnosis of Osteoporosis" provides guidelines for the clinical use of bone densitometry, while Part V provides a series of "clinical scenarios," which cover many of the situations that the clinician is likely to encounter in diagnosis as well as management.

How will this book be most useful to the clinician? First, a careful initial reading will provide primary care physicians with a general understanding of osteoporosis and alert them to considering this disorder as part of their routine evaluation of postmenopausal women and go back again and again to review the practical aspects of clinical interpretation of bone densitometry and the treatment options described here. Finally, the clinical scenarios will provide practical approaches to a number of the situations that clinicians encounter repeatedly. In using these scenarios, it is important that clinicians recognize not only the similarities, but the subtle variations in presentation among different patients and use the breadth of opinion presented here to develop an appropriate plan of management.

Though we can provide a solid basis for clinical practice, its effectiveness will depend on the commitment of primary care physicians not only to recognize this important clinical problem, but also to keep up with this rapidly changing field. This is particularly true for such topics as "Alternative Methods of Measuring Bone Mass" and "Biochemical Markers of Bone Turnover." New developments in these areas are occurring rapidly and could evolutionize our approach to screening and diagnosis.

In addition, an increasing number of therapeutic options will soon become available. New bisphosphonates and alternatives to estrogen as well as other agents are undergoing clinical trials. These fresh approaches have already resulted in novel FDA-approved drugs for the prevention and treatment of osteoporosis. Thus, throughout this text, the authors have tried to provide the basis for evaluating new as well as established approaches. Though fully confident that this first edition will be useful to its readers for some time, I nonetheless expect that it will require revision in time. The preparation of such a second edition will be guided not only by new developments in the field, but also by the comments and criticisms of our readers. Thus, we hope that everyone who uses this book will think about ways that it can be made clearer and more useful and communicate their ideas to the Editor.

PREFACE

In the mid-1990s, the ultimate challenge facing health care providers is the quest for comprehensive treatments for chronic diseases within a framework of reduced patient access and limited financial resources. Osteoporosis is one of those diseases. Basic and molecular studies of the skeletal remodeling system have produced a wealth of new information about the osteoporotic process. Clinical studies employing new "bone specific" agents have generated tremendous enthusiasm for newer therapeutic options, as well as providing a greater understanding of the spectrum of metabolic bone diseases. This expanded knowledge base has set the stage for even greater technological thrusts aimed at earlier diagnoses and cost-effective treatments.

A simultaneous revolution in the provision of American health care will crest well into the next century. This tide will produce more primary care physicians, but reduce the number of specialists and subspecialists. Additionally, because of limited financial resources, there will be less opportunity for patients to seek consultations with "bone" specialists. At the same time, the potential for universal coverage will mean that more patients will enter the medical system earlier in the course of their disease. The complexity of care inherent in our delivery system, coupled with the flourishing of primary care physicians, will present a major challenge for the proper management of chronic diseases. On the other hand, if we are to make a dent in the rising incidence of osteoporosis, the battle should be carried to the forefront of medicine—the offices of primary care providers.

The treatment of osteoporosis always begins with the message of prevention. This theme is stressed in our metabolic bone clinic, whether for an 18-year-old girl with a strong family history, or a 90-year-old man in a nursing home. To accomplish prevention on a broader scale will require a tremendous educational effort, aimed not only at patients, but also at primary care providers. Currently, little time is spent on the care and treatment of patients with osteoporosis in the medical education process. For example, in medical schools two weeks or less are committed to teaching the physiology of the musculoskeletal system. Needless to say, within that time frame, studying rare genetic and metabolic syndromes occupies a more prominent place than understanding a very common disorder. In postgraduate training programs the situation is not much better. Osteoporosis is rarely discussed since it is primarily an "outpatient" disease. Often, when studied, this disorder is considered part of the "aging" process, not as a separate pathophysiological disorder. Finally, in subspecialty training, the management of metabolic bone disease crosses many lines, thereby diluting its essence. Yet care of the osteoporotic women is the province of rheumatologists, endocrinologists, gynecologists, internists, family practitioners, physician extenders, nurse practitioners, and orthopedic surgeons.

The inspiration for *Osteoporosis: Diagnostic and Therapeutic Principles* came from discussions, consultations, and lectures with primary care providers across the country. Everywhere I traveled, providers agreed that a need existed for a clinically oriented book about osteoporosis that would provide in-depth coverage of areas not often taught or reviewed. Specifically, the sections on therapeutic intervention and interpretation of bone densitometry are a direct result of hundreds (maybe thousands) of questions from providers at grand rounds and dinner meetings. The design of the treatment section was also the result of input by family physicians and internists who felt the need, not to index drugs, but rather to work through clinical scenarios. The extensive effort focusing on quality of life and nondrug treatment options resulted from input by Drs. McClung, Stock, Miller, and Ms. Love McClung and Ovedorff, members of a "quality of life" study group. The section on clinical decision making by Dr. Guyatt represents a bold attempt to have clinicians use an evidence-based approach to treat cases of osteoporosis. The physiology and pathophysiology of this disease is complex and overwhelming. Therefore, I have added a glossary of terms in hopes of providing clarity to some very difficult issues.

Osteoporosis: Diagnostic and Therapeutic Principles is an effort to educate primary care providers, students, house staff, endocrinologists, gynecologists, rheumatologists, and orthopedic surgeons about the pathogenesis and treatment of osteoporosis. The contributors to this book were carefully chosen not for their fame or number of publications, but because they were first and foremost clinicians—doctors who see patients with osteoporosis. Yet, each author is, in his or her own right, a distinguished academician.

It is my fervent hope that *Osteoporosis: Diagnostic and Therapeutic Principles* will help ensure that the proper evaluation and treatment of patients with osteoporosis can be conducted by health care providers from all medical disciplines. Only through this mechanism can osteoporosis ultimately be prevented.

Clifford J. Rosen

CONTENTS

PART V. CASE PRESENTATIONS

CONTRIBUTORS

ROBERT A. ADLER, MD • *McGuire Veterans Affairs Medical Center; and Medical College of Virginia, Virginia Commonwealth University, Richmond, VA*

JOHN J. B. ANDERSON, PhD • *Professor of Nutrition, University of North Carolina, Chapel Hill, NC*

DANIEL T. BARAN, MD • *Professor of Orthopedic Surgery and Medicine, University of Massachusetts Medical Center, Worcester, MA*

SYDNEY LOU BONNICK, MD, FACP • *Texas Women's University, Denton, TX*

JULIE GLOWACKI, PhD • *Brigham and Women's Hospital, Boston, MA*

GORDON H. GUYATT, MD, MSc, FRCPC • *McMaster University, Hamilton, Ontario, Canada*

MICHAEL F. HOLICK, PhD, MD • *Vitamin D, Skin and Bone Research Laboratory, Endocrinology Section, Department of Medicine, Boston University Medical Center, Boston, MA*

CATHY R. KESSENICH, DScN • *Maine Center for Osteoporosis Research and Education, St. Joseph Hospital, Bangor, ME*

DOUGLAS P. KIEL, MD, MPH • *Harvard Medical School Division on Aging; and Hebrew Rehabilitation Center for Aged Research and Training Institute, Boston, MA*

MICHAEL KLEEREKOPER, MD • *Department of Internal Medicine, Wayne State University School of Medicine, Detroit, MI*

ROBERT F. KLEIN, MD • *Bone and Mineral Research Unit, Portland VA Medical Center, Oregon Health Sciences University, Portland, OR*

ROBERT M. LEVIN, MD • *Boston City Hospital, Boston, MA*

ROBERT MARCUS, MD • *The Aging Study Unit, Geriatrics Research, Education and Clinical Center, VA Medical Center, Palo Alto, CA; and Department of Medicine, Stanford University School of Medicine, Stanford, CA*

BETSY LOVE MCCLUNG, RN, MN • *Oregon Osteoporosis Center, Providence Medical Center, Portland, OR*

MICHAEL R. MCCLUNG, MD, FACE • *Oregon Osteoporosis Center, Portland, OR*

PETER S. MILLARD, MD, PhD • *Eastern Maine Medical Center, Bangor, ME*

PAUL D. MILLER, MD, FACP • *University of Colorado Health Sciences Center, Lakewood, CO*

ERIC S. ORWOLL, MD • *Bone and Mineral Research Unit, Portland VA Medical Center, Oregon Health Sciences University, Portland, OR*

JUDITH H. OVERDORF, RN, MPH • *Division of Endocrinology, The Medical Center of Central Massachusetts, Worcester, MA*

LAWRENCE G. RAISZ • *Division of Endocrinology and Metabolism, University of Connecticut Health Center, Farmington, CT*

CLIFFORD J. ROSEN, MD • *Maine Center for Osteoporosis Research and Education, St. Joseph Hospital, Bangor, ME*

KRISTI SPENCER, PT • *Wilsonville Physical Therapy, Wilsonville, OR*

JOHN L. STOCK, MD • *Medical Center of Central Massachusetts, Worcester, MA*

RICHARD WASNICH, MD • *Hawaii Osteoporosis Center, Honolulu, HI*

I

SKELETAL PHYSIOLOGY AND ITS RELEVANCE TO OSTEOPOROSIS

1

The Cellular and Biochemical Aspects of Bone Remodeling

Julie Glowacki, PhD

1. REMODELING OF BONE TISSUE

Metabolic bone diseases are fundamentally disorders of bone remodeling. Bone remodeling is the highly integrated process of resorption and successive formation of bone tissue that results in the maintenance of skeletal mass with renewal of the mineralized matrix. This is accomplished by focal cell-mediated degradation and regeneration of bone tissue without compromising the overall architecture of the anatomy of bones (Fig. 1). The remodeling sites are known as basic multicellular units (BMUs). The renewal of bone tissue occurs through orchestrated cycles of activity called Activation-Resorption-Formation (ARF). The first step is activation of quiescent osteoclasts and precursors that begin to excavate a cavity on a bony surface. After an amount of time, osteoblast precursors are activated and refill the excavation site. Under ideal conditions, the amount of bone fill equals the amount resorbed, with no net change in the volume of bone. Consequently, the molecular composition of the adult skeleton is not static, but it changes as new bone fills each excavation site.

This continuous process of internal turnover endows bone with a capacity for true regeneration in response to injury. Physiological remodeling has its counterpart in the selective resorptive and synthetic activities that occur spontaneously in injured bone. The principles of rigid fixation and compression fixation accelerate internal bridging of bone by orienting the resorptive wave and osteogenic regeneration across the fissure. In addition to and related to the bone's capacity for scarless repair, incorporation of bone

From: *Osteoporosis: Diagnostic and Therapeutic Principles*
Edited by: C. J. Rosen Humana Press Inc., Totowa, NJ

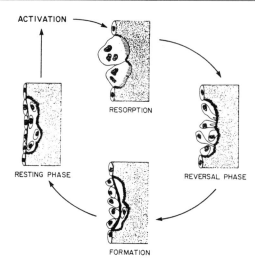

Fig. 1. Cellular events during the bone remodeling sequence. Reprinted with permission from Baron et al. (1983).

grafts and osteointegration with metallic implants rely to varying degrees on oriented tunneling and osteogenesis. The mechanisms of coupling the resorptive and synthetic processes in four dimensions are not fully understood, but they are at the heart of understanding pathophysiological states in which they are uncoupled.

The consequences of remodeling are easily appreciated by comparison with acellular (or anosteocytic) bone that many marine fish produce. In those species, bone is secreted as a nonvital structure like a hair or fingernail. Such bone lacks metabolic activity. It is capable of growth by surface accretion but does not undergo remodeling. As a result, such skeletons do not contribute to mineral homeostasis, and they are not capable of true regeneration in response to injury. These findings lend some insight into the origin and function of internal bone remodeling. A central function appears to be the acute provision of mineral for metabolic needs. The architecture and cellularity of bone are well adapted to accomplish this with great efficiency without compromising mechanical strength. The admirable Darwinian success with which cellular vertebrate bone accomplishes these tasks should not be devalued as pathophysiological mechanisms of metabolic bone diseases, such as osteoporosis, are considered.

The accurate measurement of bone turnover is fundamental for diagnosis and evaluation of treatment for disorders of bone metabolism. Bone biopsy was introduced in the 1960s as an investigative procedure for quantitative evaluation of histological parameters of resorption and formation. The anterior iliac crest is the standard biopsy site. Measures of trabecular bone volume, unmineralized osteoid volume, bone resorption and formation surfaces, and osteoclast numbers are important static indices of bone condition. Dynamic measure of mineral apposition rate requires administration of two doses of tetracycline prior to biopsy. The antibiotic binds to sites of calcification, and the width of the gap between the labels reflects the calcification rate between the two doses. Other measures of bone turnover discussed below have become useful once they have been correlated with these direct histomorphometric indices.

2. THE FUNCTIONS OF BONE

In many vertebrates, the skeleton has two unique and major functions: mechanical and metabolic. The mechanical function provides the structural framework for the organism that permits support, locomotion, and protection of organs. The metabolic function of skeletal tissue consists of storage of calcium that can be mobilized when needed for vital bodily functions, including clotting of body fluids, neuromuscular irritability, growth and regeneration, maintenance of mucous coverings, intercellular contacts, and ameboid and ciliary motion. Phosphate and other ions are also stored in bone. Another important, but not unique, function of the skeleton is as a site for hematopoiesis. Bone tissue is well suited to accomplish all these diverse functions. The mechanical properties of bone result from the combined properties of the components of its extracellular matrix. The extracellular matrix is composed of organic osteoid (primarily collagen type I) and an organic mineral phase, largely in the form of a poorly crystalline hydroxyapatite. Central to understanding metabolic bone diseases is the fact that in pathological situations, the mechanical functions of the skeleton may be sacrificed in order to maintain mineral homeostasis within the organism or to respond to factors integral to this maintenance.

Calcium homeostasis is tightly regulated in humans by parathyroid hormone (PTH), 1,25-dihydroxyvitamin D, and calcitonin (CT). These calcitropic hormones regulate calcium levels in serum by actions on bone, intestine, and kidney. Other ions, hormones, and target tissues are involved in mineral homeostasis. It is helpful to reduce this complexity to the key elements concerned with control of three ions (calcium, magnesium, and phosphate) with three hormones (PTH, CT, and 1,25-dihydroxyvitamin D) acting on three target tissues (intestine, kidney, and bone). Calcium and phosphate enter the blood from the intestine, are removed through the kidney, and are stored in bone. None of these is continuous, each is bidirectional depending on dietary intake, and each is modulated by the calcitropic hormones. Nutritional and lifestyle factors that strain this system's campaign for mineral homeostasis can increase the drain on skeletal reserves, and increase the risk of osteopenia and fracture. From the perspective of the bone tissue, decreased dietary intake of calcium, for example, would favor efflux of mineral at the expense of bone formation and renewal. Being calcium-replete, however, may not impede inevitable loss of bone with age.

PTH increases bone resorption, and it increases calcium reabsorption in the kidney. It regulates intestinal absorption of calcium indirectly by enhancing 1-hydroxylation of 25-hydroxyvitamin D in the kidney. The active hormone, 1,25-dihydroxyvitamin D, increases renal reabsorption of calcium and increases intestinal calcium absorption. It has complex effects on bone cells, increasing some functions of osteoblasts (osteocalcin and alkaline phosphatase synthesis) and decreasing others (collagen synthesis). It promotes the differentiation of osteoclasts. Calcitonin can be thought of as the antihypercalcemic hormone; it inhibits resorption of bone. It inhibits renal reabsorption of calcium and also increases the production of 1,25-dihydroxyvitamin D.

Other hormones affect calcium and skeletal homeostasis in complex ways. Growth hormone, insulin, and sex hormones have important anabolic effects on skeletal growth, whereas glucocorticoids can inhibit both formation and resorption directly. Glucocorticoids also increase resorption by direct stimulation of PTH secretion and by secondary hyperparathyroidism through impaired intestinal absorption of calcium.

Prostaglandins and cytokines stimulate bone resorption, and may mediate bone loss in inflammatory, neoplastic, and other states.

3. THE STRUCTURE OF BONES

3.1. Cortical and Cancellous (Trabecular) Bone

The long bones of the skeleton consist of a thick and dense outer layer or cortex of compact bone of which 90% by volume is calcified. The flat bones (cranial bones, scapula, mandible, ileum) are bicortical with a variable amount of space between the two layers of dense cortical bone. This type of bone is well suited for the mechanical and protective functions of the skeleton.

The internal spaces of the vertebrae, the ileum, and the ends of long bones, in particular, are filled with a network of calcified trabeculae that comprise cancellous bone. Only 15–25% of the volume of trabecular bone is calcified tissue, the remainder being marrow, connective, or fatty tissue. Thus, cancellous bone is porous, lighter than cortical bone, and contains expansive surfaces covered with cells.

3.2. Woven and Lamellar Bone

At the microscopic level, two main types of osseous tissue can be distinguished. In woven bone, there is a higher volume ratio of cells to matrix, and the matrix is either homogeneous or composed of coarse fibers condensed in angular woven patterns. It is observed during active growth periods, in fracture callus, in heterotopic osteogenesis like myositis ossificans, and in osteosarcomas. It is considered to be immature or provisional, to be replaced by more organized bone.

Lamellar bone is best appreciated with polarized light microscopy as multilayered matrix synthesized by orderly accretion in parallel sheets or as osteons, with concentric plates surrounding a blood vessel. Cell density is lower than in woven bone, but these cells are interconnected by cellular processes in radiating canaliculi that can be visualized in suitably prepared specimens. Darkly staining cement lines bounding osteons represent a unit of newly synthesized bone that has replaced older bone. Remodeling through resorption and formation around Haversian canals is the key to understanding the osteonal system. Osteons are branching interconnected structures that are the architectural units of cortical bone. This longitudinal tunneling can overlap multiple osteons, resulting in the mosaic of partial osteons and irregular pieces of interstitial bone that are the remnants of former osteons removed during remodeling. Not all osteons are equally mineralized. Quantitative microradiography shows that younger osteons can contain only 70% of the mineral in older ones. Knowing that mineral crystallinity and insolubility increase with time, one can speculate that remodeling serves to rejuvenate the more readily exchangeable mineral reserve. An alternate view is that normal bone remodeling evolved to repair microdamage inflicted on the tissue by normal wear and tear. The remarkable feature of this tissue is that it accomplishes both of these functions with precision and fidelity.

3.3. Endochondral or Membranous Development

Several mechanisms of bone development contribute to embryonic and postnatal skeletal growth. The limb bones and axial skeleton develop from a cartilaginous template within which ossification occurs. This is termed endochondral ossification. In contrast, membranous ossification is the simpler and possibly most primitive form of osteogenesis. The term refers to the embryonic condensations of fibrocellular mesenchyme that precedes the appearance of bony specules. The vault of the skull, clavicle, maxilla, mandible, and facial bones are formed in this way.

4. THE COMPOSITION OF BONE TISSUE

4.1. Cellular Components

The cells of bone are responsible for mediating the direction and magnitude of flow of minerals into and out of stored skeletal reserves. Bone is also rich in nerves, blood vessels, and marrow. The bone cell population consists of osteoblasts, osteocytes, and osteoclasts. Monocytes/macrophages and mast cells may also serve unique functions in bone. Cell division is restricted to progenitor cells that differentiate into osteoblasts and osteoclasts under appropriate stimuli.

Osteoblasts are derived from progenitor cells of mesenchymal origin. They are mononucleated cells characterized by cytoplasmic organelles that are typical of secretory cells, namely abundant rough endoplasmic reticulum and a large Golgi zone. Their major functions are to synthesize and secrete collagen and proteoglycan complexes that constitute osteoid, and to play a role in matrix mineralization. At least two products of the osteoblast, alkaline phosphatase and bone γ-carboxyglutamic acid-containing protein (BGP or osteocalcin), may be involved in mineralization. It is also likely that, because they cover many surfaces of the bony trabeculae, osteoblasts may regulate the movement of ions in and out of bone fluid. It has also been shown that the osteoblast is capable of mediating the stimulation of bone resorption by agents, such as PTH. Under certain conditions in embryogenesis, the osteoblast may resorb osteoid from bone surfaces prior to mineralization. Hormones that increase bone formation include growth hormone, thyroid hormones, androgens, insulin, vitamin D metabolites, and, under conditions of low dose and interrupted delivery, parathyroid hormone. Glucocorticoids are potent inhibitors of osteoblastic activity

Osteoblasts form a layer of cells on bone surfaces, and they are connected by tight junctions, most abundant in growing animals. The productivity of osteoblasts has been estimated in rapidly growing rats and rabbits as the rate of 170 μm of matrix/d. This is considered 170 times faster than the rate of matrix apposition in adult humans, or 100 μm^3 of matrix volume/d and 1 μm/d of appositional bone formation.

Available biochemical assays for monitoring bone formation rely on the measurement of either osteoblastic enzymes that escape into serum or fragments of structural macromolecules that are byproducts of matrix synthesis. Nondialyzable urinary hydroxyproline is an example of the latter, but is not convenient for routine use. There are several reliable serum markers of bone formation, including bone-specific alkaline phosphatase, osteocalcin (or BGP), and procollagen I extension peptides (carboxyterminal). Although these markers are byproducts of osteoblastic activity and are increased with skeletal growth, they are also increased in conditions that are characterized by increased bone turnover, such as primary and secondary hyperparathyroidism, hyperthyroidism, Paget's disease, and acromegaly. Serum osteocalcin is an index of osteoblastic activity, but also is correlated with bone loss because in these conditions, bone formation and resorption are coupled at an accelerated rate of turnover. Menopause also induces an acceleration in bone turnover that is reflected in a significant increase in serum osteocalcin.

When an osteoblast completely surrounds itself within matrix, it is called an osteocyte, residing in a lacuna within the mineralized matrix, but maintaining cytoplasmic connections with other osteocytes and with surfaced osteoblasts. This network of cells and processes in bone canaliculi provides continuity with the vascular circulation. This anatomical arrangement results in a very high surface area of interaction between the osteocytic network and bone matrix. The main function of the osteocyte is to maintain minute-to-minute exchange of mineral in the bone matrix. This function is mediated through the acres of surface area presented by their cytoplasmic extensions.

Osteocytes also serve as transducers of mechanical loading on bone. The piezoelectric property of bone matrix allows for transmission of load throughout the skeleton. How this is sensed by the osteocyte and osteoblasts is the subject of intense investigation. Simply stated, "Wolff's Law" describes the mathematical relationship between the form and function of bone. It is the cells of bone that respond to external forces, compression and tension, and effect changes in the internal architecture of bony trabeculae to provide maximum resistance to these forces. Thus, superfluous bits of bone are removed, and new bone is deposited without loss of function to transform the bone's anatomy. Functional induction of new architecture is seen clearly in the eventual smoothing of a fracture that has healed with displacement.

Osteoclasts are large, multinucleated cells found on the surface of bone and in Howship's lacunae. They are the major cells responsible for bone resorption and remodeling, containing a variable number of nuclei (often 20 or more) and vacuolated cytoplasm. The osteoclastic cytoplasm is abundant with lysosomes that contain lytic enzymes. Osteoclasts possess calcitonin receptors and are profoundly inhibited by this hormone. At the ultrastructural level, osteoclasts are characterized by membrane specializations called ruffled borders and clear zones of attachment or sealing to underlying bone matrix. This sealing ring encloses a compartment between the cell and the bone. The osteoclast progenitor cell is related to the hematopoietic stem cell, and its differentiation is similar to that of the macrophage and foreign body giant cell. Osteoclastic bone resorption is stimulated by PTH, 1,25-dihydroxyvitamin D, and by local regulators, such as interleukin-1 and prostaglandin E2. Osteoclastic bone resorption is inhibited by calcitonin.

Osteoclastic bone resorption is accomplished by the activity of four major enzyme systems: carbonic anhydrase, the proton pump, calcium-dependent ATPase, and the sodium/potassium pump. The polarized secretion of hydrogen ions into the compartment between the osteoclast and bone delineated by the clear or sealing zone of attachment promotes the solubilization of calcium from the bone surface. Once the bone has been decalcified, acid proteases can degrade the organic fraction of bone.

Because the skeleton contains approx 60% of the body collagen, the amount of collagen breakdown products in a 24-h urine sample has been taken as a measure of bone destruction. In adults, the majority of hydroxyproline in the urine is derived from degradation rather than synthesis. Gelatin-containing food must be avoided during a hydroxyproline test period. Values >21 mg/g creatinine suggest increased loss of skeletal mass. Thus, increased urinary hydroxyproline is associated with bone resorption diseases, such as hyperthyroidism, Paget's disease of bone, metastatic bone disease, and hyperparathyroidism.

Because hydroxyproline is a constituent of collagen in nonskeletal tissue, this test has limited sensitivity and specificity. Newer assays have been developed for measurement of more specific breakdown products of bone collagen crosslinks. Urinary pyridinoline and deoxypyridinoline crosslink assays have recently become widely available for diagnosis, prognosis, and monitoring response to therapies for metabolic bone diseases.

4.2. Bone Extracellular Matrix

The osteoblast produces sheets of oriented collagen in lamellae. The organic phase of bone is termed osteoid and is comprised of collagen fibers that are produced by the self-aggregation of individual collagen molecules secreted by the osteoblast. With maturation of collagen fibrils, intermolecular crosslinks covalently render the collagen fibrils less soluble. Proteoglycans and hyaluronan comprise the ground substance in the organic matrix of bone, also produced by the osteoblast. The glycoproteins of bone include osteonectin (SPARC, BM-40), osteocalcin (BGP), matrix Gla-containing protein (MGP), and the so-called RGD proteins osteopontin, fibronectin, thrombospondin, and bone sialoprotein. Minor components of the bone matrix include serum proteins, proteolipids, and growth factors. Factors or activities produced by bone or isolated from the bone matrix include insulin-like growth factor-II, transforming growth factor-β, insulin-like growth factor-I (regulated), platelet-derived growth factor, basic fibroblast growth factor (bFGF), acidic fibroblast growth factor (aFGF), bone-derived growth factor β-2 (micro-globulin), IGF-binding proteins, bone morphogenic agents, and cytokines.

The rigidity of bone is provided by the mineralized fraction. Bone hydroxyapatite is an imperfect crystal of calcium phosphate salt($Ca_{10}[PO_4]_6[OH]_2$), having substitutions by magnesium, sodium, strontium, carbonate, citrate, and fluoride. The hydroxyapatite crystal structure within bone has a high surface area capable of exchange with the extracellular fluid compartment.

There are several theories to explain the mineralization of organic matrix of bone. Several of the organic components of the bone matrix have been shown to posses nucleating sites capable of precipitating mineral in vitro: collagen, Gla-containing proteins, phosphoproteins, glycoproteins, acidic phospholipids, and proteolipids. This is considered the catalytic nucleation mechanism. Alkaline phosphatase contributes to mineralization by increasing the local concentrations of inorganic phosphate above the critical ion product to cause spontaneous precipitation of hydroxyapatite. Alkaline phosphatase also contributes to mineralization by inactivating inhibitors of crystal growth, e.g., pyrophosphate. Serum alkaline phosphatase is elevated in situations of increased bone formation, for example, Paget's disease of bone, osteoblastic carcinoma, and hypercalcemic hyperparathyroidism, and in situations of failed mineralization, for example, in rickets and in osteomalacia. Normal mineralization is impaired in vitamin D-deficiency, aluminum intoxication, fluoride intoxication, and phosphate deficiency.

Mineralization of matrix begins in two different ways. In lamellar bone and in dentin, the early mineral crystals appear within collagen fibrils. In woven bone and in cartilage, mineralization begins within membrane-bound matrix vesicles in the extracellular tissue space.

A third mechanism of biomineralization is displayed by enamel tissue. Enamel production begins with the formation of low-mol-wt amelogenins and high-mol-wt enamelin. Mineralization of enamel begins with the breakdown and selective loss of these proteins coincident with the formation of apatite crystals. Mature enamel has the least organic component, 1% by weight, of all mineralized tissues. (Dentin contains 20% organic component and bone contains 25%.) Enamel mineral is considered the most crystalline of the biological apatites, having larger and less strained crystals than in dentin or bone. As a result, dissolution of dentin and bone is relatively easier than of enamel. Mineralization of enamel is impaired in amelogenesis imperfecta.

Once formed by these nucleation processes, hydroxyapatite crystals will autocatalytically promote further crystal formation at calcium/phosphate ion products at or even below adult human levels. This point is like "Lot's Wife Problem." What prevents us from turning into pillars of hydroxyapatite? The thermodynamic answer lies in the naturally occurring ionic and macromolecular inhibitors in the extracellular fluid. Although the mechanisms regulating the composition of this fluid are not completely understood, the most important physiological substances that stop crystal growth are pyrophosphate, citrate, Mg^{2+}, and some of the proteoglycans, glycoproteins, and proteins of bone matrix. Tetracycline, Sr^{2+}, and bisphosphonates are potent nonphysiologic inhibitors of mineralization.

Several therapeutic modalities involve interactions with mineralization mechanisms. In fluoride treatment, the fluoride anion substitutes for hydroxide in the mineral crystal, thereby increasing crystal size and decreasing solubility. Bisphosphonate treatment for Paget's disease is based on the incorporation of this pyrophosphate analog into the abnormally small crystals that characterize this disease. By increasing crystal size, mineral solubility is decreased. Gallium nitrate treatment for humoral hypercalcemia of malignancy is another example of pharmacological increase in mineral crystal size and resultant decrease in mineral solubility. Another clinical problem benefited by understanding of the mechanisms of mineralization was osteomalacia associated with hemodialysis. The mystery was solved when aluminum was identified in bone biopsies from these patients. Aluminum from dialysis fluids accumulated into newly precipitated mineral crystals, preventing further mineralization. Corrective measures were introduced to monitor aluminum levels in these solutions. This example and the use of tetracycline to label acutely a new mineral point out the dynamic and continuous nature of skeletal mineralization in the adult.

5. CELLULAR PATHOPHYSIOLOGY IN METABOLIC BONE DISEASES

5.1. Diseases in Which the Primary Abnormality Is Increased Bone Resorption

5.1.1. OSTEOPOROSIS

Osteoporosis is the most frequently occurring metabolic bone disease and is particularly common in elderly women. Although a gradual decline in bone mass occurs with aging in both men and women, osteoporosis results from an exaggeration of the imbalance between resorption and formation. In 1982, Riggs characterized two distinct syndromes of involutional osteoporosis. Type I (also called high-turnover) osteoporosis occurs in postmenopausal women between the ages of 50 and 65, is associated with accelerated loss of trabecular bone and therefore with mainly vertebral fractures, and is pathogenetically related to estrogen deficiency. Type II (also called low-turnover) osteoporosis afflicts both men and women predominantly over the age of 75, involves both trabecular and cortical bone, results in hip and vertebral fractures, and is attributed to an age-related decline in osteoblast function superimposed on the lower bone mass that results from decades of imbalance between resorption and formation. It is important to note that calcium metabolism of most patients with osteoporosis is normal compared with that of normal subjects of a similar age. Calcium deficiency may be a contributory factor in some cases, but is not the sole or principal factor in most cases.

A number of hormonal factors have been implicated in the pathogenesis of osteoporosis. It is curious that, in most reports, there are no differences between postmenopausal women with osteoporosis and normal subjects in plasma concentrations of gonadal steroids and gonadotropins. In some studies, differences have been reported in levels of testosterone, progesterone, sex hormone-binding protein, and dehydroepiandrosterone.

An etiological role in osteoporosis has been postulated for PTH, 1,25 dihydroxyvitamin D, and calcitonin. Because of the lack of universal differences in these hormones, it is likely that osteoporosis comprises a heterogeneous group of skeletal disorders, and that both sex hormones and calcitropic hormones are important in pathogenesis.

What is clear is that dysregulation of balanced bone turnover by the coordinated activities of bone-producing osteoblasts and bone-resorbing osteoclasts lies at the heart of this devastating disease.

Diseases that may predispose to the development of osteoporosis are hyperthyroidism, hyperparathyroidism, Cushing's disease, Addison's disease, paralysis, chronic obstructive lung disease, intestinal malabsorption, renal dysfunction, malignancy, diabetes mellitus, pregnancy, and rheumatoid arthritis. A number of drugs are associated with osteoporosis, and include corticosteroids, thyroid hormone, anticonvulsants, aluminum-containing antacids, heparin, immunosuppressants, and some antihypertensive medications.

5.1.2. PAGET'S DISEASE

Paget's disease is characterized by excessive and abnormal remodeling of bone, usually localized in one region of the skeleton, such as the skull, pelvis, or ends of long bones, but occasionally widespread. The primary abnormality is in osteoclastic resorption. Osteoclasts are abundant in affected tissue, may assume bizarre shapes, and may contain up to 100 nuclei/cell. These cells present an advancing resorptive front with a circular form in the skull (osteoporosis circumscripta) or an arrowhead shape in long bones. An intense osteoblastic reaction follows the resorptive activity. The excessive bone that is produced has the irregular pattern of woven bone. Incomplete osteons and irregular cement lines result in a mosaic histological quality. Active sites are highly vascular, but in time, the disease process slows down, burns out, and leaves dense sclerotic bone with little evidence of cellular activity.

The stimulus for increased numbers and activity of osteoclasts has not been definitively identified, but inclusions resembling viral nucleocapsids and antigens of the measles and respiratory syncytial virus have been identified in Pagetic osteoclasts.

The architecture of Pagetic bone is not well suited for mechanical support. Although fracture healing appears to be normal, the bone is subject to deformity. Pain, degenerative arthritis, and secondary neurological abnormalities are some of the serious sequelae of Paget's disease.

The biochemical abnormalities of Paget's disease are direct consequences of increased bone turnover. The net exchange of bone calcium is usually normal however.

5.1.3. OSTEITIS FIBROSA CYSTICA

Osteitis fibrosa cystica is the bone disease resulting from parathyroid hormone excess. Increased osteoclastic activity leads to radiolucency, bone cysts, fractures, and deformities. Osteocytic lacunae appear enlarged. As a compensatory response, osteoblastic activity is increased with a patchy distribution. Increased bone turnover and hypercalcemia are found in all patients.

5.1.4. HUMERAL HYPERCALCEMIA OF MALIGNANCY (HHM)

Hypercalcemia accompanying malignant disease is more commonly the result of generalized increased bone resorption than to metastasis. Squamous carcinomas (lung, esophagus, cervix, vulva, skin, head, and neck), renal, bladder, and ovarian carcinomas, and some breast carcinomas can function as classical endocrine glands because they secrete humoral calcemic factors that act on the skeleton and kidney. Currently, HHM describes a specific clinical syndrome owing to the production of parathyroid hormone-related protein, PTHrP.

Bone lesions in HHM differ from those resulting from hyperparathyroidism in that osteoblasts are not increased in HHM. In some manner, osteoblastic activity is uncoupled from the stimulated osteoclasts. Another difference is that osteoclastic bone resorption accounts for hypercalcemia in HHM, whereas in hyperparathyroidism, hypercalcemia is the result primarily of effects on the kidney and intestine.

Tumors have been reported to produce a variety of other factors that can stimulate osteoclastic bone resorption, such as PTH itself, osteoclast activating factor (OAF or interleukin-1), prostaglandins, especially of the E2 series, and other osteolytic sterols and peptides.

5.2. Diseases in Which the Primary Abnormality Is Increased Bone Formation

Paget's disease is often diagnosed by its focal osteoclerotic changes, but this bone formation is a process secondary to the osteolytic phase. That is also the case for hyperparathyroidism.

High exposure to fluoride in water or from industrial contamination produces significant increases in bone density with coarsening and thickening of bony trabeculae, periosteal new bone formation, and spinal osteophytosis. The sclerotic bone is lamellar, with increased osteocytes and prominent cement lines. Muscles, ligaments, and tendons are also prone to calcifications. Fluorosis often affects the teeth, with mottling of the enamel.

In acromegaly, the excess of growth hormone, both directly and indirectly, produces new subperiosteal bone growth, which may not be accompanied by equivalent bone resorption.

5.3. Diseases in Which the Primary Abnormality Is Decreased Bone Resorption

5.3.1. OSTEOPETROSIS

Osteopetrosis is a rare, inherited disorder with abnormally dense bone throughout the skeleton. The autosomal recessive form is fatal, and the autosomal dominant forms are more benign. Although there may be different forms of the disease in humans, bone resorption is reduced because of either reduced numbers or reduced activity of osteoclasts. In the most severe form, the dense bone is deficient in marrow and results in anemia. Others problems include compression of cranial nerves, optic atrophy and blindness, hearing loss, and abnormal dentition. Although dense, the bones are structurally weak and they fracture readily. It is surprising that fractures heal satisfactorily. Marrow transplantation and treatment with 1,25-dihydroxyvitamin D are both designed to increase differentiation of osteoclasts, and have had some success.

5.3.2. HYPOPARATHYROIDISM

In hypoparathyroidism, deficiency of PTH results in decreased osteoclastic activity, which in turn results in decreased osteoblastic activity. Radiographic bone findings are usually normal, but decreased metabolic activity is revealed by calcium kinetic and biochemical studies.

5.4. Diseases in Which the Primary Abnormality Is Decreased Bone Formation

5.4.1 OSTEOMALACIA

In children, deficient mineralization of the skeleton is called rickets. In adults, it is called osteomalacia. In both, it can result from deficiency of the factors important in bone formation: calcium, phosphorus, 1,25-dihydroxyvitamin D, or alkaline phosphatase. There are a variety of abnormalities of vitamin D that can result in osteomalacia. Although dietary deficiency of vitamin D is rare in the US, malabsorption disorders or impairment of renal activation of vitamin D (both congenital or acquired) results in osteomalacia.

In young patients, undermineralized cartilage confers structural weakness to the skeleton. Manifestations include flattening of the skull and pelvis, bowing of the legs, and splaying of epiphyses. Cartilaginous ends of the ribs can become protuberant (called the rosary of rickets). In adults, the most common symptom is bone pain. Radiographic features are generalized osteopenia and telling lucent areas, Looser's zones, perpendicular to the long axis of the bone. Histologic examination of undecalcified biopsies reveals thick layers of osteoid on most, if not all the bone surfaces.

5.4.2. RENAL OSTEODYSTROPHY

Renal osteodystrophy occurs in chronic and advanced renal failure. It has 2 principal components: osteitis fibrosa cystica due to secondary hyperparathyroidism and osteomalacia due to deficiency of 1,25-dihydroxyvitamin D production. The pathogenesis of these features is that phosphate retention leads to secondary hyperparathyroidism and the decreased renal hydroxylation of vitamin D. Calcium supplementation and phosphate restriction are designed to suppress the parathyroid glands, whereas vitamin D supplementation corrects the deficiency of activated hormone and promotes mineralization.

6. RATIONALES OF TREATMENTS FOR OSTEOPOROSIS

The overall goal is to identify individuals at risk for osteoporosis and provide them with a safe, effective, and inexpensive intervention to prevent development of the disease. Because of the heterogeneity of factors known to contribute to osteoporosis and the unknown genetic components of disease risk, there is insufficient information available at this time to embark on such a public health plan.

Because of the importance of peak bone mass on subsequent bone mineral density with aging, attention is being paid to determining measures that can optimize bone mass in teenagers. At the present, exercise and nutritional factors are emphasized.

Preventative measures have been proposed for menopausal women at increased risk. Modifiable nutrition/lifestyle factors include reduction of alcohol, salt, caffeine, and the excessive consumption of animal protein, and elimination of cigaret consumption. Adequate calcium intake has been advocated, although there is little evidence about the effects of calcium intake on the rate of bone loss. Likewise, exercise may be a threshold issue of importance within a normally accepted range.

Some women display accelerated rates of bone loss on estrogen withdrawal by the natural menopause. The central question to be answered is why all women do not develop osteoporosis with advanced age. It appears that all women display accelerated bone loss on ovariectomy. Well-designed studies consistently show that estrogens reduce bone loss as long as treatment continues. Furthermore, it has been shown that fracture frequency is reduced with early use of estrogens. Estrogens may protect the skeleton by multiple mechanisms. One way is by stimulation of endogenous calcitonin, which is antiresorptive and inhibits osteoclastic activity. Another is by inhibition of local mediators of osteoclastic differentiation, such as interleukins 1, 6, and 11.

Simply stated, the rationale for treatment of osteoporosis is similar to that for prevention. If only bone resorption is inhibited, however, fracture risk may not be reduced for patients whose bone mass is below the hypothetical fracture threshold. It may be necessary to institute therapy with agents or regimens designed to stimulate bone formation at an earlier stage before the loss of too many osteoblasts and precursors, and before the loss of bony trabeculae on which to accrete new bone.

Many interventional studies with the very elderly have been disappointing, with transient effects, very modest effects, or unacceptable side effects, for example GI disturbances with fluoride therapy. Questions have been raised about the quality of the new bone that has been produced under the influence of fluoride and whether there is a risk of increased brittleness with close-to-effective doses. Another concern is whether fluoride promotes axial bone formation at the expense of peripheral bone. Such concerns are not restricted to fluoride, but may be raised with other agents that become incorporated into new bone.

Modulation of the bone remodeling cycle has been proposed as a strategy for increasing bone mass. It is reasoned that agents that inhibit bone resorption, for example, may be limited in effectiveness if, via the endogenous coupling mechanisms, there follows a period of inhibited bone formation. The design of a coherence treatment strategy follows from our understanding of the remodeling process. The skeleton would be pulsed with an agent to activate bone remodeling units synchronously, for example, PTH or 1,25-dihydroxyvitamin D. This would be followed by an agent to depress bone resorption (calcitonin, estrogen, or bisphosphonates) and produce shallower resorption cavities. Osteoblastic activity could then be left free or stimulated by fluoride to fill or overfill these cavities, achieving positive bone balance. The cycle would be repeated to manipulate the set points for resorption and formation. Although there is currently little evidence for the feasibility of this concept, it is biologically sound and is being tested.

Because treatment of established osteoporosis is theoretically and practically difficult, efforts are directed at preventive measures.

BIBLIOGRAPHY

Andress DL, Maloney NA, Endres DB, et al. Aluminum-associated bone disease in chronic renal failure: high prevalence in a long-term dialysis population. *J Bone Miner Res* 1986; 1: 391–398.

Baron R, Vignery A, Horowitz M. Lymphocytes, macrophages and the regulation of bone remodeling. In: Peck WA, ed. *Bone and Mineral Research Annual 2*, Elsevier, Amsterdam, 1983, pp. 175–243.

Boskey AL. Noncollagenous matrix proteins and their role in mineralization. *Bone and Miner* 1989; 6: 111–123.

Frost HM. Tetracycline-based histological analysis of bone remodeling. *Calcif Tissue Res* 1969; 3: 211–239.

Hercz G, Salusky IB, Norris KC, et al. Aluminum removal by peritoneal dialysis: intravenous vs. intraperitoneal deferioxamine. *Kidney Int* 1986; 30: 944–948.

LeGeros RZ. *Calcium Phosphates in Oral Biology and Medicine*. Basel: Karger, 1991.

Manolagas SC, Jilka RL. Emerging insights into the pathophysiology of osteoporosis. *N Engl J Med* 1995; 332: 305–311.

Mundy GR. Bone resorption and turnover in health and disease. *Bone* 1987; 8: S9–S16.

Pacifici R, Brown C, Puscheck E, et al. The effect of surgical menopause and estrogen replacement on cytokine release from human blood monocytes. *Proc Natl Acad Sci USA* 1991; 88: 5134–5138.

Parfitt AM. Osteonal and hemi-osteonal remodeling: the spatial and temporal framework for signal traffic in adult human bone. *J Cell Biochem* 1994; 55: 273–286.

Riggs BL, Wahner HW, Seeman E, et al. Changes in bone mineral density of the proximal femur and spine with aging: differences between the postmenopausal and senile osteoporosis syndromes. *J Clin Invest* 1982; 70: 716–723.

Sevitt S. *Bone Repair and Fracture Healing in Man.* New York: Churchill Livingstone, 1981.

Shapiro F. Osteopetrosis. Current clinical considerations. *Clin Orthop* 1993; 294: 34–44.

Stevenson JC, Abeyasekera G, Hillyard CJ, et al. Calcitonin and the calcium regulating hormones in postmenopausal women: effect of oestrogens. *Lancet* 1981; i: 693–695.

Wolff J. The classic: concerning the interrelationship between form and function of the individual parts of the organism. *Clin Orthop* 1988; 228: 2–11.

2

The Role of Calcium, Phosphorus, and Macronutrients in the Maintenance of Skeletal Health

John J. B. Anderson, PhD

CONTENTS

CALCIUM
PHOSPHORUS
MACRONUTRIENTS AND ENERGY
CONCLUDING REMARKS
REFERENCES

1. CALCIUM

Dietary calcium intakes by females in the US typically average considerably below the RDAs for calcium, starting at age 11 yr. The RDAs for females (and males) are 1200 mg of calcium/d from 11 through 24 yr and 800 from 25 and onward *(1)*. The NIH Consensus Conference on Calcium in 1994 suggested that calcium intakes should be 1000 mg/d for women beginning at menopause and 1500 for postmenopausal women who are not receiving any form of estrogen replacement therapy *(2)*. Probably most nutritionists are not in agreement with the NIH recommendation of 1500 mg/d because it is practically impossible to obtain compliance with such a high intake from a combination of food consumption plus additional calcium via supplements. Furthermore, the scientific evidence of skeletal benefits in support of a daily recommendation of 1500 mg of calcium alone is not convincing. (Calcium plus vitamin D may be more effective.) No harm, of course, would be anticipated from an intake of 1500 mg/d or even as high as 2000, a value now considered the upper limit of safe intake. (Neither the FDA nor the RDA Committee has published specific amounts of calcium consumption beyond which the safety of consumers would be a concern.)

The remainder of this section on dietary calcium deals with the relationships of typical calcium intakes (i.e., <800 mg a day) of females to the development of peak bone mass (PBM), to the maintenance of bone mass, and to the prevention of loss of bone mass. Issues revolving around behaviors of females relating to selecting healthy choices of calcium-containing foods are also addressed.

From: *Osteoporosis: Diagnostic and Therapeutic Principles*
Edited by: C. J. Rosen Humana Press Inc., Totowa, NJ

1.1. Relationship of Calcium Intake to the Acquisition of PBM

Bone development in early life is determined by many factors, including hereditary, endocrine, and nutritional, as well as other environmental variables, including physical activity. The timing of menarche in girls has a profound effect on bone development and the accumulation of bone mass (as measured by bone mineral content or BMC), because of the short window for growth after the regular production of sex hormones, but both calcium intake and level of physical activity also have strong influences on development of PBM following menarche *(3)*.

Early menarche is associated with high BMC and bone mineral density (BMD), whereas girls with late menarche have lower BMC and BMD values *(4)*. The age of menarche of American females and of those in affluent developed nations, such as Switzerland, has typically been lowered in the past several decades, and also average heights by age 11 yr have increased. Similarly heights achieved by age 18 have also increased, but it is probable that the net gain in height between ages 11 and 18 has improved at a lesser rate than the premenarcheal rate of growth.

Since approx 90% of female BMC and BMD is accumulated by 16 to 18 yr of age *(5,6)*, girls clearly must amass a large amount of their peak bone mass (PBM > during the period from the start of premenarche (roughly ages 9 to 11 in the US and other affluent nations) to the end of their adolescent development. This brief window of 6 yr or so is a critical time for accruing an estimated 40–50% of the PBM, as assessed at age 30. (Calcium balance data also support this timing of PBM accrual at approx age 30 [7].) Calcium intake in adequate amounts during this 6-yr time frame is clearly important, but the few published scientific reports suggest that the premenarcheal skeleton may be more responsive to higher calcium intakes then the peri- or postmenarcheal bone tissue is to calcium supplementation that brings total calcium intakes considerably above the RDA *(8)*. The BMC and BMD gains of postmenarcheal girls resulting from calcium supplements are surprisingly small *(9,10)*. Postmenarcheal girls definitely increase their values of BMC and BMD, but the same high level of calcium intake from supplements is much less effective after menarche and continuing until late in adolescence than among premenarcheal girls *(9,10)*. A prospective study of postpubertal girls from 13 to 17 yr showed gains in BMC and BMD, but not in BMAD (apparent BMD that corrects for increased dimensions or size of the measurement site) *(11)*. During this time, probably the hormones of development dominate the physiology of postmenarcheal growth and, consequently, energy and the macronutrients drive skeletal development and mineralization much more so than the intake of calcium or any other micronutrient *(12)*.

By late adolescence and early adulthood, the positive influence of calcium consumption on skeletal accumulation diminishes considerably, although adequate dietary calcium still remains important, as assessed at age 20 *(3)*. The beneficial effect of calcium intakes at or approximating the age-specific RDAs of women in their 20s and 30s continues, but again at very low rates of gain. Only one prospective investigation supports the concept of significant gains in BMC and BMD by women in the third decade of life *(13)*. Another prospective study of a small number of women demonstrated losses of bone mass as early as the 30s in control subjects, but women (experimental subjects) who received extra servings of calcium-rich foods for a period of a year lost little or no bone mass while supplemented *(14)*. A few cross-sectional studies also support the concept of continuing accrual of BMC and BMD of women during their 20s and even possibly their

30s, but the women in these studies were quite physically active and their bone mass gains could not be determined *(15–19)*.

A study of premenopausal mother–daughter pairs clearly supports the possibility of continuing incremental gains in PBM during the third and possibly even the fourth decades of life, since the mothers (mean age of 44 yr) had almost 10% greater BMC and 5% greater BMD of the radius than their daughters (mean age 18 yr) *(20)*. An explanation for the higher values of the mothers is that they have continued to be physically active after their teens, and they have delivered and raised at least one baby. It is postulated that the lifting and carrying of babies probably contributes to not only increased bone mass but also to better bone because of exercise-induced formation of new bone tissue. Therefore, the timing of PBM could possibly even be pushed back to as late as 40 yr of age in women who maintain optimal calcium intakes and modest but regular levels of physical activity. Most women, however, do not substantially increase their PBM beyond 20 or 25 yr because they do not retain a fairly physically active lifestyle. The greater benefit of exercise compared to adequate intakes of calcium on bone mass development has also been propounded by a report from the Netherlands where average calcium intakes are 300–400 mg a day higher than in the US *(21)*.

Starting at approximately age 40, BMD begins to decline at a low rate of loss in nearly all women, probably as a consequence of diminished physical activity and the decline of ovarian production of estrogens. A cross-sectional investigation of vertebral BMD changes in females between 18 and 44 yr showed no significant decline *(22)*. Starting at about age 40, however, practically all studies of women between 40 yr and the menopause demonstrate minimal declines in both bone mass and density, independent of calcium intake *(23)*. A few reports of upper body strength regimens have shown that total body BMD (or hip BMD) can be maintained by women during this time frame, but the effects of calcium supplementation alone on BMC or BMD have not yet been adequately examined in women in their 30s or 40s.

1.2. Relationship of Calcium Intakes
to the Maintenance of BMD at and Following Menopause

During the menopausal transition, the decline of ovarian estrogen production has a profound adverse effect on skeletal mass (and BMD), as first measured by hand radiogrammetry *(24)* and subsequently by absorptiometric methods. Exogenous calcium supplementation during this period has little effect on bone measurements *(25,26)*. Following the early postmenopause, however, calcium supplements administered to women do exert minimal, positive effects on BMD for periods up to 2 yr *(26–31)*. Most, but not all, studies have shown skeletal benefits of calcium supplementation in postmenopausal women, and a meta-analysis has demonstrated that the majority of investigations have reported positive effects *(32)*. One 5-yr prospective study of a large sample of older postmenopausal women (77–82 yr) on high-calcium intakes (≥RDA), however, reported that these women lost BMC and BMD at the same rate as women on low-calcium intakes (<RDA), independent of other measured variables *(33)*. The high-calcium-consuming women in this study were obtaining practically all of their calcium from foods and relatively little from supplements. Supplementation of elderly nursing home patients in France with both calcium and vitamin D resulted in improved BMD, better indices of bone metabolism, and reduced fractures compared to a control group receiving a placebo *(34)*.

It has been suggested that the act of administering calcium supplements *per se* to elderly subjects, especially in the presence of vitamin D, may stimulate new bone remodeling cycles that last for a period of only a year or so in the renewed accumulation of bone mass, but the new remodeling cycle does result in increased BMC and BMD over this period *(35)*. Whether these gains in bone of elderly women can be retained beyond this transient period, with or without calcium supplementation, remains to be determined.

1.3. Calcium in Foods

Calcium is not abundantly distributed in foods, but dairy products provide good amounts (200–400 mg) in each serving. For adolescents, 3–4 servings/d are required to meet the RDA of 1200 mg/d, whereas for adults 2–3 servings/d are sufficient to yield 800 mg, the current adult RDA.

Relatively few other foods provide calcium in substantial amounts. These foods include dark greens (except for spinach whose calcium is not bioavailable) *(36,37)*, small fish with soft bones, and breads and other baked goods prepared with calcium propionate. In the typical adult American diet, roughly 60% of all calcium is derived from dairy products, about 25% from bakery products, approx 10% from vegetables (dark greens) and fruits, and another 5% from miscellaneous foods.

In comparison to calcium, the distribution of phosphorus is widespread, i.e., in all the major food groups. In fact, calcium distribution (and occasionally availability) from foods is so limited that the food industry has voluntarily undertaken calcium fortification of new products in order to improve the intakes of females *(38)*. Calcium-fortified foods, such as breads and orange juices, are just beginning to have an impact on calcium intakes, but the extent of the benefit of calcium fortification is not yet known.

1.4. Food Habits of Adolescent Girls

The typical food habits of teenage girls supply calcium in amounts much less than the RDA of 1200 mg/d, mainly because girls do not choose dairy products as frequently as recommended (three to four servings each day) to optimize PBM. The behaviors associated with the limited selection of dairy products are complex, but several reasons are given for the avoidance of dairy products. A few of these are the following: Milk and cheese are animal foods, and many young people have become vegans (strict) or partial vegetarians. Dairy products are considered to be high in fat. Milk is not considered "cool" in comparison to cola or other nondairy drinks. Unfortunately, not enough young people understand the important contributions that low-fat dairy products make in nutritional status with respect to calcium, protein, vitamin D, riboflavin, folic acid, vitamin B_{12} (cobalamin), and several other micronutrients *(39,40)*.

The premenarcheal girls clearly need the most calcium to support their robust gains in BMC, and then peri- and postmenarcheal females need sufficient amounts of calcium to support their continued skeletal accrual of the mineral phase of bone tissue. All of these groups of females are the ones that should receive focused nutrition education in order to improve their overall nutritional consumption patterns and their specific inclusion of calcium-rich foods in their diets. Many of the late adolescent females will become pregnant prior to their 20s, and it would be highly desirable for good pregnancy outcomes for them to have good nutritional intakes well before conception.

So many low-fat, or no-fat dairy products are available in the food markets today that females (and males) can readily make healthy food choices for the provision of optimal intakes of calcium and other essential micronutrients. Unfortunately, however, too many young females either do not heed the nutritional knowledge they possess, or else they have not adequately been taught about the nutrient composition of foods, especially calcium-rich foods. Nutrition education toward improving food-related behaviors among young women is greatly deficient in the US.

1.5. Role of Calcium Supplements

Calcium supplementation, often coupled with vitamin D (400–800 IU/d), has become commonplace in the armamentarium of physicians to improve the calcium nutritional status of patients. Prior to recommending a daily dosage of 500 or 1000 mg of calcium, it would be wise to obtain either a 24-h recall of total food and drink consumption of a quick-and-dirty calcium frequency questionnaire based on the commonly consumed calcium-rich foods *(41,42)*.

Other questions of importance are the ascertainment of a "typical" pattern of eating and whether nutrient supplementation is already being used by the patient. If a dietitian-nutritionist is available to administer the questionnaire of choice and to elicit other information about usual dietary practices of the patient, better assurance of optimal dosage of supplemental calcium can be attained. For example, many elderly women on fixed incomes often consume the same foods every day, sometimes including foods designed for animal pets. Calcium-rich foods are frequently not purchased by the elderly because of their short storage time and the need to go to the market frequently.

Many choices of calcium supplements exist, but bioavailable calcium carbonate tablets, if tolerated, remain the most economical sources.

1.6. Summary

Dietary calcium intakes of most American females, and some males, are typically far too low to meet their age-specific RDAs. Recommendations of 1200 (11–24 yr olds) and 800 (>24 yr) can readily be achieved by the appropriate numbers of servings of calcium-rich foods, preferably low-fat dairy products. If these RDAs cannot be met, or even approximated by the consumption of foods, then calcium supplementation at an appropriate dose (250, 500, or 1000 mg/d), with or without vitamin D, should be instituted. Because the scientific data do not support doses higher than those for the specific age categories of the RDAs, it makes no sense to try to push 1500 or 2000 mg of calcium daily, especially to older patients. No harm should result from these extra high doses, although constipation, gagging reflex, and gastrointestinal discomfort have been reported by elderly users of calcium supplements. It should be recalled that high-calcium foods provide many other nutrients in addition to calcium that help the nutritional status of patients, whereas calcium supplements contain only calcium and an anion. Thus, the adage "foods first; supplements second" is worth adhering to in clinical practice.

In addition to adequate calcium intakes by females, a number of reports have supported the benefit of regular physical activity in conjunction with RDA levels of dietary calcium in order to enhance bone mass and to prevent the development of low bone mass *(43)*.

2. PHOSPHORUS

A dietary deficiency of phosphorus is virtually impossible, because this element is found in all foods as an anion or as part of diverse organic molecules. The problem with dietary phosphorus is that Americans consume an excess of this element in relation to calcium, thus skewing the dietary calcium-to-phosphorus (Ca:P) ratio. Although RDAs do exist for phosphorus (and they are identical to those for calcium throughout the life cycle), they are practically meaningless because daily intakes invariably exceed the RDAs *(44)*.

The most important characteristic of high dietary phosphorus consumption, including phosphate additives in many processed foods and cola drinks, is the typically low Ca:P ratio that results. Because so many American foods are processed with phosphates, women (and men) may potentially be placed at risk for the development of osteoporotic fractures because of the low Ca:P ratio of their diets *(38,45)*.

2.1. Calcium:Phosphorus Dietary Ratio and Bone

Few reports have provided data relating the estimated Ca:P ratio of intakes to measurements of BMC and BMD. One recent cross-sectional study has shown a negative contribution of dietary phosphorus to bone mass and density in young adult women, whereas calcium intake had a positive effect on bone *(18)*. Another report suggested that the phosphoric acid in cola drinks may have been responsible for bone fractures in girls who were investigated after their reported fractures *(46)*.

Other experimental investigations have shown that administration of a lower Ca:P diet or of phosphate salts alone will significantly alter calcium homeostasis, but these clinical studies were of too short a duration to demonstrate skeletal effects of the low Ca:P ratios. These reports are reviewed next.

2.2. Role of Phosphorus in Elevating Serum Parathyroid Hormone (PTH)

The human experimental studies using altered Ca:P dietary ratios illustrate how acute and rapid the PTH hormonal response is to the phosphorus (or phosphate) load administered *(47)*. In the five short-term studies reviewed here, lasting from 5 d to 8 wk, PTH concentrations in the blood were significantly elevated when measured at the end of all experiments *(48–52)*. Furthermore, other parameters of calcium homeostasis and bone resorption, when measured, were perturbed in a consistent fashion with elevated PTH concentrations in response to a high-phosphorus load or a low Ca:P ratio of the diet. Typical results (but with some inconsistencies among the studies) were as follows:

1. Plasma 1,25-dihydroxyvitamin D was elevated;
2. Urinary cyclic AMP was elevated;
3. Serum osteocalcin was elevated; and
4. Urinary hydroxyproline was elevated.

Numerous experimental investigations using rodent and other animal models have provided corroborative data on abnormally enlarged parathyroid glands, elevated PTH levels, and severely reduced bone mass following treatment with low Ca:P ratio diets.

2.3. Phosphates as Additives in Foods and Soft Drinks

Since practically all foods contain modest to large amounts of phosphorus and only a few have much calcium, it is reasonable that the dietary ratios will almost always be <1:1 from foods alone (but not if calcium supplements are taken). In fact, the optimal ratios obtained by women in the US who have good diets with respect to calcium and other nutrients range between 0.70 and 0.75. Many women consume diets with Ca:P ratios <0.50 *(45),* and some ingest these minerals at ratios even <0.25, if no dairy products are consumed. These prevalence estimates of intake ratios may be even worse because of the difficulties of accurately determining phosphorus intakes because of the widespread use of phosphate additives in processed foods and cola beverages by food manufacturers. Therefore, the monitoring of the US food supply for phosphorus consumption, with respect to calcium intake, needs to be advanced, so that nutritionists and other scientists can obtain better estimates of total phosphorus intakes from unprocessed foods, processed foods, and beverages *(38,45)*.

2.4. Summary

High-phosphorus intakes are potentially hazardous to bone health because of the development of a mild secondary hyperparathyroidism that may contribute to osteoporosis. Short-term studies have provided convincing data on the adverse effects of high-phosphorus diets on PTH and markers of bone metabolism. Long-term research findings on the effects of an abnormally low Ca:P ratio are not available yet to make strong recommendations, but it is advisable that physicians become aware of the potential adverse effects of a chronic elevation of PTH (even though within the upper level of normal hospital values) and to recommend adequate calcium intakes—at the RDA levels or modestly greater—for all females at any age to counter the high phosphorus levels in the American food supply.

3. MACRONUTRIENTS AND ENERGY

The macronutrients (carbohydrates, fats, and proteins) in foods provide the energy used by our bodies from their C—H bonds after metabolic degradation and entry of the acetyl CoA or carbon-backboned keto acids in the Krebs citric acid cycle. Foods that supply the macronutrients also generally carry the micronutrients (with the exception noted above for calcium) and nonnutrients. Only plants, however, provide the nonnutrients, such as dietary fiber and other phytochemicals.

3.1. Total Energy Intake

The typical amount of energy consumed from foods by an individual is critical for the intakes of the micronutrients in the amounts needed to support numerous cellular and extracellular roles. For example, if too little energy is consumed each day, micronutrient intakes will also be low, unless a broad-spectrum supplement is taken daily.

3.2. Carbohydrate Intake

Except for milk (lactose), almost all the carbohydrates in the diet are provided by starches or their derivatives from plant foods. When complex carbohydrates are consumed from fruits, vegetables, nuts, seeds, and whole-grain cereals, they are accompanied by large amounts of dietary fiber and often also by micronutrients. These plant foods contain fair amounts of phosphorus, but very little calcium.

3.3. Fat Intake

Animal fats and vegetable oils contain essentially no calcium and relatively small amounts of phosphorus that exist in the phospholipids, such as phosphatidylcholine.

3.4. Protein Intake—Animal vs Plant Sources

Protein-rich foods contain fair amounts of phosphorus, but very little calcium, except for dairy products. Plant proteins, such as soybeans and their products, are considered high-quality protein sources because they have protein scores that are equivalent to proteins from meats, fish, and poultry. The animal proteins, however, contain larger amounts of the amino acids, including arginine, that act as hormone (insulin and glucagon) secretagogues following a meal.

The potential adverse effects of high consumption patterns of animal proteins (but not plant proteins) has been investigated in short-term studies. A hypercalciuric action of animal protein or of protein extracts from these foods has now been well established, both acutely and over periods of a few weeks *(53)*. Long-term experimental data of high-protein (animal) dietary patterns on bone measurements are lacking, but they are required to establish with reasonable certainty any adverse role of chronic intakes of animal proteins in the development of osteoporosis. A few reports are reviewed next to illustrate the difficulty of teasing out a negative role of high protein consumption from animal sources on bone mass and density.

3.4.1. STUDIES OF ANIMAL VS PLANT FOODS ON CALCIUM

Several reports have demonstrated adverse effects of high protein intakes from animal sources on calcium retention. A type of *meta*-analysis showed that all but one study abut of almost 20 reports provided data that increases in animal protein induced hypercalciuria *(53)*. Most investigators presumed that the hypercalciuria resulted from chronic ingestion of meals containing large amounts of animal protein *(54–56)*, but one group showed that the protein effect is acute and occurs following any high-protein meal containing animal sources *(57)*. The absence of hypercalciuria after the consumption of soy protein suggests that the effect of animal protein is specific for amino acids found in good amounts in animal, but not plant proteins. The mechanism for the protein-induced hypercalciuria has not been established, but several possibilities exist, including excess acid (H+) production, stimulation of insulin and glucagon, and increased urinary sulfate excretion.

The possibility that such high consumption patterns of animal proteins could contribute to long-term bone losses has been supported by epidemiologic investigations that show adverse effects on BMC and BMD of young adult women who regularly consume high-protein diets *(18)*. One group has even hypothesized that high-protein diets contribute to hip fractures *(58)*.

3.4.2. STUDIES OF THE BONE MASS OF VEGETARIANS (VEGANS)

The role of a vegetarian diet, i.e., plant proteins, on skeletal development, the maintenance of bone mass, and the incidence of fractures, compared to omnivores, has not been thoroughly investigated. A few studies suggest that little difference exists between the late-life declines in BMC and BMD of vegetarian and omnivorous women *(33)*, but additional prospective studies are needed to confirm this observation. The overall diets of the vegetarian women, however, did seem to be healthier than those of the omnivorous women studied *(59)*. Based on the short-term studies reviewed above, one would think that it would be relatively easy to demonstrate adverse long-term effects of high-protein diets, but the critical studies probably have not yet been designed.

3.5. Summary

Of the macronutrients, only high intakes of proteins from animal sources have been implicated as adversely affecting bone mass. Short-term, but not long-term, investigations have demonstrated protein-induced hypercalciuria as a potentially deleterious factor in the development of low bone mass and osteoporosis. Further long-term experiments using specific proteins (e.g., meat, egg white, or lactalbumin) are needed to establish whether a long-term deleterious skeletal effect results from high animal protein consumption pattern.

4. CONCLUDING REMARKS

Several dietary factors, such as excessive intakes of phosphorus and animal protein, may have potential adverse effects on bone development and maintenance, whereas others, especially calcium and vitamin D, have beneficial effects on bone tissue and measurements of BMC and BMD at almost every stage of the life cycle. In addition, several other essential micronutrients probably also are needed at reasonable intake levels on a daily basis for the growth and maintenance of the skeleton. These other nutrients, including vitamins, such as vitamin K, and trace elements, such as fluoride, have not been adequately studied to make any recommendations other than to follow the RDAs for intake guidelines. Finally, the forces impinging on the skeleton from physical activities, including the lifting and handling of infants and children as well as other upper-body-strength exercises, may have strong independent effects on bone measurements throughout life.

REFERENCES

1. Subcommittee on Dietary Allowances, Food and Nutrition Board, National Research Council, *Recommended Dietary Allowances,* 10th ed., Washington, DC: National Academy Press, 1989.
2. NIH Consensus Conference, *Optimal Calcium Intake.* Bethesda, MD, 1995; 272: 1942–1948 (*Also see JAMA,* Dec. 31, 1994).
3. Tylavsky FA, Anderson JJB, Talmage RV, Taft T. Are calcium intakes and physical activity patterns during adolescence related to radial bone mass of white college-age females? *Osteoporosis Int* 1992; 2: 232.
4. Ito M, Yamada M, Hayashi K, Ohki M, Uetani M, Nakamura T. Relation of early menarche to high bone mineral density. *Calcif Tissue Int* 1995; 57: 11–14.
5. Bonjour JP, Theintz G, Buchs B, Slosman D, Rizzoli R. Critical years and stages of puberty for spinal and femoral bone mass accumulation during adolescence. *J Clin Endocrinol Metab* 1991; 73: 555.
6. Theintz G, Buchs B, Rizzoli R, Bonjour J-P. Longitudinal monitoring of bone mass accumulation in healthy adolescents: evidence for a marked reduction after 16 years of age at levels of lumbar spine and femoral neck in female subjects. *J Clin Endocrinol Metab* 1992; 75: 1060.
7. Matkovic V, Heaney RP. Calcium balance during human growth: evidence for threshold behavior. *Am J Clin Nutr* 1992; 55: 992.
8. Johnston CC Jr, Miller JZ, Slemenda CW, Reister TK, Christian JC, Peacock M. Calcium supplementation and increases in bone mineral density in children. *N Engl J Med* 1992; 327: 82.
9. Matkovic V, Fontana D, Tomineac C, Goel P, Chesnut CH III. Factors that influence peak bone mass formation: a study of calcium balance and the inheritance of bone mass in adolescent females. *Am J Clin Nutr* 1990; 52: 878.
10. Lloyd T, Andon MB, Rollings N, Martel JK, Landis JR, Demers LM, Eggli DF, Kieselhorst K, Kulin HE. Calcium supplementation and bone mineral density in adolescent girls. *JAMA* 1993; 270: 841.
11. Katzman DK, Bachrach L, Carter DR, Marcus R. Clinical and anthropometric correlates of bone mineral acquisition in healthy adolescent girls. *J Clin Endocrinol Metab* 1991; 73: 1332–1339.
12. Anderson JJB. The role of nutrition in the functioning of skeletal tissue. *Nutr Rev* 1992; 50: 388.
13. Recker RR, Davies M, Hinders SM, Heaney RP, Stegman MR, Kimmel DB. Bone gain in young adult women. *JAMA* 1992; 268: 2403.
14. Baran D, Sorensen A, Grimes J, Lew R, Karellas A, Johnson B, Roche J. Dietary modification with dairy products for preventing vertebral bone loss in premenopausal women: a three-year study. *J Clin Endocrinol Metab* 1989; 70: 264.
15. Kanders B, Dempster DW, Lindsay R. Interaction of calcium nutrition and physical activity on bone mass in young women. *J Bone Miner Res* 1988; 3: 145.
16. Halioua L, Anderson JJB. Lifetime calcium intake and physical activity habits: independent and combined effects on the radial bone of healthy premenopausal Caucasian women. *Am J Clin Nutr* 1989; 49: 534.

17. Fehily AM, Coles RJ, Evans WD, Elwood PC. Factors affecting bone density in young adults. *Am J Clin Nutr* 1992; 56: 579.
18. Metz J, Anderson JJB, Gallagher PN Jr. Intakes of calcium, phosphorus, protein and level of physical activity are related to radial bone mass in young adult women. *Am J Clin Nutr* 1993; 58: 537.
19. Picard D, Ste.-Marie LG, Coutu D, Carrier L, Chartrand R, Lepage R, Fugere P, D'Amour P. Premenopausal bone mineral content relates to height, weight and calcium intake during early adulthood. *Bone Miner* 1988; 4: 299.
20. Tylavsky FA, Bortz AD, Hancock RL, Anderson JJB. Familial resemblance of radial bone mass between premenopausal mothers and their college-age daughters. *Calcif Tissue Int* 1989; 45: 265.
21. Welten, DC, Kemper HCG, Post GB, Van Mechelen W, Twisk J, Lips P, Teule GJ. Weight-bearing activity during youth is a more important factor for peak bone mass than calcium intake. *J Bone Miner Res* 1994; 9: 1089.
22. Rosenthal DI, Mayo-Smith W, Hayes CW, Khurana JS, Biller BMK, Neer RM, Klibanski A. Age and bone mass in premenopausal women. *J Bone Miner Res* 1989; 4: 533–538.
23. Riggs BL, Wahner HW, Melton LJ Jr, Richelson LS, Judd AJ, O'Fallon WM. Dietary calcium intake and rates of bone loss in women. *J Clin Invest* 1987; 80: 979.
24. Lindsay R, Hart DM, Aitken JM, MacDonald EB, Anderson JB, Claeke AC. Long-term prevention of postmenopausal osteoporosis by oestrogen. *Lancet* 1976; I: 1038–1041.
25. Riis B, Thomsen K, Christiansen C. Does calcium supplementation prevent postmenopausal bone loss? *N Engl J Med* 1987; 316: 173.
26. Dawson-Hughes B, Dallal GE, Krall EA, Sadowski L, Sahyoun N, Tannenbaum S. A controlled trial of the effect of calcium supplementation on bone density in postmenopausal women. *N Engl J Med* 1990; 323: 878–888.
27. Ettinger B, Genant HK, Cann CE. Postmenopausal bone loss is prevented by low-dose estrogen with calcium. *Ann Int Med* 1987; 106: 40.
28. Ooms ME, Lips L, Van Lingen A, Valkenburg HA. Determinants of bone mineral density and risk factors for osteoporosis in healthy elderly women. *J Bone Miner Res* 1993; 8: 669–676.
29. van Beresteijn ECH, Dekker PR, van der Heiden-Winkeldermaat HJ, van Schaik M, Visser RM, de Waard HE. The habitual calcium intake from milk products and its significance for bone health: A longitudinal study. In: Burckhardt P, Heaney RP, eds. *Nutritional Aspects of Osteoporosis,* New York: Raven, 1991, pp. 206–212.
30. Aloia JF, Vaswani A, Yeh JK, Ross PL, Flaster E, Dilmanian FA. Calcium supplementation with and without hormone replacement therapy to prevent postmenopausal bone loss. *Ann Int Med* 1994; 120: 97.
31. Prince RL, Smith M, Dick IM, Price RL, Webb PG, Henderson NK, Harris MM. A comparative study of exercise, calcium supplementation, and hormone-replacement therapy. *N Engl J Med* 1991; 325: 1189.
32. Cumming RG. Calcium intake and bone mass: a quantitative review of the evidence. *Calcif Tissue Int* 1990; 47: 194.
33. Reed JA, Anderson JJB, Tylavsky FA, Gallagher PN Jr. Comparative changes of radial bone density of elderly female lactoovovegetarians and omnivores. *Am J Clin Nutr* 1994; 59(Suppl.): 1197s–1202s.
34. Chapuy MC, Arlot ME, Duboeuf F, Brun J, Crouzet B, Arnaud S, Delmas PD, Meunier PJ. Vitamin D3 and calcium to prevent hip fractures in elderly women. *N Engl J Med* 1992; 327: 1637–1642.
35. Heaney RP. The bone-remodeling transient: implications for the interpretation of clinical studies of bone mass change. *J Bone Miner Res* 1994; 4: 1515–1523.
36. Heaney RP, Weaver CM, Recker RR. Calcium absorbility from spinach. *Am J Clin Nutr* 1988; 47: 707–709.
37. Weaver CM, Martin BR, Heaney RP. Calcium absorption from foods. In: Burckhardt P, Heaney RP, eds. *Nutritional Aspects of Osteoporosis,* Serono Symposium No. 85, New York: Raven, 1991, pp. 133–139.
38. Anderson JJB, Barrett CJH. Dietary phosphorus: the benefits and the problems. *Nutr Today* 1994; 20(No. 2): 29–34.
39. Barger-Lux MJ, Heaney RP, Packard PT, Lappe JM, Recker RR. Nutritional correlates of low calcium intake. *Clin Appl Nutr* 1992; 2(4): 39.
40. Miller GD, Jarvis JK, McBean LD. *Handbook of Dairy Foods and Nutrition.* Boca Raton, FL: CRC, 1995.
41. Musgrave KO, Leclerc H, Rosen CJ, et al. Validation of quantitative food frequency questionnaire for calcium consumption. *J Am Diet Assoc* 1989; 89: 1484–1488.
42. Hertzler AH. Assessment of calcium intakes of adults and the elderly. Department of Nutrition and Foods, and Virginia Cooperative Extension, Virginia Polytechnical Institute and State University, Blacksburg, VA, 1993 (mimeograph).

43. Anderson JJB, Metz JA. Contributions of dietary calcium and physical activity to primary prevention of osteoporosis in females. *J Am Coll Nutr* 1993; 12: 378–385.
44. Anderson JJB. Dietary calcium and bone mass through the lifecycle. *Nutr Today* 1990; 25(No. 2): 9.
45. Calvo MS. Dietary phosphorus, calcium metabolism, and bone. *J Nutr* 1993; 123: 1627–1633.
46. Wyshak G, Frisch RE. Carbonated beverages, dietary calcium, the dietary calcium-phosphorus ratio and bone fractures in boys and girls. *J Adolesc Health* 1994; 15: 210–215.
47. Reiss E, Canterbury JM, Bercovitz MA, Kaplan EL. The role of phosphate in the secretion of parathyroid hormone in man. *J Clin Invest* 1970; 49: 2146–2149.
48. Calvo MS, Kumar R, Heath H III. Elevated secretion and action of serum parathyroid hormone in young adults consuming high phosphorus, low calcium diets assembled from common foods. *J Clin Endocrinol Metab* 1988; 66: 823–829.
49. Calvo MS, Kumar R, Heath H III. Persistently elevated parathyroid hormone secretion and action in young women after four weeks of ingesting high phosphorus low calcium diets. *J Clin Endocrinol Metab* 1990; 70: 1334–1340.
50. Portale AA, Halloran BP, Murphy MM, Morris CM Jr. Oral intake of phosphorus can determine the serum concentration of 1,25-dihydroxyvitamin D by determining its production rate in humans. *J Clin Invest* 1986; 77: 7–12.
51. Silverberg SJ, Shane E, Clemens TL, Dempster DW, Segre GV, Lindsay R, Bilezikian JP. *J Bone Miner Res* 1986; 1: 383–388.
52. Barger-Lux J, Heaney RP. Effects of calcium restriction on metabolic characteristics of premenopausal women. *J Clin Endocrinol Metab* 1993; 76: 103.
53. Kerstetter JE, Allen LH. Dietary protein increases urinary calcium. *J Nutr* 1990; 120: 134–136.
54. Margen S, Chu J-Y, Kaufman NA, Calloway DH. Studies in calcium metabolism. I. The calciuretic effect of dietary protein. *Am J Clin Nutr* 1974; 27: 540–549.
55. Hegsted MS, Schuette SA, Zeroed MB, Linkswiler HM. Urinary calcium and calcium balance in young men as affected by level of protein and phosphorus intake. *J Nutr* 1981; 111: 553–562.
56. Schuette SA, Linkswiler HM. Effects on Ca and P metabolism in humans by adding meat, meat plus milk, or purified proteins plus Ca and P to a low protein diet. *J Nutr* 1982; 112: 338.
57. Anderson JJB, Thomson K, Christiansen C. High protein meals, insular hormones and urinary calcium excretion in human subjects. In: Christiansen C, Johansen JS, Riis BJ, eds. *Osteoporosis 1987*. Copenhagen: Osteopress ApS, 1987, pp. 240–245.
58. Abelow BJ, Holford TR, Insogna KL. Cross-cultural association between dietary animal protein and hip fracture: a hypothesis. *Calcif Tissue Int* 1992; 150: 14.
59. Tylavsky FA, Anderson JJB. Dietary factors in bone health of elderly lactoovovegetarian and omnivorous women. *Am J Clin Nutr* 1988; 48: 842–850.

ADDITIONAL REFERENCES NOT CITED

Anderson JJB. Nutritional biochemistry of calcium and phosphorus. *J Nutr Biochem* 1991; 2: 300–309.
Anderson JJB, ed. Symposium: Nutritional advances in human bone metabolism. *J Nutr* 1996; 126 (4S) (April): in press.
Anderson JJB, Tylavsky FA, Halioua L, Metz JA. Determinants of peak bone mass in young adult women: a review. *Osteoporosis Int* 1993; 3(Suppl. 1): S32.
Burckhardt P, Heany RP, eds. *Nutritional Aspects of Osteoporosis '94*. Ares-Serono Symposia, Rome, 1995.
Chapuy MC, Arlot ME, Duboeuf F, Brun J, Crouzet B, Arnaud S, Delmas PD, Meunier PJ. Vitamin D3 and calcium to prevent hip fractures in elderly women. *N Engl J Med* 1992; 327: 1637–1642.
Heaney RP. Calcium, bone health and osteoporosis. *Bone Miner Res* 1986; 4: 255.
Heaney RP, Burckhardt P. Nutrition and bone health. *Challenges Modern Med* 1995; 7: 419–424.
Hu F, Zhao XH, Jia JB, Parpia B, Campbell TC. Dietary calcium and bone density among middle-aged and elderly women in China. *Am J Clin Nutr* 1993; 58: 219–227.
Matkovic V, Kostial K, Simonovic I, Buzina R, Brodarec A, Nordin BEC. Bone status and fracture rates in two regions of Yugoslavia. *Am J Clin Nutr* 1979; 32: 540.
Nieves JW, Golden AL, Kelsey JL, Lindsay R. Teenage and current calcium intake are related to bone mineral density of the hip and forearm of women 30–39. *Am J Epidemiol* 1995; 141: 342–351.
Sentipal JM, Wardlaw GM, Mahan J, Matkovic V. Influence of calcium intake and growth indexes on vertebral bone mineral density in young females. *Am J Clin Nutr* 1991; 54: 425–428.

3   Vitamin D in Health and Prevention of Metabolic Bone Disease

Michael F. Holick, PhD, MD

1. INTRODUCTION

Vitamin D is not in the strict sense a vitamin, but a hormone. Vitamin D is synthesized in the skin by the action of sunlight. Once vitamin D is formed in the skin or ingested in the diet, it journeys to the liver and kidney, where it is hydroxylated sequentially on carbons 25 and 1, respectively, to form its biologically active form 1,25-dihydroxyvitamin D (1,25[OH]$_2$D). The major physiologic function of vitamin D is to maintain the extracellular and blood concentrations of calcium within the physiologic range in order to maintain cellular activities and neuromuscular function. Vitamin D is not only important for the skeletal health in healthy growing children, but this hormone is also essential for maintaining a healthy skeleton throughout our lives. Vitamin D insufficiency and deficiency are now being recognized as a major health problem for the elderly.

2. FACTORS THAT INFLUENCE THE PRODUCTION OF VITAMIN D$_3$ IN THE SKIN

It is casual everyday exposure to sunlight that provides humans of all ages with their vitamin D requirement *(1)*. During exposure to sunlight, the solar high energy ultraviolet B

From: *Osteoporosis: Diagnostic and Therapeutic Principles*
Edited by: C. J. Rosen Humana Press Inc., Totowa, NJ

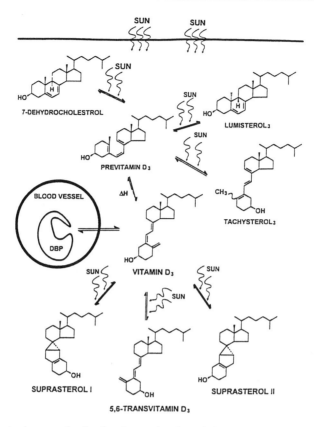

Fig. 1. Photochemical events that lead to the production of vitamin D_3 and the regulation of vitamin D_3 in the skin. Reproduced with permission from ref. *1*.

(UVB; 290–315 nm) photons are absorbed by the precursor of cholesterol, 7-dehydro-cholesterol, in the skin. This absorption process causes a transformation of 7-dehydro-cholesterol (provitamin D_3) to previtamin D_3. Previtamin D_3 is unstable and over several hours is converted to vitamin D_3 *(1)*. Once formed, vitamin D_3 exits the skin into the circulation bound to the vitamin D-binding protein (Fig. 1).

There are a variety of factors that can markedly influence the vital cutaneous synthesis of vitamin D_3. Melanin is a natural sunscreen, and people with increased melanin content in their skin require longer exposures to sunlight to produce an adequate amount of vitamin D_3 *(2)*. Similarly, the topical use of a sunscreen will act like melanin and absorb the sunlight responsible for making vitamin D_3 in the skin *(3)*. The proper use of sunscreen with a sun protection factor (SPF) of 8 will diminish by >95% the cutaneous production of vitamin D_3. Chronic use of sunscreens by the elderly can result in vitamin D insufficiency and deficiency *(4)*. Clothing is a very effective sunscreen and will absorb vitamin D_3-producing photons, thereby preventing the cutaneous production of vitamin D_3 in skin covered with clothing *(5)*. Glass and most plastics efficiently absorb UVB radiation explaining why exposure to sunlight indoors will not result in any production of vitamin D_3 in the skin *(1)*.

The stratospheric ozone layer is responsible for absorbing most of the damaging high-energy uv photons, but permits some of the vitamin D_3-producing UVB radiation to reach

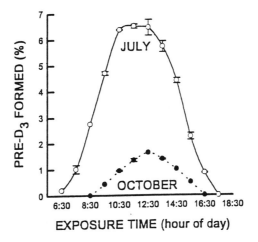

Fig. 2. Photosynthesis of previtamin D_3 at various times on cloudless days in Boston in October (●) and July (○). Adapted from Lu Z, Chen T, Holick MF. Influence of season and time of day on synthesis of vitamin D_3. In: Holick MF, ed. *Biological Effects of Light,* Berlin: Walter de Gruyter, 1992, pp. 53–56. Reproduced with permission from ref. *1.*

the earth. The zenith angle of the sun plays a crucial role in determining the number of vitamin D_3-producing UVB photons that are able to penetrate through the ozone layer and reach the earth's surface. In Boston (42°N), exposure to sunlight will produce vitamin D_3 in the skin during the spring, summer, and fall months. However, as the sun's position migrates south of the equator, the zenith angle of the sun is markedly increased causing the sunlight to strike the atmosphere at a more oblique angle, giving an opportunity for the ozone layer to absorb efficiently the UVB photons. This explains why during the months of November through February exposure to sunlight throughout the day in Boston will not produce any significant quantities of vitamin D_3 in the skin *(6)*. In Edmonton Canada (52°N), vitamin D_3 production in the skin is halted between the months of October and March. However, in more southern latitudes, such as in Los Angeles (34°N), Puerto Rico (18°N), and Buenos Aries (35°S), enough UVB photons penetrate the earth's stratospheric ozone layer to permit the synthesis of vitamin D_3 in the skin throughout the year *(1).* Similarly, the time of day determines how many UVB photons reach the earth's surface. Thus, during the summer in Boston, exposure to sunlight will promote vitamin D_3 synthesis from approx 7:00 AM Eastern Daylight Time (EDT) until 4:00 PM EDT, whereas in the fall, vitamin D_3 synthesis occurs much later in the morning ~9:00 AM EDT and ceases after ~3:00 PM *(1)* (Fig. 2).

Aging is associated with a decrease in the skin's concentration of 7-dehydrocholesterol. As a result, an elderly 70+-yr-old person will make approx 25–30% of the amount of vitamin D_3 that a younger person can *(7)* (Fig. 3).

Excessive exposure to sunlight will not result in vitamin D intoxication. During the initial exposure to sunlight, 7-dehydrocholesterol is converted to previtamin D_3. However, once previtamin D_3 is formed, it can either thermally isomerize to vitamin D_3 or be photochemically degraded to two biologically inert photoproducts, lumisterol and tachysterol *(1)* (Fig. 1). Similarly, when vitamin D_3 is made in the skin, it also can absorb energy from sunlight resulting in its degradation to biologically inert photoproducts *(1,8)* (Fig. 1).

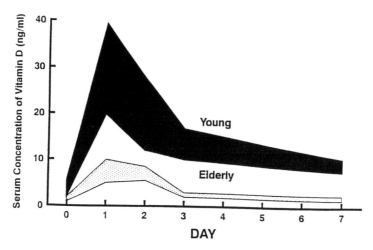

Fig. 3. Circulating concentrations of vitamin D in response to a whole-body exposure to 1 minimal erythemal dose in healthy young and elderly subjects. Reproduced with permission from ref. *1.*

3. DIETARY AND SUPPLEMENTAL SOURCES OF VITAMIN D

There are very few foods that naturally contain vitamin D. Those foods containing variable amounts of vitamin D include fatty fish, such as mackerel and salmon, and fish liver oils, such as cod liver oil. There are several foods that are fortified with vitamin D, including milk, some cereals, and some bread products. Although milk is considered to be a major food source of vitamin D, three separate studies have shown that <20% of milk samples evaluated from all sections of the United States and in western Canada contain the amount of vitamin D stated on the label. Approximately 50% of the milk samples did not contain 50% of the amount stated on the label and 14% of skim milk samples contained no detectable vitamin D at all *(9–11).* No other dairy products, such as cheese, yogurt, ice cream, and so forth, are fortified with vitamin D. Multivitamin preparations containing 400 IU of vitamin D and pharmaceutical preparations of vitamin D (50,000 IU/capsule) contain at least the amount stated on the label.

4. METABOLISM AND BIOLOGIC ACTIVITY OF VITAMIN D

Vitamin D_3 is the naturally occurring vitamin D that is produced in the skin. Vitamin D_2 comes from the uv irradiation of the fungal and plant sterol ergosterol. Both vitamin D_3 and vitamin D_2 are considered to be equally biologically potent in humans. Once vitamin D_3 is made in the skin or vitamin D_2 and vitamin D_3 (vitamin D without a subscript represents either vitamin D_2 or vitamin D_3) are ingested from the diet, the vitamin D is transported to the liver, where it is metabolized to its major circulating form, 25-hydroxyvitamin D (25-OH-D) *(12–14)* (Fig. 4).

At physiologic concentrations, 25-OH-D is biologically inert on calcium metabolism. The vitamin D metabolite requires a further hydroxylation in the kidney to form its biologically active metabolite $1,25(OH)_2D$ (Fig. 4). 25-OH-D and $1,25(OH)_2D$ can be further metabolized on carbon 24 to form 24,25-dihydroxyvitamin D and 1,24,25-tri-hydroxyvitamin D, respectively. It is thought that this 24-hydroxylation step is the initiation step for the degradation of 25-OH-D and $1,25(OH)_2D$. $1,25(OH)_2D_3$ continues to

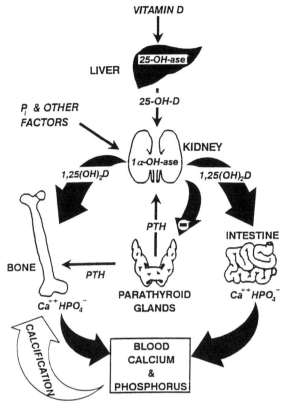

Fig. 4. Metabolism of vitamin D and the biologic actions of 1,25(OH)$_2$D. Reproduced with permission from ref. *1*.

undergo further hydroxylation in the side chain followed by a cleavage between carbons 23 and 24 to form the water-soluble excretory product calcitroic acid *(12,13)*.

It is 1,25(OH)$_2$D that is responsible for the major biologic functions of vitamin D in maintaining the serum calcium within the normal physiologic range. This hormonal form of vitamin D is recognized by a specific vitamin D receptor (VDR) in the small intestine that results in an increase in the efficiency of intestinal calcium absorption. Separately, 1,25(OH)$_2$D$_3$ stimulates stem cells within the bone marrow to become mature osteoclasts, which, in turn, mobilize calcium stores from the bone (Fig. 4).

Any decrease in the blood-ionized calcium concentrations stimulates the parathyroid glands to increase the synthesis and secretion of parathyroid hormone (PTH) *(12,14)*. PTH not only increases tubular reabsorption of calcium in the kidney and mobilizes stem cells to become osteoclasts, but it also stimulates the renal metabolism of 25-OH-D to 1,25(OH)$_2$D. Thus, PTH indirectly regulates intestinal calcium absorption through its influence on the renal production of 1,25(OH)$_2$D. PTH and 1,25(OH)$_2$D act in concert to mobilize monocytic stem cells in the bone marrow to become osteoclasts, thereby increasing calcium removal from the bones. The net effect of PTH and 1,25(OH)$_2$D$_3$ is to raise serum-ionized calcium concentrations in order to preserve neuromuscular function and cellular activity. Once the ionized calcium concentrations are within the normal range, the calcium sensor in the parathyroid glands *(15)* signals the parathyroid glands to decrease the production and secretion of PTH. Separately, 1,25(OH)$_2$D also independently interacts with a vitamin D receptor in the parathyroid glands, resulting in an inhibition of the transcription of the PTH gene and a decrease in the secretion of PTH *(16)*.

5. BIOLOGIC FUNCTION OF VITAMIN D IN THE BONE

Vitamin D deficiency in children results in the bone-deforming disease rickets *(1,12,17,18)*. In adults, the epiphyseal plates are closed, and therefore, the skeletal signs of rickets, including widening of epiphyseal plates and deformed long bones especially of the legs and rib cage, are not apparent. Instead, vitamin D deficiency causes a mineralization defect in the skeleton of adults resulting in the metabolic bone disease osteomalacia *(1,12,18)*. Osteomalacia cannot be easily distinguished on X-ray from osteoporosis, since both are recognized as osteopenia, i.e., a decrease in the opacity of skeleton on X-ray *(1,12,18)*. Osteomalacia, unlike osteoporosis, can cause isolated or generalized deep bone pain and, like osteoporosis, increases the risk of skeletal fractures *(1,12,19–21)*.

6. USE AND INTERPRETATION OF VITAMIN D ASSAYS

There are no commercial assays available to measure vitamin D in the blood. To determine the vitamin D status of a person, the measurement of 25-OH-D is recommended. The normal range for 25-OH-D is variable depending on which commercial assay is used. However, a level of <10 ng/mL is considered to be vitamin D deficiency. Although the upper limit of normal is approx 55 ng/mL, blood levels of up to 100 ng/mL as seen in lifeguards are not considered to be vitamin D intoxication *(12,22)*. However, 25-OH-D levels of >125–150 ng/mL would be considered, in face of hypercalcemia, to be vitamin D intoxication *(12,22,23)*. It is now recognized, especially for the elderly, that 25-OH-D levels need to be at least 20 ng/mL in order to satisfy their body's requirement for vitamin D. There is strong suggestive evidence that, for the elderly, 25-OH-D levels below 20 ng/mL result in an increase in circulating levels of PTH that are not necessarily outside of the normal range. When these patients receive vitamin D supplementation or sunlight in the summer and their 25-OH-D levels increase above 20 ng/mL, the PTH levels often fall by as much as 25–50%, and the bone mineral density in the spine and hip increases *(1,24–26)* (Fig. 5). Thus, vitamin D insufficiency occurs when the 25-OH-D falls between 10 and 20 ng/mL and vitamin D deficiency when 25-OH-D is below 10 ng/mL.

There are a several acquired and inherited disorders in the metabolism of 25-OH-D to 1,25(OH)$_2$D that are associated with a variety of hypo- and hypercalcemic disorders and metabolic bone diseases *(12,17,18,22,27)*. There are three circumstances whereby a renal deficiency in the production of 1,25(OH)$_2$D$_3$ can cause metabolic bone disease and exacerbate osteoporosis in the elderly. The elderly who often have mild or moderate renal failure can have a decreased capacity to produce 1,25(OH)$_2$D. The normal range for 1,25(OH)$_2$D is 16–65 pg/mL. These patients often have circulating concentrations of 1,25(OH)$_2$D <20 pg/mL.

Elderly osteoporotic patients may have a decreased ability to upregulate the renal production of 1,25(OH)$_2$D in response to PTH (Fig. 6) *(28,29)*. A very rare disorder known as oncogenic osteomalacia is associated with severe hypophosphatemia and very low circulating concentrations of 1,25(OH)$_2$D *(12,18,22)*. This disease causes severe osteomalacia and can result in deep unrelenting bone pain.

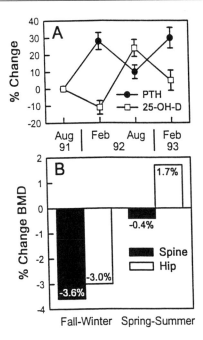

Fig. 5. Seasonal changes (as percentage of previous measurement) in: **(A)** serum parathyroid hormone (PTH) and 25-OH-D over 18 mo, and **(B)** changes in bone mineral density (BMD) of the lumbar spine during 12 mo in women living in rural Maine. Results are ± SEM. Reproduced with permission from ref. *24*.

7. CAUSES OF VITAMIN D DEFICIENCY

Vitamin D deficiency can be caused by a decrease in the synthesis of vitamin D_3 in the skin owing to:

1. Clothing of all sun-exposed areas;
2. Excessive sunscreen use over all sun-exposed areas;
3. Aging;
4. Changes in the season of the year and time of day; and
5. Increase in latitude.

For the elderly who are institutionalized, it is often the lack of any exposure to sunlight that is the principal cause of vitamin D insufficiency and deficiency for them.

Malabsorption of vitamin D is associated with fat malabsorption syndromes, including Crohn's disease, sprue, Whipple's disease, and hepatic dysfunction *(12,22,30)*. Dilantin and phenobarbital can alter the kinetics for the metabolism of vitamin D to 25-OH-D, requiring that these patients received two to five times the RDA for vitamin D in order to correct this abnormality *(12,22)*. It is rare to have a deficiency of 25-OH-D owing to liver dysfunction because of the large capacity that the liver has to produce 25-OH-D. It is often the fat malabsorption associated with liver failure that causes vitamin D deficiency. Patients with nephrotic syndrome who excrete >4 gm of protein/24 h can be vitamin D-deficient because the 25-OH-D, which is bound to vitamin D-binding protein, is lost in the urine along with albumin *(12,22,31)*.

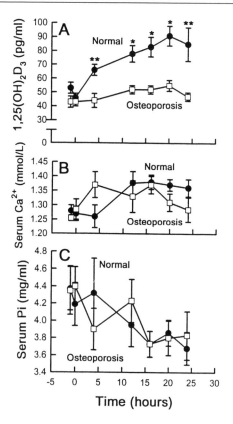

Fig. 6. **(A)** Effect of synthetic parathyroid hormone (hPTH-[1-34]) on levels of 1,25(OH)$_2$D in normal subjects (solid circles) and patients with untreated osteoporosis (open squares). All values are expressed as the mean ± SEM. The single asterisk denotes significant differences at $p < 0.01$, and the double asterisk at $p < 0.05$, between the level in the patients and that in the controls at corresponding time-points. Asterisks also refer to significant differences between the preinfusion baseline levels and levels at particular time-points. **(B)** Effect of hPTH-(1-34) on serum levels on ionized calcium (Ca^{2+}), and **(C)** inorganic phosphate (P$_i$) in normal subjects (solid circles) and patients with osteoporosis (open squares). All values are expressed as mean ± SEM. There was no significant difference between the levels in the two groups. Modified and reproduced with permission from ref. *28*.

A decrease in the renal production of 1,25(OH)$_2$D$_3$ in the kidney can be a cause for a vitamin D-deficient state in the elderly. Replacement with 1,25(OH)$_2$D$_3$ (0.25 μg once or twice a day) usually corrects this abnormality.

8. RECOMMENDATIONS FOR MAINTAINING A NORMAL VITAMIN D STATUS IN THE ELDERLY

Casual exposure to sunlight provides all of us with most, if not all of our vitamin D requirement. The elderly who are often indoors, and especially those who are institution-alized and not exposed to sunlight, are very prone to developing vitamin D deficiency and vitamin D insufficiency. Although the elderly have less capacity to produce vitamin D

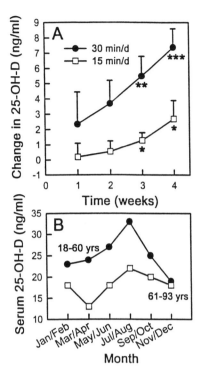

Fig. 7. (A) Change in serum 25-OH-D levels from baseline in elderly rest home residents in Auckland, New Zealand (37°C) spending 15 or 30 min/d outdoors in the spring who exposed their heads, necks, forearms, and lower legs to sunlight. $n = 5$ each group; $*p < 0.06$, $**p < 0.02$, and $***p < 0.005$ adapted from ref. *32*. **(B)** Seasonal variation in serum 25-OH-D levels in Denmark adapted from ref. *33*.

in their skin, exposure to as little as 15–30 min on a verandah of hands, face, and forearms several times a week will result in increasing circulating concentrations of 25-OH-D (Fig. 7) *(32)*. For a healthy young person, a whole-body exposure to one minimal erythemal dose of sunlight results in an increase in circulating levels of vitamin D_3 comparable to taking between 10,000 and 25,000 IU of vitamin D a day *(1)*. Extrapolating to the elderly a whole-body exposure of sunlight causing a minimum skin redness is equal to taking, orally, approx 2500 and 16,000 U of vitamin D. Therefore, the elderly will benefit from having their face, forearms, and hands exposed to suberythemal amounts of sunlight two to three times a week during the spring, summer, and fall in far northern and southern latitudes (Fig.7) *(33)*. People who are at latitudes nearer the equator need less exposure throughout the year to promote vitamin D_3 synthesis in their skin *(1,6)*. If an elderly person wishes to stay outside for a longer period of time, they can use a sunscreen with a sun protection factor of 15 or greater after the initial beneficial exposure. Therefore, by using this practice, the elderly can take advantage of the beneficial effect of sunlight while preventing the damaging effects caused by excessive exposure of unprotected skin to sunlight.

Since foods cannot be depended on for a guaranteed source of vitamin D, an excellent alternative is to provide a multivitamin that contains 400 IU *(1)* of vitamin D each day.

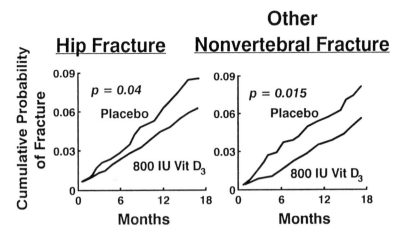

Fig. 8. Cumulative probability of hip fracture and other nonvertebral fracture in the placebo group and the group treated with 800 IU of vitamin D_3 and 1200 mg of calcium, estimated by the life-table method and based on the length of time to the first fracture. Modified and reproduced with permission from ref. *20.*

Although the RDA for adults over the age of 24 yr is 200 IU *(34),* there is mounting evidence that in the absence of exposure to sunlight, the body's requirement for vitamin D is closer to three to four times the RDA or between 600 and 800 IU of vitamin D each day *(1,20,25,35).* When healthy ambulatory women with a mean age of 84 ± 6 yr received 1.2 gm of calcium with 800 IU (20 µg) of vitamin D_2, they had a 43 and 32% lower number of hip and nonvertebral fractures compared to a similar group of women who were not supplemented with either calcium or vitamin D (Fig. 8) *(20).* It is not recommended that the elderly take two multivitamin pills to increase their vitamin D intake because of the risk of vitamin A intoxication.

An alternative to supplement quickly a patient with vitamin D insufficiency and vitamin D deficiency is to give him or her 50,000 IU of vitamin D once a week for 8 wk. The 25-OH-D increases rapidly and after 8 wk is in the midnormal range of 25–45 ng/mL. After this 8-wk treatment, a multivitamin containing 400 IU of vitamin D will help maintain a normal vitamin D status. It has been suggested for the elderly that are infirm and unable to be outdoors that they receive an im injection of 150,000 IU of vitamin D once a year. This therapy was shown to maintain the serum 25-OH-D throughout the year and decrease the incidence of skeletal fractures *(36).* This may be a cost-effective alternative to help prevent vitamin D deficiency in this susceptible group of patients.

Only rarely is there a need to provide elderly patients with $1,25(OH)_2D_3$ (calcitriol; Rocaltrol). Patients with moderate renal failure and oncogenic osteomalacia clearly benefit from receiving 0.25–0.5 µg of $1,25(OH)_2D_3$ once or twice a day *(18,22).* Care must be taken to make certain that the patients do not develop hypercalciuria or hypercalcemia. Patients with osteoporosis and who may have a defect in the PTH-mediated renal production of $1,25(OH)_2D$, may also benefit from $1,25(OH)_2D_3$ therapy. In a group of over 300 elderly women receiving 0.25 µg of $1,25(OH)_2D_3$ twice/d with a variable amount of calcium intake from their diet had a significant increase in bone mineral density, and decrease in vertebral and nonvertebral fractures compared to a control group of subjects taking 1000 mg of calcium *(37)* (Fig. 9).

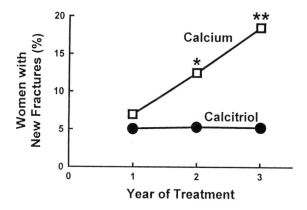

Fig. 9. Percent of new fractures in women who took either 0.25 μg of 1,25(OH)$_2$D$_3$ twice a day or supplemental calcium (1 g/d). Modified and reproduced with permission from ref. *37.*

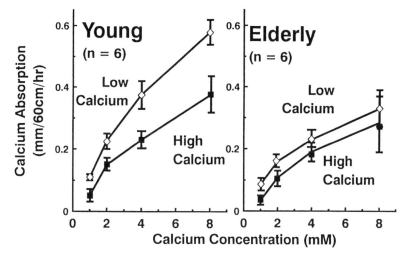

Fig. 10. Intestinal calcium absorption as a function of luminal calcium concentration in healthy young and old adults, studied after their adaptation to low or high dietary calcium intakes. The illustrated measurements were made in the jejunum using a triple-lumen intestinal intubation technique. The postprandial luminal calcium concentrations on low-calcium diets normally range from 0.3 to 2.0 mM/L, and from 3.0 to 8.5 mM/L on very high dietary calcium intakes. Modified and reproduced with permission from ref. *38.*

9. THE ROLE OF THE VITAMIN D RECEPTOR IN BONE HEALTH

It is recognized that aging alters the efficiency of the intestine to absorb dietary calcium. Young adults who are on a low-calcium intake can increase the efficiency of intestinal calcium absorption from 15 to up to 60% when switched from a high- to low-calcium diet *(38)* (Fig. 10). The mechanism for this increase is thought to be owing to the increased production of 1,25(OH)$_2$D and/or an increase in the number of vitamin D receptors in the intestinal absorptive cells. The elderly are unable to increase the efficiency of intestinal calcium absorption when on a low-calcium intake (Fig. 10). Although

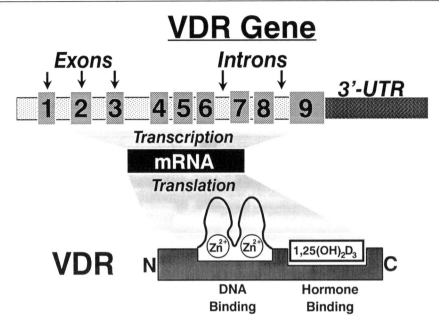

Fig. 11. Structure of the vitamin D receptor (VDR) gene showing the nine exons and interviewing introns and untranslated region. The nine exons are transcribed into the VDR mRNA, which, in turn, is translated into the VDR, which contains a DNA and a hormone-binding domain.

the exact mechanism for this lack of adaptability is unknown, there is evidence that there may be a small decrease in the number of vitamin D receptors in the small intestine that could account for this *(39)*. Alternatively, a decrease in the PTH-stimulatory production of $1,25(OH)_2D$ may play a role *(28,29)* (Fig. 6). There are no significant differences in circulating levels of $1,25(OH)_2D$ whether you are 20 or 80 yr of age *(40)*.

Recently, it has been suggested that there are several polymorphisms in the vitamin D receptor gene *(41)*. The vitamin D receptor gene is composed of nine exons, which are sequences of DNA that are transcribed and the mRNAs are spliced together to form the messenger RNA for the vitamin D receptor (Fig. 11). In between the nine exons are intervening DNA sequences known as introns. An alteration in the nucleotide sequence of an intron, although not directly affecting the amino acid structure of the vitamin D receptor, may play a role in the stabilization of the mRNA for the VDR, and therefore, the translation of its mRNA to the vitamin D receptor. There are two polymorphism's somewhere within the intron and exon sequences between exon 7 and the 3'-untranslated region. Some reports have suggested that a polymorphism of the VDR gene detected with the endonuclease *Bsm*I is associated with bone mineral density of the hip and spine *(41,42)*. Homozygotes without a cut site for *Bsm*I designated as BB have a lower bone density than homozygotes with both DNA strands having this restriction site and designated as bb (Fig. 12). It has been suggested that the genetic composition of the VDR gene may be responsible for the number of VDRs present in the intestine, and bone that could ultimately affect intestinal calcium absorption and peak bone mass. Several other investigators have been unable to demonstrate this association; and therefore, this concept is somewhat controversial at this time *(43)*.

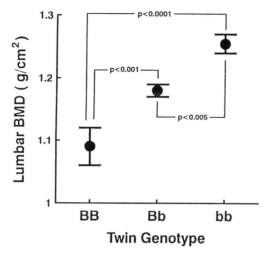

Fig. 12. Higher bone density is associated with the b allele of the VDR gene of the lumbar spine. Modified and reproduced with permission from ref. *41*.

10. CONCLUSION

Vitamin D insufficiency and deficiency in men and women over the age of 60 yr is now being recognized as a significant health risk for fractures. In a nursing home setting, residents not receiving a vitamin D supplement are especially at risk for vitamin D deficiency. In one study, 56 and 83% of elderly residents who did not receive a vitamin D supplement had 25-OH-D levels below 20 ng/mL at the end of the summer and middle of the winter, respectively *(44)*. An insufficiency and deficiency of vitamin D cause a marked decrease in the efficiency of calcium absorption. With an inadequate supply of vitamin D, the efficiency of the intestine to absorb dietary calcium is no greater than 15–20%. In the presence of vitamin D, the efficiency can be increased substantially (up to 60–80%). The lack of vitamin D causes secondary hyperparathyroidism, resulting in the mobilization of precious stores of calcium from the bone. This process can greatly exacerbate osteoporosis. Therefore, vitamin D insufficiency and deficiency not only causes osteomalacia, but will also worsen osteoporosis resulting, in decreased bone mass and increased risk of fracture.

It is reasonable to obtain a measurement of serum 25-OH-D along with calcium and phosphorus when evaluating a patient for osteoporosis. A serum $1,25(OH)_2D$ may also be valuable at times to detect insufficient renal production of this hormone.

Vitamin D deficiency is easily corrected with sunlight exposure, a vitamin D supplement, or a vitamin D pharmaceutical preparation. With the recent popularity of using bisphosphonates for treating osteoporosis, it is especially important to make certain that the patient is vitamin D-sufficient before bis-phosphonates are contemplated, since bisphosphonates can cause osteomalacia.

ACKNOWLEDGMENT

Support was provided in part by NIH grant RR00533, AR 36963, Teaching Nursing Home Grant AG 04390, and NASA grant #9501-0356.

REFERENCES

1. Holick MF. Vitamin D: new horizons for the 21st century. *Am J Clin Nutr* 1994; 60: 619–630.
2. Clemens TL, Henderson SL, Adams JS, Holick MF. Increased skin pigment reduces the capacity of skin to synthesise vitamin D_3. *Lancet* 1982; 1: 74–76.
3. Matsuoka LY, Ide L, Wortsman J, MacLaughlin J, Holick MF. Sunscreens suppress cutaneous vitamin D_3 synthesis. *J Clin Endocrinol Metab* 1987; 64: 1165–1168.
4. Matsuoka LY, Wortsman J, Hanifan N, Holick MF. Chronic sunscreen use decreases circulating concentrations of 25-hydroxyvitamin D: a preliminary study. *Arch Derm* 1988; 124: 1802–1804.
5. Matsuoka LY, Wortsman J, Dannenberg MJ, Hollis BW, Lu Z, Holick MF. Clothing prevents ultraviolet-B radiation-dependent photosynthesis of vitamin D. *J Clin Endocrinol Metab* 1992; 75: 1099–1103.
6. Webb AR, Kline L, Holick MF. Influence of season and latitude on the cutaneous synthesis of vitamin D_3: exposure to winter sunlight in Boston and Edmonton will not promote vitamin D_3 synthesis in human skin. *J Clin Endocrinol Metab* 1988; 67: 373–378.
7. Holick MF, Matsuoka LY, Wortsman J. Age, vitamin D, and solar ultraviolet radiation. *Lancet* 1989; November 4: 1104, 1105.
8. Webb AR, DeCosta BR, Holick MF. Sunlight regulates the cutaneous production of vitamin D_3 by causing its photodegradation. *J Clin Endocrinol Metab* 1989; 68: 882–887.
9. Holick MF, Shao Q, Liu WW, Chen TC. The vitamin D content of fortified milk and infant formula. *N Engl J Med* 1992; 326: 1178–1181.
10. Chen TC, Heath H, III, Holick MF. An update on the vitamin D content of fortified milk from the United States and Canada. *N Engl J Med* 1993; 329: 1507.
11. Tanner JT, Smith J, Defibaugh P. Survey of vitamin content of fortified milk. *J Assoc Off Anal Chem* 1988; 71: 607–610.
12. Holick MF. Vitamin D: photobiology, metabolism, and clinical applications. In: DeGroot L, ed. *Endocrinology,* 3rd ed. Philadelphia: W.B. Saunders, 1995, pp. 990–1013.
13. Darwish H, DeLuca HF. Vitamin D-regulated gene expression. *Crit Rev Eukaryotic Gene Express* 1993; 3: 89–116.
14. Reichel H, Koeffler HP, Norman AW. The role of the vitamin D endocrine system in health and disease. *N Engl J Med* 1989; 320: 981–991.
15. Brown EM, Gamba G, Riccardl D. Cloning and characterization of an extracellular Ca^{2+}-sensing receptor from bovine parathyroid. *Nature* 1993; 366: 575–580.
16. Naveh-Many T, Silver J. Regulation of parathyroid hormone gene expression by hypocalcemia, hypercalcemia, and vitamin D in the rat. *J Clin Invest* 1990; 86: 1313–1319.
17. Demay MB. Hereditary defects in vitamin D metabolism and vitamin D receptor defects. In: DeGroot LJ, ed., Cahil GF Jr, Martini L, Nelson DH, consulting eds. *Endocrinology,* vol. 2, 13th ed. Philadelphia: Saunders, 1995: pp. 1173–1178.
18. Krane S, Holick MF. Metabolic bone disease. In: Isselbacher KJ, Braunwald E, Wilson JD, eds. *Harrison's Principles of Internal Medicine,* 13th ed. New York: McGraw-Hill, 1994, pp. 2172–2183.
19. Aaron JE, Gallagher JC, Anderson J. Frequency of osteomalacia and osteoporosis in fractures of the proximal femur. *Lancet* 1974; 7851: 230–233.
20. Chapuy MC, Arlot M, Duboeuf F. Vitamin D3 and calcium to prevent hip fractures in elderly women. *N Engl J Med* 1992; 327: 1637–1642.
21. Doppelt SH, Neer RM, Daly M, Bourret L, Schiller A, Holick MF. Vitamin D deficiency and osteomalacia in patients with hip fractures. *Orthop Trans* 1983; 7: 512, 513.
22. Holick MF, Krane S, Potts JR Jr. Calcium, phosphorus, and bone metabolism: calcium-regulating hormones. In: Isselbacher KJ, Braunwald E, Wilson JD, eds. *Harrison's Principles of Internal Medicine,* 13th ed. New York: McGraw-Hill, 1994, pp. 2137–2151.
23. Jacobus CH, Holick MF, Shao Q, Chen T, Holm IA, Kolodney JM, El-Hajj Fuleihan G, Seely E. Hypervitaminosis D associated with drinking milk. *N Engl J Med* 1992; 326: 1173–1177.
24. Rosen CJ, Morrison A, Zhou H, Storm H, Hunter S, Musgrave K, Chen T, Wen-Wei L, Holick MF. Elderly women in northern New England exhibit seasonal changes in bone mineral density and calciotropic hormones. *Bone Miner* 1994; 25: 83–92.
25. Lips, Wiersinga A, van Ginkel FC. The effect of vitamin D supplementation on vitamin D status and parathyroid function in elderly subjects. *J Clin Endocrinol Metab* 1988; 67: 644–650.
26. Krall E, Sahyoun N, Tannenbaum S, Dallal G, Dawson-Hughes B. Effect of vitamin D intake on seasonal variations in parathyroid hormone secretion in postmenopausal women. *N Engl J Med* 1989; 321: 1777–1783.

27. Potts JT Jr. Diseases of the parathyroid gland and other hyper- and hypocalcemic disorders. In: Isselbacher KJ, Braunwald E, Wilson JD, eds. *Harrison's Principles of Internal Medicine,* 13th ed. New York: McGraw-Hill, 1994, pp. 2151–2172.

28. Slovik DM, Adams JS, Neer RM, Holick MF, Potts JT. Deficient production of 1,25-dihydroxyvitamin D in elderly osteoporotic patients. *N Engl J Med* 1981; 305: 372–374.

29. Riggs BL, Hamstra A, DeLuca HF. Assessment of 25-hydroxyvitamin D 1a-hydroxylase reserve in postmenopausal osteoporosis by administration of parathyroid extract. *J Clin Endocrinol Metab* 1981; 53: 833–835.

30. Bengoa JM, Sitrin MD, Meredith S. Intestinal calcium absorption and vitamin D status in chronic cholestatic liver disease. *Hepatology* 1984; 4: 261–265.

31. Pietrek J, Kokot F. Serum 25-hydroxyvitamin D in patients with chronic renal disease. *Eur J Clin Invest* 1977; 7: 283–287.

32. Reid IR, Gallagher DJA, Bosworth J. Prophylaxis against vitamin D deficiency in the elderly by regular sunlight exposure. *Age Ageing* 1985; 15: 35–40.

33. Lund B, Sorensen OH. Measurement of 25-hydroxyvitamin D in serum and its relation to sunshine, age and vitamin D intake in the Danish population. *Scand J Clin Lab Invest* 1979; 39: 23–30.

34. Food and Nutrition Board. Recommended dietary allowances. In: Anonymous Subcommittee on the tenth edition of the RDAs. Washington, DC: National Academy Press, 1989, pp. 92–99.

35. Dawson-Hughes B, Dallal GE, Krall EA, Harris S, Sokoll LJ, Falconer G. Effect of vitamin D supplementation on wintertime and overall bone loss in healthy postmenopausal women. *Ann Int Med* 1991; 115: 505–512.

36. Heikinheimo RJ, Ubjivaaram JA, Jantti PO, Maki-Jokela PL, Rajala SA, Sievanen H. Intermittent parenteral vitamin D supplementation in the elderly in nutritional aspects of osteoporosis. In: Burckhard P, Heaney RP, eds. *Challenges of Modern Medicine.* Rome, Italy: Ares-Serono Symp. Publ, 1994, pp. 335–340.

37. Tilyard MW, Spears GFS, Thomson J, Dovey S. Treatment of postmenopausal osteoporosis with calcitriol or calcium. *N Engl J Med* 1992; 326: 357–362.

38. Ireland P, Fordtran JS. Effect of dietary calcium and age on jejunal calcium absorption in humans studied by intestinal perfusion. *J Clin Invest* 1973; 52: 2672–2681.

39. Ebeling PR, Sandgren ME, DiMagno EP, Lane AW, DeLuca HF, Riggs BL. Evidence of an age-related decrease in intestinal responsiveness to vitamin D: relationship between serum 1,25-dihydroxyvitamin D3 and intestinal vitamin D receptor concentration in normal women. *J Clin Endocrinol Metab* 1992; 75: 176–182.

40. Sowers MR, Wallace RB, Hollis BW, Lemke JH. Parameters related to 25-OH-D levels in a population-based study of women. *Am J Clin Nutr* 1986; 43: 621–628.

41. Morrison NA, Qi JC, Tokita A. Prediction of bone density from vitamin D receptor alleles. *Nature* 1994; 367: 284–287.

42. Krall EA, Parry P, Lichter JB, Dawson-Hughes B. Vitamin D receptor alleles and rates of bone loss: influences of years since menopause and calcium intake. *J Bone Miner Res* 1995; 10: 978–984.

43. Hustmyer FG, Peacock M, Hui S, Johnston CC, Christian J. Bone mineral density in relation to polymorphism at the vitamin D receptor gene locus. *J Clin Invest* 1994; 94: 2130–2134.

44. Webb AR, Pilbeam D, Hanafin N, Holick MF A one-year study to evaluate the roles of exposure to sunlight and diet on the circulating concentrations of 25-OH-D in an elderly population in Boston. *J Clin Nutr* 1989; 125: 1692–1697.

II   THE PATHOPHYSIOLOGY OF OSTEOPOROSIS

4

The Pathophysiology of Osteoporosis

Cathy R. Kessenich, DScN
and Clifford J. Rosen, MD

Contents

1. OVERVIEW OF OSTEOPOROSIS

Osteoporosis is a clinical syndrome of reduced bone mass and increased fracture susceptibility. In most cases, the disease is characterized by back pain from recurrent vertebral compressions, although fractures of the distal tibia, hip, ribs, or wrist can be the initial presentation. The vast majority of cross-sectional and longitudinal studies in men and women now confirm an increased risk for fracture if bone mineral density (BMD) (spine, hip, wrist, or total body) is more than 1 SD below predicted for a healthy 35-yr-old person. The relative risk/U SD is approx 2.5, and increases exponentially with the number of previous vertebral fractures and the extent of reduction in BMD *(1,2)*.

Despite the strong and independent predictive value of bone mass measurements, trauma occupies a central role in the pathophysiology of osteoporotic fractures (Fig. 1). It has been estimated that about one-third of white community dwelling individuals over age 75 will fall at least once per year, with about 6% of those falls resulting in fracture *(3)*. Several etiologic factors (muscle mass, balance, use of neuroleptics, fraility, angle of the fall, and so on) predispose elderly "fallers" to fracture. However, a low bone density means that the force (stress) required to produce a fracture is less. Hence, minimal trauma (e.g., sneezing, coughing, lifting a window against resistance, twisting, or slipping) in a woman with a very low BMD can result in a compression fracture of the spine or a catastrophic hip fracture.

2. FACTORS THAT AFFECT BONE MASS

This chapter will focus on the multitude of factors that affect bone mass. All interact through three common pathways, which determine fracture susceptibility:

From: *Osteoporosis: Diagnostic and Therapeutic Principles*
Edited by: C. J. Rosen Humana Press Inc., Totowa, NJ

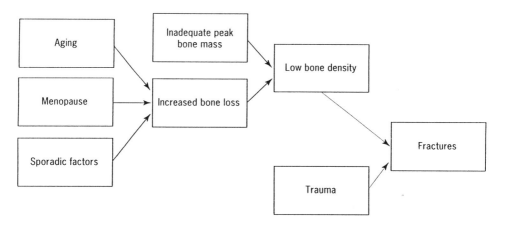

Fig. 1. The pathophysiology of an osteoporotic fracture includes low bone mass and trauma. Both are equally important in determining relative risk. Low bone density is a function of either inadequate peak bone mass or accelerated bone loss.

1. The metabolic control over bone turnover;
2. Bone strength (a function of both the density and the mechanical properties of bone); and
3. The number and type of falls sustained over a given period (a complete discussion of the etiologies of falls and their prevention in age-related osteoporosis is found in Chapter 18). This discussion will focus on how specific nutritional, metabolic, hormonal, and environmental factors affect bone turnover.

At any given point in a person's life, adult bone mass represents the sum of two events: (1) acquisition of peak bone mass between the ages of 15 and 25 and (2) age-related bone loss (Fig. 2). Several cross-sectional and longitudinal studies have demonstrated that age is one of the strongest risk factor for fracture at any site *(4–6)*. However, numerous other etiologic factors affect bone mass and, therefore, contribute to fractures during several junctures in life. The periods in a person's life that appear to be the most vulnerable to these factors include:

1. Acquisition of bone mass during adolescence (Fig. 2: period "a");
2. Maintenance of peak bone mass from age 20 to 50 (Fig. 2: period "b" + "c");
3. Bone loss associated with estrogen deprivation (ages 50–65) (Fig. 2: period "d"); and
4. Age-associated bone loss (ages 65–100) (Fig. 2: periods "e" + "f").

For example, estrogen deprivation in the sixth decade accelerates age-related bone loss, but its severity may vary from individual to individual depending on other pathogenetic factors (Fig. 2: different slopes during period "d"). The "slope" of bone loss is determined by the sum of genetic, hormonal, and environmental factors that act in the absence of estrogen to accelerate bone turnover. In a similar manner, it is a combination of various factors that govern the state of the senescent and adolescent skeleton (various rates of acquisition or loss are noted in Fig. 2). In sum, BMD is the single best predictor of future fracture. Etiologic factors influence BMD by acting through a final common pathway, the bone remodeling unit.

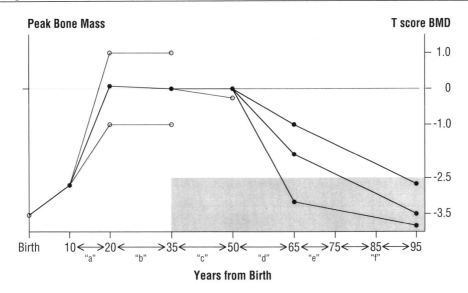

Fig. 2. The acquisition and maintenance of bone mass are essential to skeletal health over a lifetime. The y-axis represents the T score, a measure of the units of standard deviation from a normal healthy 35-yr-old control. Bone density below 1 SD is considered "osteopenic" and below 2.5 SD is classified as osteoporotic. In period "a," bone mass is acquired; the rate of acquisition during phase "a" is genetically and hormonally determined. The light lines represent theoretical rates of acquisition, which would have a future (positive or negative) impact on fracture risk. Periods "b + c" represent a time when bone mass is consolidated. It is thought that some bone loss might occur in susceptible individuals during phase "c." In period "d," bone loss during menopause may be rapid or slow, depending on environmental and possibly genetic factors. During phases "e + f," bone loss may plateau or continue its downward spiral, depending on calcium intake, sunlight exposure, estrogen use, and other factors.

3. BONE REMODELING AND THE PATHOPHYSIOLOGY OF OSTEOPOROSIS

The bone remodeling cycle is a tightly coupled physiologic process where bone resorption equals bone formation and net bone mass is maintained (Fig. 3 *[7]*). The basic remodeling unit consists of several cell types intimately associated with the bone marrow compartment (*see* Chapter 1). Remodeling is the predominant adult skeletal metabolic process serving two major functions: (1) to provide a constant and rapid source of calcium for homeostatic processes; and (2) to enhance strength and elasticity of the skeleton. Remodeling during late adolescence is especially important and unique because it represents the only time when bone formation exceeds resorption (Fig. 2 "a"). Factors that limit bone acquisition (dotted lines in Fig. 2: period "a") figure prominently in final adult bone density and, therefore, could become important risk factors for future osteoporosis (e.g., a 10% reduction in peak bone mass would mean that BMD would fall into a theoretical "fracture" range [shaded area <2.5 SD from mean] much earlier than expected: *see* Fig. 2).

The remodeling cycle begins when a quantum of bone is resorbed by activated osteoclasts (i.e., the resorption phase). This is followed by recruitment of osteoblasts, which secrete collagenous osteoid and other matrix proteins to fill the resorption lacunae. Min-

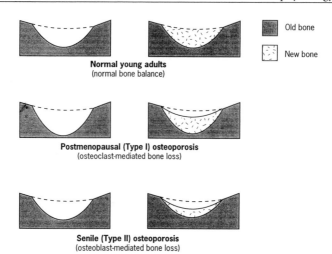

Fig. 3. Bone remodeling represents the coupling of resorption to formation. In general, Type I osteoporosis is associated with enhanced resorption, whereas Type II osteoporosis (also called "senile") is related to reduced bone formation with normal or increased bone resorption. The net effect is a reduction in bone mass with Type I or Type II osteoporosis.

eralization of osteoid completes this cycle in 100 d. In the adult skeleton, trabecular bone sites (vertebrae, distal radius, parts of the femur) are remodeled more frequently than areas where cortical bone predominates (e.g., long bones), primarily because of the greater surface area-to-volume ratio. In healthy adults, as many as two million remodeling sites may be active at any one time, and nearly 25% of trabecular bone is resorbed and reformed each year *(7)*. On the other hand, cortical bone is metabolically less active; hence, its remodeling frequency is eightfold lower than trabecular bone.

As a general rule, during remodeling, the amount of bone resorbed equals the amount of bone formed, thereby preserving bone mass. This balance is maintained because activation of the osteoclast cannot occur in the absence of the osteoblast. In fact, the initiating event in the remodeling cycle is signaling of the osteoblast to generate osteoclast-active cytokines. Hence, remodeling proceeds in cycles that begin and end with the osteoblast. This ensures that the coupling process remains intact. Uncoupling of the remodeling cycle occurs when resorption exceeds formation, either because of enhanced recruitment of osteoclasts or impaired osteoblastic activity. Since osteoclast-mediated bone resorption is a relatively rapid process (3–13 d) compared to formation (90–110 d), repetitive activation of the remodeling cycle ultimately leads to an imbalance with osteoclastic activity exceeding osteoblastic function for a period of months to years.

Involutional (or primary) osteoporosis can be classified according to uncoupling defects in the remodeling unit. Type I (postmenopausal) osteoporosis is caused by acceleration in bone turnover as a result of hormonal deprivation. Although the entire remodeling unit is activated by estrogen deprivation, bone resorption exceeds bone formation because of time constraints on osteoblast activity. The result is a net loss of bone. In Type II (senile or age-related) osteoporosis, the capacity of the osteoblast to form new bone is impaired, even though resorption is either normal or enhanced (Fig. 3). Thus, chronic imbalances in remodeling lead to persistent deficits in bone mass which eventually translate into increased fracture susceptibility.

The classification of osteoporosis permits a relatively straightforward interpretation of bone loss in involutional osteoporosis (i.e., both Types I and II). However, it may be too simple. For example, elderly women with low calcium intakes exhibit significant bone loss (Fig. 2: e + f) approximately equal to the rate of decline in bone mass during the perimenopausal period (Fig. 2: d) *(8)*. In this scenario, the mechanism of bone loss is an abnormal mix of resorption and formation. In calcium-deficiency states, PTH secretion is enhanced. This secondary hyperparathyroidism results in increased bone resorption with subsequent liberation of calcium from its skeletal stores. In order to conserve intravascular calcium, however, bone formation must be suppressed. Therefore, imbalances in the remodeling cycle in Type II osteoporosis result from a combination of increased bone resorption and decreased bone formation.

Irrespective of the type of osteoporosis, identifying etiologic factors that adversely affect the basic multicellular unit and thereby increase an individual's risk for fracture will remain a major goal both in the prevention and treatment of osteoporosis.

4. ETIOLOGIC FACTORS IN OSTEOPOROSIS

4.1. Genetic Regulation

The risk of an osteoporotic fracture is dependent on BMD, which in turn is related to: (1) the acquisition of peak bone mass and (2) the net rate of bone loss. The effects of hormonal and environmental factors on bone loss have been examined in detail at both the molecular and cellular level. Recently, the importance of bone acquisition in the pathogenesis of osteoporosis has emerged. In turn, the role of genetic determinants in that process has been underscored. It is now estimated that as much as 70% of the variation in peak bone mass can be accounted for by genetic factors *(9)*. Genetic regulation of bone loss after hormonal deprivation has also been theorized, although to date evidence to substantiate that hypothesis has not been forthcoming. In this section, comments will be confined to studies that suggest that genes regulate peak bone mass and therefore are important etiologic factors in the osteoporotic syndrome.

A family history of osteoporosis has always been considered a risk factor for future bone disease. Recent evidence from clinical studies provides some support for this contention. McKay et al. studied mother–daughter and mother–grandmother pairs, and found a very strong family resemblance at the proximal femur and lumbar spine *(10)*. Hansen et al. noted in a cross-sectional study of mother–daughter pairs that premenopausal bone densities at the spine, hip, and distal forearm were very closely related *(11)*. Because of the diverse extent of genetic and environmental variability within parent–child cohorts, these data alone are insufficient to conclude there is a significant genetic regulatory component in the acquisition of bone mass.

Human twin studies afford stronger support for the genetic hypothesis. Smith et al. were the first to recognize significantly greater variation in radial bone mass and width in dizygotic than in monozygotic twins *(12)*. More recently, other groups have demonstrated that bone densities of the spine and hip in young adult monozygotic twins are subject to much less variation than those in dizygotic twins *(9,13,14)*. However, studies in older (>age 50) monozygotic twin population have shown less concordance, suggesting that environmental and hormonal effects become more pronounced over the life of an individual. In fact, common environmental factors (diet, exercise, sunlight exposure, and others) shared by adult twins make definitive conclusions about the precise genetic contribution to bone mass difficult. Still, it is likely that there are certain genes that control peak bone mass.

To define further potential candidate genes that regulate bone acquisition, investigators have begun to study genomic control over synthesis of bone-specific proteins. Kelly et al. recently reported a strong genetic effect on serum osteocalcin (*see* Chapter 11), a noncollagenous skeletal protein synthesized by osteoblasts *(15)*. In that study, within-pair differences in osteocalcin in dizygotic twins predicted within pair differences in bone density at the lumbar spine and femoral neck. This finding suggested that genetic effects on bone formation were related to bone density.

Osteocalcin (also called bone Gla-protein [BGP]) synthesis in osteoblasts is regulated by $(1,25[OH]_2D_3)$, a critical steroid for the bone remodeling unit (as well as for absorption of calcium). Therefore, research efforts have focused on the role of vitamin D in the regulation of bone mass. Morrison et al. first reported the presence of several restriction fragment length polymorphisms (RFLPs) (i.e., differences in DNA sequences in coding [exon] or noncoding [intron] regions of a particular gene) for the vitamin D receptor (VDR) in humans, which predicted the variance in serum osteocalcin *(16)*. Subsequently, these investigators demonstrated that specific alleles in the vitamin D receptor gene were important contributors to the genetic variation in bone density among twins and osteoporotic women from Australia *(17)*. Similar findings have recently been reported in premenopausal North American women by one research group, although no relationship between VDR genotype and BMD was noted by two other investigative teams *(18–20)*.

The vitamin D receptor is only one of many factors that regulate skeletal homeostasis. Other genes that affect bone mass will almost certainly be found. Indeed, bone mass acquisition is likely a polygenic trait regulated by a host of genes at various locations in the human genome. Although this polygenicity might limit the usefulness of one approach (RFLP) for determining markers of low bone mass, it does provide a guarantee that clinicians can eventually define specific genes that regulate components of the acquisition of bone density. Currently, experimental animal models are being utilized to screen for such candidate genes.

For the practitioner, the significance of these efforts cannot be understated, even though its relevance in 1996 may be obscure. Figure 2 illustrates the importance of peak bone mass in determining future fracture risk. For example, the higher the bone mass at adolescence, the longer it would take for bone density to fall to a level where fractures would be more apt to occur. On the other hand, a peak bone mass that is lower than expected would predispose an individual to a higher risk of future fracture. Several lines of evidence illustrate this point. Significant differences in peak bone mass have been reported in black males and females vs similarly aged white men and women *(21)*. These racial differences are also associated with differences in serum parathyroid hormone (PTH) levels, osteocalcin and $(1,25[OH]_2D_3)$ *(21)*. Taken together, these data might explain the lower prevalence of osteoporosis in black women across all age groups compared to whites. Genetic factors are clearly an important cause for racial differences in bone mass. Still, preliminary studies of black vs white premenopausal women have failed to reveal that bone acquisition rates are related to polymorphisms in the VDR gene. This again reinforces the polygenic nature of this disorder and the difficulty inherent in searching for a single genetic defect *(18)*.

In contrast to enhanced acquisition, failure to attain optimal bone mass is associated with lower bone density later in life and therefore probably represents a major risk factor for osteoporotic fractures. For example, boys with delayed puberty (late onset of test-osterone production) tend to have lower bone mass in their 30s than age-matched men who went through puberty between ages 12 and 15 *(22)*. Similarly, women with primary amenorrhea have reduced bone density in their 30s and 40s even after hormone replacement *(23)*. Thus a critical period exists in the acquisition phase that is related to nutritional, environmental, hormonal, and genetic effects.

If, in the future, clinicians are able to screen adolescents for those at the greatest risk for osteoporosis, then preventive measures to optimize bone mass could be undertaken in time to capitalize on the accelerated formation phase of remodeling. For example, in a large monozygotic twin study, calcium supplementation for 3 yr to prepubertal boys increased radial bone mass by 5% *(24)*. Although 5 % does not seem like a large number, changes in bone density of that proportion translate into a significant reduction in fracture risk. Therefore, even though genetic determinants cannot be reversed, optimization of environmental and hormonal factors during adolescence could make a significant difference over the lifetime of an individual. Hence, the search for genetic factors that determine peak bone mass will have major implications for the prevention of osteoporosis well into the next century.

4.2. Hormonal Factors in the Pathogenesis of Osteoporosis

Systemic hormones are the major regulators of bone remodeling and therefore represent powerful determinants of bone mass. The presence of gonadal steroids (androgens and estrogens) are critical in the acquisition of bone mass, whereas the cessation of sex steroid production in middle life triggers bone loss Adequate growth hormone (GH) secretion is a necessity for optimal bone mass and could be very important in the maintenance of adult bone mass. PTH is the principal regulator of calcium homeostasis within the remodeling unit, and during calcium deficiency, PTH has major pathogenetic effects on bone. Abnormalities in these hormones can lead to the development of osteoporosis. However two caveats about these regulatory factors are important: (1) None of these hormones acts solely on the bone remodeling unit, but rather work in concert with other autocrine paracrine, and endocrine factors; and (2) calciotropic hormones work through intermediary factors to provide the signals necessary to activate the multicellular unit (e.g., gonadal steroids act via the interleukins and other cytokines; GH works through insulin-like growth factor-I; PTH action is mediated through insulin-like growth factor-I and certain cytokines).

4.2.1. GONADAL STEROIDS

The importance of estrogen in maintaining calcium homeostasis was first noted by Fuller Albright more than 50 yr ago. In 1941, he established that estrogen replacement to postmenopausal women reduced urinary calcium excretion, thereby promoting calcium balance *(25)*. Although knowledge about the remodeling unit is much greater now than in the 1940s, investigators are only just beginning to understand the mechanisms of estrogen action on bone. Furthermore, recent attention to peak bone mass has only served to highlight further the importance of gonadal steroids in the acquisition and maintenance of bone mass (*see* Chapter 14).

Both androgens and estrogens are essential for acquiring optimal bone mass during adolescence. In anorexia nervosa, especially in older teenagers, BMD at all sites is reduced primarily because of amenorrhea *(26)*. It is not certain whether progesterone and estrogen are both necessary for optimization of peak bone mass, although luteal-phase abnormalities (without amenorrhea) in female athletes may contribute to osteopenia at an early age *(27,28)*. Similarly, males with delayed puberty or secondary hypothalamic hypogonadism have low bone mass even in their 20s *(29)*.

As noted previously, the two major determinants of adult bone mass are acquisition and loss. Recent work has focused on the cellular and molecular mechanism of postmenopausal bone loss *(7)*. In women during and immediately after menopause, the rate of bone loss is 10-fold higher than the rate of decline in bone mass from the ages of 35 to 50 (Fig. 2: period "c"). The withdrawal of estrogens in experimental animals and humans leads to an immediate upregulation of interleukin-6 (IL-6) synthesis in bone marrow stromal and osteoblastic cells (*see* Chapter 1) *(7)*. IL-6 (and IL-11), in turn, stimulates osteoclastogenesis, which results in accelerated bone resorption *(7)*. This process is completely inhibited by 17-β estradiol. A similar scenario holds for androgen deprivation and replacement *(7)*. However, the precise mechanism and the time course for enhanced sensitivity of osteoclastic precursor cells to these cytokines have not been determined. Still these findings open up endless possibilities for using natural and synthetic antagonists to specific cytokines in order to rebalance the remodeling unit.

Originally the beneficial effects of estrogen replacement on bone were thought to be only operative in women who were early in their postmenopausal lives. Now several studies have shown that almost all women (irrespective of time after menopause) respond to estrogen treatment by maintaining their bone density *(30)*. Therefore, estrogen deprivation may be an important pathophysiologic component of bone loss over the entire postmenopausal life of a woman. Further proof of that assumption comes from the Framingham study where investigators have demonstrated that only current exposure to estrogen protects against hip fractures (i.e., past use of estrogen is not considered to have beneficial effects on relative fracture risk) *(31)*. In fact, cessation of postmenopausal estrogen use at any age leads to the prompt acceleration of bone remodeling at a rate that approximates that during the perimenopausal period of the individual.

The effects of androgen deprivation on osteoclastogenesis in males are similar to withdrawal of 17-β estradiol and almost certainty represent the major mechanism of bone loss for adult hypogonadal males (*see* Chapter 20) *(7)*. However, men do not spontaneously undergo cessation of gonadal function, making it much more difficult to discern the in vivo effects of gradual testosterone diminution on bone mass. In fact, most males with spinal osteoporosis are not hypogonadal. Larger and longer longitudinal studies in males will be needed to define the precise role of testosterone in age-related bone loss.

4.2.2. GH

GH secretion reaches its height during adolescence, and is critical to both longitudinal growth and acquisition of peak bone mass. GH deficiency in animals and humans is associated with small bones and low BMD, even after correction for size *(32)*. Since GH secretion is positively affected by enhanced sex steroid production, its role in the attainment of adult bone mass has been examined. In one recent study, serum GH concentrations were higher in black men than whites, suggesting a possible link between GH secretion and peak bone mass *(33)*. In that study, serum IGF-I levels, a more integrated measure of GH secretion, did not differ between groups. More studies are needed to determine the precise role of GH in the acquisition of bone mass after longitudinal growth ceases.

The effects of GH secretion on the maintenance of adult bone mass have received considerable attention over the last several years. Part of this focus can be attributed to one preliminary study that suggested that GH deficiency was responsible for the fraility of aging *(34)*. Newer assay methods and sampling techniques have permitted a closer examination of GH secretion profiles during aging. Pulses of GH secretion continue throughout life, although the frequency and amplitude of secretion are lower during the eighth and ninth decades *(35)*.

For the most part, attempts to link the decline in GH secretion in elders with age-related bone loss have been relatively unsuccessful. However, several lines of evidence suggest that GH does play an important role in maintenance of adult bone mass. First, acquired GH deficiency (owing to pituitary humors or infiltrative disease of the pituitary/hypothalamus) is associated with mean bone densities, which are lower than age-matched controls even after replacement of other hormones *(36,37)*. Second, acromegalics (patients with excess GH secretion) have bone densities that are either normal or increased despite hypogonadism *(38)*. Third, serum insulin-like growth factor binding protein-3 (IGFBP-3), a carrier protein for IGF-I, which is induced by GH, correlates closely with total body bone density in adult males *(39)*. Fourth, GH replacement for 1 yr to GH-deficient adults produces a significant rise in BMD *(40)*. On the other hand, except for one study, GH therapy to elderly men and women has not been shown to have significant effects on bone mass, other than activation of remodeling sequences *(34)*. Further studies will be needed to determine the role of GH in the acquisition and maintenance of bone mass.

4.2.3. PTH

A nearly constant concentration of serum calcium is essential for free-living organisms. PTH controls extracellular calcium balance by mobilizing this cation from the skeleton through osteoclast-mediated bone resorption. PTH secretion from the parathyroid gland occurs in response to a fall in serum calcium. Although diseases related to calcium sensing have been known for more than 50 yr, only in the last two years has the physiologic mechanism responsible for regulation of PTH secretion been clarified. Brown et al. were the first group to clone a calcium sensing receptor from bovine parathyroid tissue *(41)*. These G-protein surface receptors on the parathyroid gland are responsive to changes in extracellular calcium, so that a decreased serum calcium triggers a cascade of second messages, which lead to increased PTH secretion. Mutations in this receptor produce genetic conditions, such as familial hypocalcuric hypercalcemia or neonatal hyperparathyroidism, where the set point for PTH secretion is altered *(42)*. It is likely, although not proven, that alterations in this receptor may play a role in other disorders of the parathyroid gland.

Chronic states of calcium deficiency lead to an upregulation of PTH secretion (via the calcium sensing receptor), which in turn stimulates bone resorption, thereby maintaining serum calcium within a narrow physiologic range. Serum PTH levels increase with age as a result of impaired calcium absorption (owing to reduced 25-hydroxyvitamin D [25-OH-D] and age-related alterations in renal function (leading to reduced synthesis of $[1,25(OH)_2D]$) *(43)*. Such perturbations have prompted investigators to speculate that secondary hyperparathyroidism is a major pathogenetic factor in age-related bone loss. However, prospective data to support that hypothesis are limited. In most studies of elderly subjects, serum PTH is inversely related to serum 25-OH-D *(8,44,45)*. However, the relationship between PTH and BMD or change in bone density is less convincing, especially when age is held constant *(8,46,47)*. Meunier et al. demonstrated a weak relationship between PTH and femoral neck BMD ($r = -0.21$) after age adjustment in older institutionalized women from France *(48)*. In contrast, several studies have shown that calcium or calcium and vitamin D supplementation prevents bone loss at the hip and suppresses serum PTH, even though changes in PTH do not predict changes in bone density *(8,45,46)*.

The precise mechanism whereby increased PTH could cause bone loss in the elderly is not well understood. There is no doubt that sustained excesses of PTH can be catabolic to bone (e.g., primary hyperparathyroidism). Moreover, recent evidence derived from biochemical markers of bone turnover in elders with low vitamin D levels supports the thesis that bone resorption is increased in secondary hyperparathyroidism *(49)*. On the other hand, in calcium-deficiency states, bone formation is either suppressed or unchanged, leaving the remodeling unit uncoupled (i.e., increased bone resorption compared to formation). Whether this type of uncoupling represents a defect in the senescent osteoblast or PTH induction of a skeletal inhibitor of bone formation remains to be determined *(50)*. Hence, the mechanism of PTH-induced bone loss continues to be undefined.

4.2.4. THYROID HORMONE

Thyroid hormone can stimulate bone remodeling by activating receptors on the osteoblast *(51)*. In general, thyroxine shortens the remodeling cycle, so that resorption exceeds formation and the unit becomes imbalanced. Severe untreated thyrotoxicosis can lead to increased serum calcium and accelerated bone loss (*see* Fig. 4). Biochemical markers of bone turnover are generally increased in the serum and urine of patients with thyrotoxicosis (*see* Chapter 11) *(52)*. Moreover, anectodal cases of thyroid hormone excess associated with low bone mass and fractures have been reported for more than 100 yr. Still, no studies to date have documented a higher incidence of osteoporotic fractures in hyperthyroid patients, although a previous history of hyperthyroidism may represent an independent risk factor for hip fractures in elderly subjects *(53)*. In general, thyrotoxic bone disease is completely reversible once the hyperthyroidism has been treated *(54)*. In fact, hypothyroidism is associated with a marked reduction in the bone remodeling frequency, allowing osteoblasts to "catch-up" with osteoclasts, thereby recoupling the remodeling cycle. More clinically relevant, however, is the question of whether exogenous thyrotoxicosis or chronic suppressive thyroxine therapy has a deleterious effect on bone.

Early cross-sectional studies suggests that women on thyroid hormone had lower bone densities in the femur and radius than age-matched controls (pre- and postmenopausal) *(55,56)*. However, some of the patients in those studies had a previous history of thyrotoxicosis thereby complicating interpretation of the results. A more recent study reported that suppressive doses of levothyroxine (TSH < 0.05 µU/mL, but adjusted to the lowest possible dose) given to premenopausal women were not associated with bone loss from either the spine or hip *(57)*. On the other hand, postmenopausal women overtreated with thyroxine may be at risk for bone loss *(58)*. A recent report suggests that estrogen replacement therapy may negate the risk of bone loss in these patients, again suggesting that increased bone resorption from any etiology can be suppressed by hormone replacement therapy *(59)*.

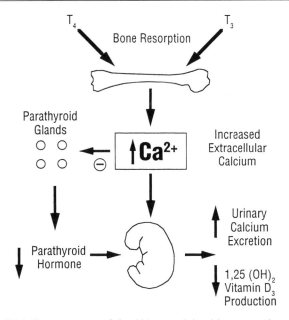

Metabolic consequences of thyroid-hormone-induced bone resorption
include decreased parathyroid hormone levels and 1,25-dihydroxyvitamin
D_3 production and increased urinary calcium excretion.

Fig. 4. The metabolic consequences of thyroid hormone-induced bone resorption.

In summary, thyroid disease and thyroid hormone replacement are very common in the general population, as is postmenopausal osteoporosis. However, bone loss from thyrotoxicosis is reversible with treatment, and there is little evidence to date suggesting that thyroid hormone replacement causes osteoporotic fractures. On the other hand, judicious use of thyroxine is indicated, especially in postmenopausal women who may be at higher risk for developing osteoporosis because of imbalances in the remodeling unit. Newer biochemical markers of bone turnover (osteocalcin, urinary collagen crosslinks) may provide evidence of increased bone turnover, allowing the clinician to make the proper dose adjustments net essary to minimize bone loss. As with all chronic disorders, prudent observation of the patient remains the cornerstone of successful therapy.

4.3. Environmental Factors

Several environmental factors are involved in the etiology and progression of osteoporosis. Smoking, alcoholism, and various medications have been noted as causative factors in the pathophysiology of osteoporosis.

4.3.1. SMOKING

Tobacco smoking has been linked to a reduction in bone density, although the exact mechanism by which smoking facilitates bone loss is unclear. Some studies indicate that women who smoke have lower levels of serum estrogen compared to nonsmokers, and that smoking may be associated with early menopause *(60,61)*. Smokers have been noted to have higher rates of vertebral fractures and greater rates of bone loss following menopause *(61–63)*. In a recent study of female twins, it was concluded that a woman who smokes one pack of cigarets each day throughout adulthood will, by the time of menopause, have an average deficit of 5–10% in bone density, which is sufficient to increase the risk of fracture *(63)*. Differences in spinal bone density between members of a pair of twins in this study were associated with differences in the serum concentrations of PTH, calcium, and urinary pyridinoline.

Several researchers have investigated the relationship between smoking and decreased bone density. Johnston et al. hypothesized that women and men who smoke are more slender than their nonsmoking counterparts and therefore have lower bone density because of less stress and strain imposed on their skeletons *(64)*. The association between cigaret smoking and BMD has been examined prospectively in a population-based study of older Caucasian men and women *(65)*. Smoking patterns and BMD measurements were determined at a baseline evaluation and, again 16 yr later in a group of 544 men and 822 women. Smoking was positively and significantly associated with decreased hip bone density and increased risk of hip fracture in old age.

The exact mechanism by which smoking reduces bone mass and increases the risk of osteoporotic fractures remains unclear, and several possibilities are currently being investigated. Cigaret smoking may be related to altered production of sex steroids, aberrant mineral metabolism, or changes in PTH *(66,67)*.

4.3.2. ALCOHOLISM

Alcohol is known to be toxic to osteoblasts and thereby disruptive to the bone remodeling cycle *(68)*. Bone loss is severe in those that abuse alcohol, in that both men and women alcoholics exhibit bone mass values similar to those found in individuals of the same sex, but 40 yr older *(69)*. Chronic excessive alcohol consumption may result in dietary deficiencies, reduced intestinal absorption or increased urinary loss of nutrients, hyperparathyroidism, liver damage, and hypogonadism *(70)*.

Abuse of alcohol disrupts bone metabolism and can ultimately cause osteoporosis. Unfortunately, the confounding factors associated with excessive intake of alcohol have complicated the investigation of the effect of alcohol on bone . Several avenues of biochemical research have yielded information about the relationship between alcohol intake and bone metabolism. Laitinen et al. investigated the direct effect of alcohol on bone and noted an elevation of serum PTH levels *(71)*. In 1994, Laitinen et al. concluded that in alcohol-intoxicated subjects, the parathyroid glands do not respond normally to a hypocalcemic stimulus, and that bone formation is uncoupled from accelerated bone resorption. A correlation between serum bone Gla-protein levels, low levels of serum vitamin D_3, and BMD in chronic alcoholics has been found, suggesting that alcohol directly depresses bone formation *(72,73)*. Finally, magnesium (mg) deficiency (owing to renal Mg-wasting, dietary deprivation, and gastrointestinal losses) in alcoholics has been noted to contribute to bone loss by its effects on mineral homeostasis. In Mg depletion, there is often hypocalcemia resulting from impaired parathyroid secretion, low levels of serum $1,25(OH_2)D_3$, as well as renal and skeletal resistance to PTH action. These changes are seen with even mild degrees of Mg deficiency and may contribute to the metabolic bone disease seen in chronic alcoholics *(74)*.

The effect of "social drinking" (1–2 drinks/d) on bone density is less clear. Numerous studies have failed to find associations between alcohol consumption and bone loss, although this may reflect the modest levels of consumption by the women in these studies

(75). Alcoholism is undoubtedly associated with increased fracture risk, but the basis for this association may be owing to the excessive falls and nutritional deficiencies that accompany excessive alcohol intake, rather than the effects of alcohol on bone.

4.3.3. GLUCOCORTICOIDS

Abnormally high levels of glucocorticoids interfere with the bone remodeling process and calcium regulation in a variety of ways. Glucocorticoids decrease the amount of calcium absorbed from foods and increase urinary excretion, leading to an increase in PTH and concomitant removal of calcium from bone *(76)*. Glucocorticoids act on calcium metabolism at many levels to produce osteoporosis, the major pathogenic effect probably being an inhibition of bone formation *(77)*. Glucocorticoids stimulate osteoclasts and inhibit osteoblasts, causing a disturbance in the bone remodeling cycle. Glucocorticoid action on osteoblasts can be direct, by activating or repressing osteoblast gene expression, or indirect by altering the expression or activity of osteoblast growth factors *(78)*. Finally, the production of estrogen in women and testosterone in men is reduced by glucocorticoids, leading to an exacerbation of bone loss. Glucocorticoids affect the areas of the skeleton containing the greatest proportion of trabecular bone, and early changes in BMD can be noted in the spine and femoral neck of patients on glucocorticoid therapy *(79)*.

Despite the well-known detrimental effects of glucocorticoid excess, no effective means of treating or avoiding steroid-induced bone loss is currently available. It is clear that the risk of bone loss is dose-related, and therefore, the lowest effective dose of glucocorticoid therapy should be a constant goal *(80)*. Inhaled glucocorticoids have gained widespread recognition as a means of avoiding the systemic effects of oral glucocorticoids. Unfortunately, studies of inhaled glucocorticoids have yielded conflicting results with some data suggesting that inhaled glucocorticoids may have less deleterious effects on skeletal metabolism *(81–83)*.

4.3.4. OTHER MEDICATIONS

Immunosuppressive drugs, such as Cyclosporine A, may be associated with bone loss after long-term treatment. Studies in animal models have demonstrated that immunosuppressive drugs alter calcium homeostasis by stimulating bone resorption *(84,85)*. The treatment and prevention of bone loss in these patients are further complicated by the fact that immunosuppressive drugs are frequently used in combination with glucocorticoids, which cause osteoporosis by increasing bone resorption and decreasing bone formation.

Long-term use of heparin for anticoagulation may lead to bone loss and spontaneous fractures *(86)*. Heparin has been noted to decrease the stability of lysosomes and release lysosomal enzymes that may be responsible for bone loss *(87)*. Heparin-induced osteoporosis is a relatively rare occurrence, but one that should be considered, particularly in postmenopausal women.

REFERENCES

1. Cummings SR, Black DM, Rubin SM. Lifetime risks of hip, Colles' or vertebral fracture and coronary heart disease among white postmenopausal women. *Arch Intern Med* 1989; 149: 2445–2448.
2. Ross PD, David JW, Epstein RS, Wasnich RD. Preexisting fractures and bone mass predict vertebral fracture incidence in women. *Ann Int Med* 1991; 114: 919–923.
3. Tinetti, ME, Speechley M, Gunter SF. Risk factors for falls among elderly persons living in the community. *N Engl J Med* 1988; 319: 1701–1707.

4. Melton LJ, Chrishilles EA, Cooper C, Lane AW, Riggs BL. Perspective: how many women have osteoporosis? *J Bone Miner Res* 1992; 7: 1005–1010.
 5. Melton LJ III, Atkinson EJ, O'Fallon WM, Wahner HW, Riggs BL. Long term fracture prediction by bone mineral assessed at different skeletal sites. *J Bone Miner Res* 1993; 8: 1227–1233.
 6. Hui SL, Slemenda CS, Johnston CC. Age and bone mass as predictors of fracture in a prospective study. *J Clin Invest* 1988; 81: 1804–1809.
 7. Manolagas SC, Jilka RL. Bone marrow, cytokines and bone remodeling. *N Engl J Med* 1995; 332: 305–311.
 8. Rosen CJ, Morrison AM, Zhou H, Storm D, Hunter SJ, Musgrave KO, Chen T, Wen Wei T, Holick MF. Elderly women in northern New England exhibit seasonal changes in bone mass and calciotropic hormones. *Bone Miner* 1994; 25: 83–92.
 9. Pocock NA, Eisman JA, Hopper JL, Yeates MG, Sambrook PN, Eberl S. Genetic determinants of bone mass in adults: a twin study. *J Clin Invest* 1987; 80: 706–710.
10. McKay HA, Bailey DA, Wilkinson AA, Houston CS. Familial comparison of bone mineral density at the proximal femur and lumbar spine. *Bone Miner* 1994; 24: 95–107.
11. Hansen MA, Hassager C, Jensen SB, Christiansen C. Is heritability a risk factor for postmenopausal osteoporosis. *J Bone Miner Res* 1992; 9: 1037–1043.
12. Smith DM, Nance WE, Kang KW, Christian JC, Johnston CC. Genetic factors in determining bone mass. *J Clin Invest* 1973; 52: 2800–2808.
13. Slemenda CW, Christian JC, Williams CJ, Norton JA, Johnston CC. Genetic determinants of bone mass in adult women: a reevaluation of the twin model and the potential importance of gene interaction on heritability estimates. *J Bone Miner Res* 1991; 6: 561–567.
14. Slemenda CW, Christian JC, Reed T, Reister TK, Williams CJ, Johnston CC. Long term bone loss in men: effects of genetic and environmental factors. *Ann Int Med* 1992; 117: 286–291.
15. Kelly PJ, Hopper JUL, Macaskill GGT, Pocock NA, Sambrook PH, Eisman JA. Genetic factors in bone turnover. *J Clin Endocrinol Metab* 1991; 72: 808–814.
16. Morrison N, Yeomans R, Kelly PJ, Eisman JA. Osteocalcin levels define functionally different alleles of the human vitamin D receptor. *Proc Natl Acad Sci* 1992; 89: 6665–6669.
17. Morrison NA, Qi JC, Tokita A, Kelly PJ, Crofts L, Nguyen TV, Sambrook PN, Eisman JA. Prediction of bone density from vitamin D receptor alleles. *Nature* 1994; 367: 284–287.
18. Fleet JC, Harris SS, Wood RW, Dawson-Hughes B. The BsmI Vitamin D receptor restriction fragment length polymorphism (BB) predicts low bone density in premenopausal black and white women. *J Bone Miner Res* 1995: 10: 985–990.
19. Riggs BL, Nguyen TV, Melton L, Morrison NA, O'Fallon WM, Kelly P, Egan KS, Sambrook PN, Muhns JM, Eisman JA. The contribution of vitamin D receptor gene alleles to the determination of bone mineral density in normal and osteoporotic women. *J Bone Miner Res* 1995; 10: 991–996.
20. Hustmeyer FG, Peacock M, Hui S, Johnston CC, Christian J. Bone mineral density in relation to polymorphism at the vitamin D receptor gene locus. *J Clin Invest* 1994; 94: 2130–2134.
21. Bell NH, Shary J, Stevens J, Garza M, Grodon L, Edwards J. Demonstration that bone mass is greater in black than in white children. *J Bone Miner Res* 1991; 6: 719–723.
22. Finklestein JS, Neer RM, Biller BMK, Crawford JD, Klibanski A. Osteopenia in men with a history of delayed puberty. *N Engl J Med* 1992; 326: 600–604.
23. Stepan JJ, Musilova J, Pacovsky V. Bone demineralization, biochemical indices of bone remodeling and estrogen replacement therapy in adults with Turner's syndrome. *J Bone Miner Res* 1989; 4: 193–198.
24. Johnston CC, Miller JZ, Slemenda CW, Reister TK, Hui S, Christian JC, Peacock M. Calcium supplementation and increases in bone mineral density in children. *N Engl J Med* 1992; 327: 82–87.
25. Albright F. Postmenopausal osteoporosis. *JAMA* 1941; 116: 2465–2474.
26. Bachrach LK, Guido D, Katzman D, Litt IF, Marcus R. Decreased bone density in adolescent girls with anorexia nervosa. *Pediatrics* 1990; 86: 440–447.
27. Prior JC, Vigna Y, Schechter MT, Burgess AE. Spinal bone loss and ovulatory disturbances. *N Engl J Med* 1990; 323: 1221–1227.
28. Bonen A, Calcastro AN, Ling WY, Simpson AA. Profiles of selected hormones during menstrual cycles of teenage athletes. *J Appl Physiol: Respir Environ Exerc Physiol* 1981; 50: 545–551.

29. Finkelstein JS, Klibanski A, Neer RM, Greenspan SL, Rosen DI, Crowley WFJ. Osteoporosis in men with idiopathic hypogonadotropic hypogonadism. *Ann Int Med* 1987; 106: 354–361.
30. Lindsay R, Tohme J. Estrogen treatment of patients with established postmenopausal osteoporosis. *Obstet Gynecol* 1990; 76: 290–300.
31. Felsen DT, Zhang Y, Hannan MT, Kiel DP, Wilson PWF, Andersonn JJ. The effect of postmenopausal and later life estrogen therapy on bone density in elderly women. *N Engl J Med* 1993; 329: 1141–1145.
32. Donahue LR, Beamer WG. Growth hormone deficiency in little mice results in aberrant body composition, reduced IGF-I and IGFBP-3, but does not affect IGFBP-2,-4,-1. *J Endocrinol* 1993; 136: 91–104.
33. Wright NM, Renault J, Pandey J, Willi S, Veldius JD, Gordon L, Key LL, Bell NH. Greater secretion of GH in black than in white men: possible factor in great bone mineral density. *J Clin Endocrinol Metab* 1995; 80: 2291–2297.
34. Rudman D, Feller AG, Nagraj HS, Gergens GA, Lalitha PY, Goldberg AF, Schlenker RA, Chn L, Rudman IW, Mattson DE. Effects of human GH in men over 60 years of age. *N Engl J Med* 1990; 323: 1–8.
35. Borst SE, Millard WJ, Lowenthal DT. Growth hormone, exercise and aging: the future of therapy for the frail elderly. *J Am Geriatr Soc* 1994; 42: 528–535.
36. Bing-you RG, Denis MC, Rosen CJ. Low bone density in adults with previous hypothalamic-pituitary tumors: correlations with serum growth hormone response to GHreleasing hormone, IGF-I and IGFBP-3. *Calcif Tissue Int* 1993; 52: 183–187.
37. Johansson G, Burman P, Westermark K, Ljunghall S. The bone mineral density in acquired GH deficiency correlates with circulating levels of IGF-I. *J Int Med* 1992; 232: 447–452.
38. Diamond T, Nery L, Posen S. Spinal and peripheral bone mineral densities in acromegaly: the effects of excess GH and hypogonadism. *Ann Intern Med* 1989; 11: 567–573.
39. Johansson AG, Forslund A, Hambraeus L. Blum WF, Ljunghall S. GH dependent IGFBP is a major determinant of bone mineral density in healthy men. *J Bone Miner Res* 1994; 9: 915–921.
40. Rosen T, Johannsson G, Hallgren P, Caidahl K, Bosaeus I, Bengtsson B-A. Beneficial effects of 12 months replacement therapy with rh GH to GH deficient adults. *Endocrinol Metabol* 1994; 1: 55–66.
41. Brown EM, Gamaba G, Riccardi D. Cloning and characterization of an extracellular Ca^{2+}-sensing receptor from bovine parathyroid. *Nature* 1993; 366: 575–580.
42. Brown EM, Pollak M, Seidman CE, et al. Calcium ion sensing cell surface receptors. *N Engl J Med* 1995; 333: 234–238.
43. Nussbaum SR, Zahradnick RJ, Lavigne JL. Highly sensitive two site immunoradiometric assay of parathyrin and its clinical utility in evaluating patients with hypercalcemia. *Clin Chem* 1987; 33: 1364–1367.
44. Quesada JM, Coopmans W, Ruiz B, Aljiama P, Jans I, Bouillon R. Influence of vitamin D on parathyroid function in the elderly. *J Clin Endocrinol Metab* 1992; 75: 494–501.
45. Chapuy MC, Arlot ME, Duboeuf F, Brun J, Crouzet B, Arnaud S, Delmas PD, Meunier PJ. Vitamin D and calcium to prevent hip fractures in elderly women. *N Engl J Med* 1992; 327: 1637–1642.
46. Dawson-Hughes B, Harris S, Krall E, et al. Rates of bone loss in postmenopausal women randomly assigned to one of two dosages of vitamin D. *Am J Clin Nutr* 1995; 61: 1140–1145.
47. Martinez ME, Delcampo MJ, Sanchez-Calbezudo, MJ. Relation between serum calcidiol levels and bone mineral density in post menopausal women with low bone density. *Calcif Tiss Int* 1994; 55: 253–256.
48. Meunier PJ, Chapuy MC, Arlot ME, Delmas PD, Duboeuf F. Can we stop bone loss and prevent hip fractures in the elderly. *Osteoporosis Int* 1994; 4(S1), S76–78.
49. Kamel S, Brazier M, Picar C, Boitte F, Sarzason L, Desmet G, Sebert JL. Urinary excretion of pyridinoline cross-link measured by immunoassay and HPLC techniques in normal subjects and elderly patients with vitamin D deficiency. *Bone Miner* 1994; 26: 197–208.
50. Rosen CJ, Donahue LR, Hunter SJ, Holick MF, Kavookjian H, Kirshenbawnn A, Mohan S, Baylink DJ. The 24/25 kd serum IGFBP is increased in elderly women with hip and spine fractures. *J Clin Endocrinol Metab* 1992; 74: 24–28.
51. Allain TJ, McGregor AM. Thyroid hormones and bone. *J Endocrinol* 1993; 139: 9–18.
52. Harvey RD, McHardy KC, Reid IW. Measurement of bone collagen degradation in hyperthyroidism and during thyroxine replacement therapy using pyridinium cross-links as specific urinary markers. *J Clin Endocrinol Metab* 1991; 72: 1189–1194.

53. Solomon BL, Wartofsky L, Burman KD. Prevalence of fractures in postmenopausal women with thyroid disease. *Thyroid* 1993; 3: 1723.

54. Rosen CJ, Adler RA. Longitudinal changes in lumbar bone density among thyrotoxic patients after attainment of euthyroidism. *J Clin Endocrinol Metab* 75: 1531–1534.

55. Ross DS, Neer RM, Ridgeway EC, Daniels GH. Subclinical hyperthyroidism and reduced bone density as a possible result of prolonged suppression of the pituitary–thyroid axis with L-30 thyroxine. *Am J Med* 1987; 82: 1167–1170.

56. Paul LT, Kerrigan J, Kelly AM, Braverman LE, Baran DT. Long term thyroxine therapy is associated with decreased hip bone density in premenopausal women. *JAMA* 1988; 259: 31373141.

57. Marcocci C, Golia F, Bruno-Bossio G, Vignali E, Pinchera A. Carefully monitored levothyroxine suppressive therapy is not associated with bone loss in premenopausal women. *J Clin Endocrinol Metab* 1994; 78: 818823.

58. Stall GM, Harris S, Sokoll LJ, Dawson-Hughes B. Accelerated bone loss in hypothyroid patients overtreated with l-thyroxine. *Ann Intern Med* 1990; 113: 265–269.

59. Schneider DL, Barrett-Connor EL, Morton DJ. Thyroid hormone and bone mineral density in elderly women. *J Bone Miner Res* 1993; 8(S1): 259.

60. Jensen J, Christiansen C, Rodbro P. Cigarette smoking, serum estrogens, and bone loss during hormone replacement therapy early after menopause. *N Engl J Med* 1985; 313: 107–129.

61. Krall EA, Dawson-Hughes B. Smoking and bone loss among postmenopausal women. *J Bone Miner Res* 1991; 6: 331–338.

62. Daniell HW. Osteoporosis of the slender smoker. *Arch Int Med* 1976; 136: 298–304.

63. Hopper JL, Seeman E. The bone density of female twins discordant for tobacco use. *N Engl J Med* 1994; 330: 387–392.

64. Johnston JD. Smokers have less dense bones and fewer teeth. *J Res Soc Health* 1994; 114: 265–269.

65. Hollenbach KA, Barrett-Connor E, Edelstein SL, Holbrook T. Cigarette smoking and bone mineral density in older men and women. *Am J Public Health* 1993; 83: 1266–1270.

66. Landin-Wilhelmsen K, Wilhelmsen L, Lappas G, Rosen T, et al. Serum intact parathyroid hormone in a random population sample of men and women: relationship to anthropometry, life-style factors, blood pressure, and vitamin D. *Calcif Tiss Int* 1995; 56: 104–108.

67. Ortego-Centeno N, Munoz-Torres M, Hernandez-Quero J, Jurado-Duce A, de la Higuera Torres-Puchol J. Bone mineral density, sex steroids, and mineral metabolism in premenopausal smokers. *Calcif Tiss Int* 1994; 55: 403–407.

68. Labib M, Abdel-Kader M, Ranganath L. Bone disease in chronic alcoholism: the value of plasma osteocalcin measurement. *Alcohol* 1989; 24: 924–928.

69. Heaney R. Prevention of osteoporotic fracture in women. In: Avioli LV, ed., *The Osteoporotic Syndrome*, 3rd ed. New York: Wiley-Liss, 1993, pp. 89–107.

70. Bunker VW. The role of nutrition in osteoporosis. *Br J Biomed Sci* 1994; 51: 228–240.

71. Laitinen K, Tahtela R, Luomanmaki K, Valimaki MJ. Mechanisms of hypocalcemia and markers of bone turnover in alcohol-intoxicated drinkers. *Bone Miner* 1994; 24: 171–179.

72. Gonzalez-Calvin JL, Garcia-Sanchez A, Bellot V, Munoz-Torres M, et al. Mineral metabolism, osteoblastic function and bone mass in chronic alcoholism. *Alcohol* 1993; 28: 571–579.

73. Peris P, Pares A, Guanabens N, Pons F, et al. Reduced spinal and femoral bone mass and deranged bone mineral metabolism in chronic alcoholics. *Alcohol* 1992; 27: 619–625.

74. Abbott L, Nadler J, Rude RK. Magnesium deficiency in alcoholism: possible contribution to osteoporosis and cardiovascular disease in alcoholics. *Alcohol Clin Exp Res* 1994; 18: 1076–1082.

75. Slemenda CW. Adult bone loss. In: Marcus R, ed., *Osteoporosis*. Boston: Blackwell Scientific, 1994, pp. 107–124.

76. Raisz L, Kream BE. Regulation of bone formation. *N Engl J Med* 1983; 30: 83–89.

77. Reid IR, Veale AG, France JT. Glucocorticoid osteoporosis. *J Asthma* 1994; 31: 7–18.

78. Delaney AM, Dong Y, Canalis E. Mechanisms of glucocorticoid action in bone cells. *J Cell Biochem* 1994; 56: 295–302.

79. Fitzpatrick LA. Glucocorticoid-Induced osteoporosis. In: Marcus R, ed., *Osteoporosis*. Boston: Blackwell Scientific, 1994, pp. 202–226.

80. Bachrach L. Bone acquisition in childhood and adolescence. In: Marcus R, ed., *Osteoporosis*. Boston: Blackwell Scientific, 1994, pp. 69–106.

81. Boe JE, Skoogh BE. Is long-term treatment with inhaled steroids in adults hazardous? *Eur Respir J* 1992; 5: 1037–1039.

82. Boulet LP, Giguere MC, Milot J, Brozazn J. Effects of long-term use of high dose inhaled steroids on bone density and calcium metabolism. *J Allergy Clin Immunol* 1994; 94: 796–803.

83. Barnes PJ. Inhaled glucocorticoids for asthma. *N Engl J Med* 1995; 332: 868–875.

84. Movsowitz C, Epstein S, Ismall F, Fallon M, Thomas S. Cyclosporin A in the oophorectomized rat: unexpected severe bone resorption. *J Bone Miner Res* 1989; 5: 393–398.

85. Schlosberg M, Movsowitz C, Epstein S, Ismall F, Fallon M, Thomas S. The effect of cyclosporin A administration and its withdrawal on bone mineral metabolism in the rat. *Endocrinology* 1989; 124: 2179–2184.

86. Kaplan FS. Prevention and management of osteoporosis. *Clin Symp* 1992; 47(1): 2–32.

87. Riggs BL. Overview of osteoporosis. *West J Med* 1991; 154: 63–77.

5

The Epidemiology of Osteoporosis

Michael Kleerekoper, MD

CONTENTS

1. INTRODUCTION

Not very many years ago, osteoporosis was not considered a specific disease process worthy of attention, but was regarded simply as part of the natural aging process. Over the past two decades, improved diagnostic modalities and therapeutic options have dramatically focused attention on this disease, almost to a point where statements about prevalence, incidence, health care costs to society, and so forth, border on hyperbole. This chapter will attempt to summarize the increasing amount of carefully derived epidemiologic data from a number of sources, separating fact from fiction. However, the reader should be aware that much of our knowledge base, particularly as it relates to the prevalence and incidence of osteoporotic fractures, particularly at sites other than the proximal femur, remains speculative. This is simply because national data bases for fractures other than those requiring hospitalization, such as hip fractures, are either nonexistent or have substantial logistic biases with respect to ascertainment and verification of the data. Perhaps in recognition of these difficulties, a World Health Organization (WHO) Study Group has recently developed diagnostic criteria for osteoporosis based solely on measured bone mass *(1),* with fracture no longer being required for the diagnosis. For population-based activity, which is the principal role of the WHO, this is very appropriate and certainly makes it an easier task to compose a chapter such as this. At the same time, it is important to point out that population-based diagnostic criteria may not necessarily translate directly to diagnostic criteria in individual patients.

2. PREVALENCE OF OSTEOPOROSIS

The prevalence of osteoporosis, (i.e., the number of individuals in a defined group in whom bone mass is >2.5 SD below the mean of peak adult bone mass) has been estimated to be 30% of all postmenopausal white women in the US *(2).* Site-specific estimates are

From: *Osteoporosis: Diagnostic and Therapeutic Principles*
Edited by: C. J. Rosen Humana Press Inc., Totowa, NJ

16.5% for osteoporosis at the lumbar spine, 16.2% at the hip, and 17.4% for the midradius. Other data place the site-specific prevalence at the hip at 23% *(3)*, so that between one in five and one in seven white women >50 yr of age in the US have osteoporosis of the hip, at least by this definition. It is of course difficult to develop similar prevalence data using the past occurrence of an osteoporotic hip fracture as the definition.

One rationale for using bone mass and not fracture to define osteoporosis for prevalence studies in osteoporosis is the extremely difficult task of ascertaining the relationship between skeletal fragility and the severity of trauma that resulted in a fracture, in addition to the difficulty of ascertaining just how many individuals in a given population have had a fracture in the past. Additionally, it has been well established from cross-sectional and prospective studies that the risk of fracture increases as bone mass decreases, with doubling of the risk for each standard deviation decrement in bone mass *(4)*. Given this, it is assumed that the prevalence of osteoporosis will be lower in populations known to have higher bone mass than white women in the US, including US males and US blacks of both sexes, but actual prevalence data have not been estimated. Some estimates for vertebral fracture prevalence have included 27% of women in Minnesota at age 65 *(5)* and 21% of Danish women at age 70 *(6)*, but there are several important limitations on these data, as detailed in the following section.

3. INCIDENCE OF NEW FRACTURES RESULTING FROM OSTEOPOROSIS

Almost all fractures of the proximal femur require hospitalization with or without surgical intervention. Thus, hospital discharge data provides a very firm base for assessing the true incidence (i.e., the number of new cases in a defined period of time) of these fractures. Given what is known about the increasing likelihood of fracture with advancing age, the Medicare data base that focuses on people age 65 or older can be regarded as a very reliable guide to the true incidence of hip fractures that result from osteoporosis. The most recent figures that have been published set this figure at approx 275,000 new osteoporotic hip fractures each year in the US *(7)*. The female:male ratio for this incidence is 2:1, with African-Americans, both female and male having a much lower incidence (Fig. 1).

A discussion of incidence rates for hip fractures is straightforward, because a fractured neck of femur is a fractured neck of femur. Several factors markedly limit our ability to document rigorously the true incidence of osteoporotic vertebral fractures. First, it is believed by most authorities that such fractures may occur spontaneously in the absence of both an identifiable traumatic event, no matter how trivial, and in the complete absence of acute symptoms. This is in sharp contrast to hip fractures, where an identifiable traumatic event, such as a fall, is present in more than 95% of the cases, and in the absence of a sensory deficit, these fractures are always symptomatic. Second, there continues to be considerable debate about what vertebral abnormality constitutes a true vertebral fracture (*see* Chapter 7). Most patients who present for acute medical care because they think they might have sustained a long bone fracture (arm, leg, digit, clavicle, and so on) are usually correct in their assumption, and the presence of a new fracture is relatively easy to confirm by history, physical examination, and plane radiograph. Vertebral fractures result in permanent deformity of the vertebral body, so that without a previous radiograph for direct comparison, it is impossible to be certain that any deformity is clearly new. Radiographic technique is also more critical when attempting to detect vertebral fractures, particularly when the vertebrae are markedly demineralized.

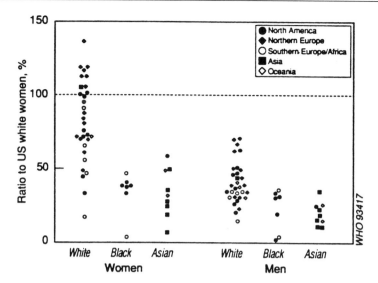

Fig. 1. Hip fracture incidence around the world as a ratio of the rates observed in various populations to those expected for white women in USA. ●, North America; ◆, Northern Europe; ○, Southern Europe/Africa; ■, Asia; ◇, Oceania.

To overcome these technical problems, several groups have devised rigorous protocols for obtaining plane radiographs of the spine in a true lateral projection, avoiding any magnification errors from one radiograph to the next, and then quantifying vertebral body dimensions. This techniques has been referred to as vertebral morphometry, and a new (incident) vertebral fracture is defined as a reduction in vertebral body height between one radiograph and the next. There is no consensus concerning how much of a reduction must be present to qualify as a new fracture (as opposed to measurement imprecision), but most authorities favor a 20–25% reduction of measured vertebral height. One additional caveat is that when determining fracture incidence, it is important to standardize the time interval between radiographs, since vertebral fractures, again unlike peripheral fractures, are not all or none events, but may be graded phenomena with a 25% or greater reduction occurring in several smaller steps, none of which would be counted as fractures as just defined, but clearly in retrospect, all contributing to the vertebral deformity.

This lengthy, somewhat technical discussion of the detection and quantitation of vertebral fractures underscores the difficulty in accurately reporting the incidence of vertebral fractures. It also assumes importance when discussing the impact of therapy on vertebral fracture rate where it becomes important to understand precisely what method was used to define a fracture when comparing studies from different sources. For example, the reported fracture rate in osteoporotic subjects given placebo in different clinical trials, which should be a fairly constant figure, varies by at least one order of magnitude *(8)*. Finally, although it is easy to use hospital discharge data to determine the denominator for hip fracture incidence, and be reasonably assured that one can compare rates in different communities and countries, the same is not quite true for vertebral fractures, since the rate will vary markedly with the population being studied. All subjects must be able to have at least two spine radiographs separated by a fixed period of time, and this has potential to introduce bias by excluding those not able to meet this minimal criterion for inclusion in the survey. The older the population or the lower the bone mass, the

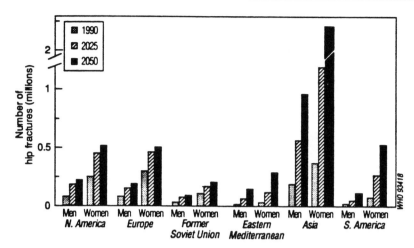

Fig. 2. Estimated number of fractures for men and women in different regions of the world in 1990, 2025, and 2050. Modified from ref. *9.*

greater the likelihood of fracture, so these aspects must be considered when determining the incidence of vertebral fracture. Furthermore, studies have demonstrated that the presence of a vertebral fracture or deformity at the baseline radiograph increases the subsequent likelihood of new fractures, independent of bone mass *(10).*

4. TRENDS IN THE PREVALENCE
AND INCIDENCE OF OSTEOPOROSIS

The risk of sustaining an osteoporotic fracture increases with age and with decreasing bone mass. As the populations of the world age, one can anticipate a dramatic increase in the prevalence of both osteoporosis and osteoporotic fractures, even if the incidence in any given population decreases over time. The greatest impact is likely to be seen in currently underdeveloped countries, where the greatest increase in life expectancy is anticipated (Fig. 2).

REFERENCES

 1. Assessment of fracture risk and its implication to screening for postmenopausal osteoporosis. WHO Technical Report Series #843, Geneva, Switzerland, 1994.
 2. Melton LJ III. How many women have osteoporosis now? *J Bone Miner Res* 1995; 10: 175–177.
 3. Kanis JA, Melton LJ III, Christiansen C, Johnston CC, Khaltaev N. The diagnosis of osteoporosis. *J Bone Miner Res* 1994; 9: 1137–1141.
 4. Cummings SR, Black DM, Nevitt MC, Browner W, Cauley J, Ensrud K, Genant HK, Palermo L, Scott J, Vogt TM. Bone density at various sites for prediction of hip fractures. *Lancet* 1993; 341: 72–75.
 5. Melton LJ III. Epidemiology of vertebral fractures in women. *Am J Epidemiol* 1989; 129: 1000–1011.
 6. Jensen S, Christiansen C, Boesen J, Hegedus V, Transbol I. Epidemiology of postmenopausal spinal and long bone fractures. *Clin Orthop* 1982; 166: 75–81.
 7. Jacobsen SJ, Goldberg J, Miles TP, Brody JA, Stiers W, Rimm AA. Regional variation in the incidence of hip fracture: US white women aged 65 years and older. *JAMA* 1990; 264: 500–502.
 8. Seeman E, Tsalamandris C, Bass S, Pearce G. Present and future of osteoporosis. *Bone* 1995; 17: 23S–29S.
 9. Cooper C, Campion G, Melton LJ III. Hip fractures in the elderly: a worldwide protection. *Osteoporosis Int* 1992; 2: 285–289.
10. Ross PD, Davis JW, Epstein R, Wasnich RD. Pre-existing fractures and bone mass predict vertebral fracture incidence in women. *Ann Intern Med* 1991; 114: 919–923.

6

Psychosocial Aspects of Osteoporosis

Betsy Love McClung, RN, MN
and Judith H. Overdorf, RN, MPH

CONTENTS

1. INTRODUCTION

Osteoporosis is defined as a reduction in bone mass associated with increased skeletal fragility. By far, fractures are the most clinically significant aspect of the osteoporotic syndrome. Compression fractures in the midthoracic and upper lumbar region of the spine lead to chronic back pain, reduction in physical activity, body deformity, muscle weakness, and fatigue. In general, the principal therapeutic end point for judging the efficacy of treatment is a reduction in fracture rate. Perhaps of more importance, however, to the patient is a diminution of symptoms associated with the consequences of fracture. These changes would be expected to lead to an improvement in quality of life for that individual *(1,2)*. Not all individuals are symptomatic from osteoporotic compression fractures of the spine, and the proportion of patients with vertebral osteoporosis who suffer morbid consequences is unknown *(3)*. Women with severe osteoporosis are at consistently higher risk of having any symptoms, compared with women with mild osteoporosis or no osteoporosis *(4)*. The risk of pain and disability increases with the number and severity of fractures, and individuals with prevalent fractures have an increased risk of back pain and physical disability, which persists for 3 years or more on average *(4,5)*. To what degree the severity of osteoporotic symptoms affects the psychosocial status of patients is not well understood. Because patients may not openly discuss their emotions and concerns about living with this disease, the psychosocial status of all patients needs to be assessed. A key therapeutic strategy is to identify and address the individual psychosocial needs of each patient, so a renewed sense of life satisfaction might be achieved while coping with a chronic, painful disease.

From: *Osteoporosis: Diagnostic and Therapeutic Principles*
Edited by: C. J. Rosen Humana Press Inc., Totowa, NJ

Table 1
Consequences of and
Psychological Responses to Osteoporosis

Consequences of Osteoporosis
    Pain
    Reduction in physical activity
    Body deformity
    Muscle weakness
    Fatigue
    Social isolation
    Loss of independence

Psychological Responses to Osteoporosis
    Stress
    Depression
    Feelings of worthlessness
    Fear
    Anxiety
    Poor self-image
    Anger
    Feelings of hopelessness

The consequences of vertebral osteoporotic fractures have profound effects on patients' lives (3). A woman hearing the diagnosis of osteoporosis for the first time may feel frightened and anxious about how this condition will affect her now and in the future. The psychological responses of patients who suffer from symptomatic vertebral osteoporosis arise largely as a result of their pain and disability. In a study evaluating the impact of spinal fractures on the general well-being in elderly women, it was found that women with spine fractures complained of back pain well beyond the time of acute fracture (6). These women had significant levels of depression, anxiety, and sleeplessness associated with a decline in vitality, general health, and self-control (6). It is important for clinicians to address the psychological responses of stress, depression, anxiety, anger, and fear, which are clearly evident in the majority of patients who have symptomatic vertebral osteoporosis (Table 1).

Back pain, ranging in degree of severity, duration, and frequency in individual patients, is the most common consequence of vertebral osteoporosis. This type of pain is usually aggravated by sitting, standing, or reaching forward for any length of time. Patients with back pain experience stress, which is related to the increased need for coping mechanisms necessary to adjust to daily living activities (7). Patients who have led active, independent lives may have to give up driving, performing traditional household chores, shopping, and recreational activities. Often older individuals find it difficult to ask for help in coping with an altered lifestyle (8). Becoming dependent on others to do what one has always done for oneself contributes to feelings of worthlessness and depression. Signs of depression include increased somatization, poor sleep patterns, appetite disturbances, lack of concentration, and reduced interest in social activities. Isolation and withdrawal from family and friends often become a defense mechanism against the perceived loss of ability to maintain control and self-confidence in social interactions.

Although symptomatic back pain may be the most common symptom of vertebral osteoporosis, other consequences of this disorder can cause psychological responses leading to diminished sense of well-being. Reduction in physical activity can be the result of fear of new fractures. Newly diagnosed patients as well as patients with established osteoporosis often view themselves as fragile, and may become frightened at the prospect of engaging in physical activities that they perceive would put them at risk for a new fracture and new episodes of acute back pain. Fear of falling creates anxiety, and these patients develop a sedentary lifestyle, which contributes to isolation *(9)*. Patients, even in the absence of symptoms, perceive themselves as having a disabling disease that can negatively affect their self image.

Consequences of vertebral osteoporosis that lead to changes in physical appearance have an emotional impact. Women who previously enjoyed fashionable clothes and shoes have difficulty finding clothes that "camouflage" a humped back and a protruding abdomen. High-heeled shoes are no longer an option because of changes in balance and fear of falling. Changes in physical appearance and the need to adjust clothing styles often contribute to a woman's perception of feeling "old and ugly."

Anger that such a circumstance has befallen them is a psychological response of many women. They have never heard of osteoporosis, do not understand its causes, nor have they been informed of anything that could be done to improve their discomfort, disability, and physical appearance.

2. WHAT PATIENTS SAY
ABOUT HOW OSTEOPOROSIS HAS AFFECTED THEIR LIVES

Esther, 82 Years Old, on Lifestyle Changes and Adaptation

"One of the hardest things for me is getting in and out of the car. I cannot shop very long like I used to be able to. To put my arms up while I am looking through a clothes rack really hurts me. When I walk, I am looking around all the time with my face looking down at the sidewalk. I cannot go up and down curbs because of the jolting and hurting my back. When you cannot look at the flowers for fear of falling, walking is not nearly as much fun. One of the things I love to do and cannot do anymore is sit at my sewing machine, because I am stooped over and I have too much pain when I do that. I have learned to do Hardanger, which is Norwegian embroidery. I sit back in my easy chair. I have no back pain at all, and I have something to do with my hands. Now I am teaching classes in Hardanger. Teaching classes makes me feel worthy. That is something I enjoy." (9)

Pearl, 85 Years Old, on Loss of Independence

"After I got acquainted with osteoporosis, everything seemed to change. I lost six inches in height from it. Being unsure of myself in setting around and having to depend on someone else has been the hardest thing for me. It has affected my lungs and heart, crowding them up from the fractures. It pushes my organs, down. When you were young, you went out to go to work. You had to become independent, do for yourself, and help others along the way. When you do that all your life, and along toward the end you get slapped down [from osteoporosis] you have to ask for help. It really makes it hard." (9)

Carol, 81 Years Old, on Depression

"I think the frustration and efforts to keep things as they were, and knowing that you cannot in the end lead you to get very depressed. You realize you are no longer in control. Family members and people you know expect you to be like you always were. One tries to live up to that. Those of us who have always taken care of everyone else and

have invested a great deal of time with friends and family need to let them take their turn. Maybe it is time to give up a facet of your personality that wants to have everything under control all the time. There is a certain amount of growth involved, and it is very painful at the time. But once you realize this, it can be easy and you can grow." (9)

Beatrice, Age 77, on Fear, Anger, and Resolve

"I am alone in the world. I worked in a factory on an assembly line until I was 70. Then I could no longer lean over trays because of back pain. Finding out that I had osteoporosis was very frightening. I was so afraid that eventually I could not take care of myself. I am still worried about that. I am angry that this has happened to me, but now I figure I need to learn all I can do to help myself. I have always considered myself pretty tough and even this [osteoporosis] does not change my mind about that!"

3. CLINICAL INTERVENTIONS TO ENHANCE PSYCHOSOCIAL WELL-BEING

Education about osteoporosis, the symptoms that may be experienced, the possible complications, and current approaches to management will improve patients' understanding of the disease, and enhance their ability to cope with the long-term nature of this chronic disease *(10)*. Decreased anxiety, reduced fear, less depression, and improved future outlook are positive results of an ongoing educational program. When there is meaningful change in patients' understanding of the disease, they are more apt to take responsibility for self-management and to avoid harmful activities *(11)*.

A patient education program that addresses osteoporosis management and related psychosocial issues can be initiated by the physician, but requires consistent reinforcement by the entire health care team, including nurses, social workers, physical therapists, and nutritionists. The idiosyncratic nature of osteoporosis (i.e., each patient responds differently to fracture pain), role changes, and the stress of coping with an irreversible, debilitating disease demand that educational goals be individualized *(12)*. Enlisting the patient and family members as partners with the health care team is critically important. Only when patients and family members understand the etiology and prognosis of the disease can they be expected to carry out medication, exercise, and dietary recommendations faithfully *(13)*. The patient–family–physician partnership also helps to avoid situations where caring family members may hinder outcomes, such as when a support giver out of empathy or concern reinforces a behavior that is incompatible with an optimal outcome. For example, a daily exercise regimen may demand that the patient exercise to the point of feeling discomfort, and a sympathetic caregiver, who does not understand the ultimate goal, may place immediate comfort before long-term gain and discourage the required activity.

Although the health care team prospective is ideal, time and cost may necessitate that a physician in a solitary setting enlist the patient and accompanying family members as partners at the first evaluation visit. A key component of this partnership is sharing the elements of an osteoporosis education program.

Elements of this program should include:

An explanation of:
    What osteoporosis is;
    Why the disease occurs;
    How it affects physical function;

What can be done to treat osteoporosis; and

How symptoms of fractures can be relieved.

An offer of professional support:

Recognition that symptoms are real; and

Validation of emotional responses to living with a chronic disease.

Repeated planned contact with the physician and other members of the health care team is important. This is based on the fact that older people do not ask for help as readily as younger individuals, and need regular encouragement and support to do so. Frequent updates of factual knowledge prevent incorrect perceptions on the part of patients and families, prevent "information overload" when too much material is shared at one time, and promote timely changes to interventions as patients progress. Regular follow-up visits allow the physician and other team members to assess current psychosocial status, and help patients feel more hope and optimism.

Educational strategies for patients with osteoporosis may include:

- Enlisting patients and families as partners at initial visit;
- Providing written instructions on individualized treatment regimens;
- Addressing the patient's and family's questions, concerns, compliance issues, and psychosocial needs on subsequent visits;
- Presenting supportive, topic-oriented, formal educational programs for patients and families;
- Conducting self-management training classes;
- Sponsoring workshops and seminars;
- Making available educational pamphlets and newsletters;
- Providing telephone support;
- Offering nutritional consultation;
- Establishing group exercise classes;
- Providing referrals for individual counseling; and
- Encouraging attendance at peer support groups.

4. OSTEOPOROSIS SUPPORT GROUPS

Meeting other patients who have experienced similar problems or events in the course of their disease is especially helpful (14). An educational peer support group provides a forum in an unthreatening atmosphere, which encourages patient information sharing, legitimizes the acceptance of available social and community support services, and gives the physician and health care team members an opportunity to update the group on new advances in the management of osteoporosis.

Support groups vary widely in their nature, purpose, and goals. They may be community-based and organized by a committed patient, or located in an osteoporosis center and staffed by members of the health care team. There is clear evidence that patients improve their sense of control and independence by gaining information about their chronic disease, and thus, improve their ability to understand and follow advice where self-management is important (15).

As our population grows older, the problems posed by chronic and disabling conditions increasingly demand our attention. Although a cure for osteoporosis may be years away, we now have the means to manage not only a patient's physical condition, but also the opportunity to improve the quality of life for the "whole" person. Osteoporosis information resources are listed in Table 2. Providing education and professional support

Table 2
Osteoporosis Information Resources

National Osteoporosis Foundation
1150 17th Street, NW
Washington, DC 20036
(202) 223-2226 or (800) 223-9994
    Publication on osteoporosis
    Contacts for local support groups

Administration on Aging
330 Independence Avenue, SW
Washington, DC 20201
(202) 619-0641

American Association of Retired Persons
601 E Street, NW
Washington, DC 20201
(202) 434-2277
    Publications *(Modern Maturity)*
    Advocacy

National Center for Nutrition and Dietetics
American Dietetic Association
216 West Jackson Blvd.
Chicago, IL 60606-6995
(800) 366-1655 consumer nutrition hotline

National Chronic Pain Outreach Association
7979 Old Georgetown Road
Bethesda, MD 20814
(301) 652-4948

National Daily Council
6300 North River Road
Rosemont, IL 60018-4233
(312) 696- 1020

National Institute on Aging Information Center
PO Box 8057
Gaithersburg, MD 20898-8057
(800) 222-2225
Publishes
    Resource Directory for Older People
    Who? What? Where? Resources far Women's Health and Aging
    Age Pages (fact sheet series)

National Women's Health Network
514 10th Street NW, Suite 402
Washington, DC 20004
(202) 347-1140
Member-based educational organization

continued

Table 2 *(continued)*

Older Women's League
666 Eleventh Street NW, Suite 700
Washington, DC 20001
(202) 783-6686 or 1-800-TAKE-OWL
Published Status Report on osteoporosis, fact sheets, resource guides

Women's Health America
429 Gammon Place
PO 9690
Madison, WI 53715
(608) 833-9102
Educational materials

State and Regional Offices on Aging
Area and town councils provide community support, transportation,
    and "meals on wheels"

to help patients and their families cope with their physical, emotional, and social needs can make a significant contribution to a patient's life satisfaction *(16)*.

REFERENCES

1. Ryan PJ, Blake G, Herd R, et al. A clinical profile of back pain and disability in patients with spinal osteoporosis. *Bone* 1994; 15(1): 27–30.
2. Kanis JA, Minne WH, Meunier PJ, et al. Quality of life and vertebral osteoporosis. *Osteoporosis Int* 1992; 2: 161–163.
3. Kanis JA. Osteoporosis and its consequences. In: *Osteoporosis*. Oxford, England: Blackwell Science, 1994, pp. 1–21.
4. Ettinger B, Black DM, Nevitt MC, et al. Contribution of vertebral deformities to chronic pain and disability. *J Bone Miner Res* 1992; 7: 449–456.
5. Ross PD, Davis JW, Epstein R, et al. Pain and disability associated with new vertebral fractures and other spinal conditions. *J Clin Epidemiol* 1994; 47(3): 231–239.
6. Rosen CJ, Linnell P, McClung M, et al. The impact of spinal fractures on general well being in elderly women. *J Bone Miner Res* 1992; 7(Suppl. 1): S175 abstract.
7. McClung M. Nonpharmacologic management of osteoporosis. In: Marcus R, ed. *Osteoporosis*. Boston: Blackwell Scientific, 1994, pp. 336–353.
8. Gold DT, Lyles KW, Bales CW, et al. Teaching patients coping behaviors: an essential part of management of osteoporosis. *J Bone Miner Res* 1989; 4(6): 799–801.
9. Quality of Life Focus Group. Osteoporosis: vertebral fractures and symptoms. Portland, OR: Osteoporosis Research Center, March 31, 1994.
10. Moneyham L, Scott CB. Anticipatory coping in the elderly. *J Gerontol Nurs* 1995; 21(7): 23–28.
11. Gold DT, Stagmaier K, Bales CW, et al. Psychosocial functioning and osteoporosis in late life: results of a multidisciplinary intervention. *J Women's Health* 1993; 2(2): 149–155.
12. Riordan ME, Bales C, Drezner MK. A preventive and therapeutic program for osteoporosis: a multifaceted approach to care. *Health Values* 1987; 11(4): 51–56.
13. Roberto KA. Women with osteoporosis: the role of the family and service community. *Gerontology* 1988; 28: 224–228.
14. Gold DR, Bales CW, Lyles KW, et al. Treatment of osteoporosis: the psychological impact of a medical education program on older patients. *J Am Geriatr Soc* 1989; 37: 417–422.
15. Wallston KA, Maides S, Wallston B. Health-related information seeking as a function of health-related locust of control and health value. *J Res Pers* 1976; 10: 215–222.
16. Hallal JC. Life satisfaction in women with postmenopausal osteoporosis of the spine. *Health Care for Women Int* 1991; 12: 99–110.

III   THE DIAGNOSIS OF OSTEOPOROSIS

7 What Is an Osteoporotic Fracture?

Richard Wasnich, MD

CONTENTS

1. INTRODUCTION

Hypertension would be nothing but a physiologic variant, of no practical, medical importance, save for the fact that it leads to symptoms and adverse outcomes, such as stroke. Likewise, there would be little medical interest or concern about osteoporosis were it not for the associated fractures. It is the fracture outcome, along with the related pain, disability, cost, morbidity, and mortality, that ultimately defines osteoporosis. All public health and medical efforts are aimed at preventing fractures. Therapeutic trials are ultimately based on a fracture outcome. For these reasons, it is important to define osteoporotic fracture as precisely as possible.

2. DEFINITION

Fracture. A break, breach, cleft, crack, split. A break in a bone, or occasionally a tear in a cartilage.

The clinical diagnosis of fracture is usually straightforward, and is based on clinical and radiographic criteria. However, as discussed below, fracture definition and diagnosis are not always simple, particularly with regard to vertebral fractures.

A recent consensus conference defined osteoporosis as a metabolic bone disease "characterized by low bone mass and microarchitectural deterioration of bone tissue, leading to enhanced bone fragility and a consequent increase in fracture risk" *(1)*. Therefore, a fracture, in order to be classified as osteoporotic, should occur in a patient meeting the above definition.

From: *Osteoporosis: Diagnostic and Therapeutic Principles*
Edited by: C. J. Rosen Humana Press Inc., Totowa, NJ

Table 1
Nonosteoporotic Fracture Etiologies

Traumatic fractures in childhood and adolescence
Occupation-related trauma
Severe trauma from any source
Other metabolic bone diseases
    Hyperparathyroidism, primary and secondary
    Osteomalacia
    Osteoporosis Imperfecta
Malignancy
    Multiple myeloma
    Primary bone malignancy
    Metastatic bone malignancy

However, in clinical practice, the diagnosis of osteoporotic fracture is also a diagnosis of exclusion. For example, traumatic fractures in childhood and adolescence are non-osteoporotic; these include skull fractures among infants and long bone fractures in adolescents. Another class of nonosteoporotic fractures are occupation-related fractures, frequently involving the hands and feet. Finally, there are other metabolic bone diseases that must be excluded (Table 1).

3. CHARACTERISTICS OF OSTEOPOROTIC FRACTURES

Normal, healthy bones can be fractured by trauma of sufficient force. Thus, osteoporotic fractures are those that either occur spontaneously, or as the result of mild or moderate trauma. Mild or moderate trauma is usually defined as a fall to the ground from a sitting or standing position. Such trauma would not ordinarily cause fractures in a healthy, 30-yr-old woman. In actual practice, it is often not possible to classify fractures by the degree of trauma involved. There are an infinite variety of falls and resulting forces on bone; there are also multiple protective mechanisms involved. Also, the incidence of falls does not begin to explain the exponential increases of fractures with aging. Although severe traumas (e.g., auto accident, falls from heights) are usually obvious, it is often not possible to determine precisely the amount of force involved with lesser degrees of trauma. For these reasons, a finding of low bone mass is usually used to confirm the diagnosis of suspected osteoporotic fracture.

Although osteoporosis is the most common etiology of low bone mass or density, there are other diseases that can also be manifested by osteopenia. These include osteomalacia, hyperparathyroidism, and multiple myeloma These conditions in particular may need to be excluded.

Nevertheless, the most useful clinical characteristic of an osteoporotic fracture is its association with low bone mass. Many prospective and cross-sectional studies have shown an association between low bone density and increased fracture risk (2–5). Vertebral fracture incidence increases by a factor of 2.0–2.4 for each standard deviation (SD) decrement in bone density (6). A 1 SD decrease in bone density is comparable to a 17-yr increase in age (7). Nonspine fractures are also inversely related to bone density, with relative risks of 1.5–2.7 for each 1 SD decrease in bone density.

Table 2
Comparison of Methods
for Classifying a Type of Fracture Associated with Low Bone Mass

Fracture type	Bone mass[a]	Classified by minimal/moderate trauma[b]	Age[c]
Humerus	+	+	+
Hip	+	+	+
Vertebral	+	+	+
Pelvic	+	+	+
Wrist	+	+	−
Rib	+	+	−
Leg	+	+	−
Hand	+	+	−
Foot	+	−	−
Toe	+	−	−
Clavicle	+	−	−
Patella	−	+	+
Ankle	−	+	−
Elbow	−	+	−
Face	−	+	−
Finger	−	−	−

[a]Based on significant ($p < 0.05$) relation with at least two measures of appendicular bone mass.
[b]More than 50% of fractures at the site preceded by fall from standing height or less, or spontaneous.
[c]Based on significant ($p < 0.05$) relation with age.

Seeley et al., in the study of osteoporotic fractures, concluded that low bone mass resulted in the most consistent classification of osteoporotic fracture (8). Fractures of the ankle, elbow, finger, and face were not associated with bone mass at any measurement site (Table 2). Employment of age or trauma-related criteria, in this study, led to inconsistent fracture classifications. A more recent study suggests that many ankle fractures are associated with low bone mass and, therefore, would be considered of osteoporotic etiology (9).

4. CURRENT FRACTURE RISK

Because the relationship between bone density and fracture risk is continuous, the level of bone density that represents osteoporosis is necessarily arbitrary. There have been two general approaches used to define an osteoporotic threshold or cutoff level. The first is based on the current level of bone mass. A World Health Organization (WHO) Study Group has recommended that the mean bone density of healthy young adults be considered the reference level (10). The SD variations above and below the young adult mean level are also described as T-scores. (Approaches employing age-matched reference ranges, i.e., the Z-score, were not considered useful.) Normal values are those not more than 1 SD below the young adult mean value (Fig. 1). Osteoporosis is represented by values that are more than 2.5 SD below the young adult level. Severe or established

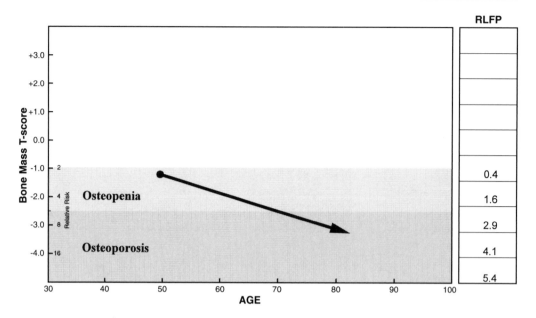

Fig. 1. WHO classification of osteoporosis based on bone density T-scores. The light-gray area denotes women with osteopenia and the dark-gray area, osteoporosis. This represents current fracture risk. An approach to future cumulative fracture risk has been incorporated into a standardized fracture risk report, which is based on RLFP *(12)*.

osteoporosis is defined as T-scores of more than –2.5, occurring in the presence of one or more fragility fractures. These proposed thresholds conform reasonably well to the actual life-time risks of fracture.

The problem area involves those women who have lesser degrees of bone density reduction, but who would benefit from therapies to prevent bone loss. The WHO Study Group recommended that density values that lie between 1 and 2.5 SD below the young adult mean value be considered osteopenic. It is this group in whom prevention of bone loss may be most useful. However, as illustrated below, an 80-yr-old woman whose T-score is –1.0 ("osteopenic") might receive less benefit from treatment than a 50-yr-old woman with a T-score of –0.9 ("normal").

5. CUMULATIVE, FUTURE FRACTURE RISK

The alternative approach is based on the concept of life-time fracture risk. For a population of 50-yr-old women with average bone density, there is a 15% life-time risk of hip fracture *(11)*. For a population at 2 SD below average at age 50, the life-time risk is about 60%. However, life-time risks for populations are difficult to translate into clinical guidelines for individual patients.

The concept of remaining lifetime fracture probability (RLFP) incorporates initial age, life expectancy, anticipated bone loss, and initial bone density to estimate the future probability of any fracture *(12)*. Since bone loss can be altered by therapeutic intervention, the RLFP model also facilitates objective therapeutic decisions. For example, consider two women with identical bone density T-scores of –1.0 (Table 3). The 80-yr-old, with more limited life expectancy (and future bone loss) has an estimated RLFP of 0.4;

Table 3
Comparison of RLFP for 50- and 80-Yr-Old Women with Identical T-Scores

Age	Initial T-score	RLFP without Rx[a]	RLFP with Rx[b]
50	−1.0	3.1	0.4
80	−1.0	0.4	0.2

[a]Assumes average life expectancy and future bone loss rates.
[b]Assumes complete prevention of future bone loss.

even with treatment that prevents all bone loss, her RLFP is only reduced by 0.2 to 0.2. However, the 50-yr-old has an RLFP of 3.1, and complete prevention of bone loss lowers her RLFP by 2.7 to 0.4. Thus, individual risk/cost/benefit decisions can be improved by incorporating information other than current bone density levels alone. Models, such as RLFP, are also capable of incorporating other major risk factors, such as existing (prevalence) fractures.

6. FRACTURES PREDICT FRACTURES

There is one additional characteristic of osteoporotic fractures that is worthy of discussion. Independent of bone density, existing osteoporotic fractures are strong predictors of future fragility fractures (13). Women with a single, prevalent vertebral fracture at baseline experience subsequent vertebral fractures at a rate 2.6–3.0 times greater than women without prevalent fractures, independent of bone mass (6). Women with two or more prevalent fractures developed new fractures at about seven to nine times the rate of women without prevalent fractures. Thus, each prevalent spine fracture had an effect on fracture risk slightly greater than a 1 SD decrease in bone mass.

The mechanism of this phenomenon is of interest. One possibility is that prevalent fractures serve as a surrogate indicator of defective bone quality (which is not reflected by bone mass or density). Another possibility is more mundane; women with fractures may fall more frequently than women without fractures. A third hypothesis is based on mechanical factors; deformation of one vertebral body may alter the load distribution on other vertebrae, particularly those adjacent to the original fracture. This hypothesis would help to explain the "clustering" of spine fractures in the T7-T9 and T11-L1 regions (14).

Opposing the mechanical hypothesis is the finding that existing, nonspine fractures also increase the risk of subsequent spine fractures (15). Women with prevalence nonspine fractures had a threefold greater risk of subsequent spine fractures, independent of the known association between existing spine fractures and subsequent spine fractures (Fig. 2). Women with both an existing nonspine fracture and low bone mass (50th percentile or lower) had an eightfold greater risk of new spine fractures, compared to women above the 50th percentile of bone mass and no existing fractures. Finally, women with existing fractures at both nonspine and spine locations, and low bone mass had a 16-fold greater risk of subsequent spine fractures.

7. FRACTURE DIAGNOSIS

Most patients with acute fractures will complain of pain at the fracture site. Physical examination may reveal swelling, tenderness to palpation, and pain with movement or weightbearing.

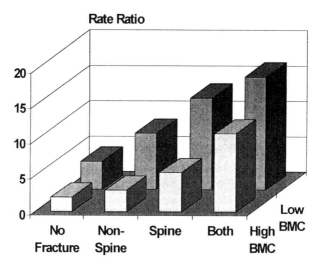

Fig. 2. Age-adjusted rate ratios for new spine fractures for women with low heel bone density (≤50th percentile) compared with women with high bone density, and further categorized according to the presence or absence of prevalent fractures.

Radiographs are the primary diagnostic tool; most fractures will exhibit characteristic displacement or a discontinuous bone contour. Nondisplaced fractures may not be radiographically apparent. Of the alternative imaging methods, radionuclide bone scintigraphy may be most useful when the radiograph is negative or equivocal. Computed tomography may be helpful in some circumstances.

7.1. Nonvertebral Fractures

Fractures of the distal radius ("Colles' Fracture") are a typical osteoporotic fracture. This injury usually results from a forward fall on an outstretched hand The distal fragment of the radius is tilted backward, displaced posteriorly, and often impacted. Distal radius fractures demonstrate a significant association with bone density of the distal radius, in addition to bone density measured elsewhere in the skeleton (8).

Fractures of the proximal humerus also occur frequently from a fall on an outstretched hand. Displaced fractures are frequent, and there are often several fragments. Proximal humerus fractures, unlike fractures of the shaft or distal humerus, increase with age, and three-fourths of such fractures occur in women.

Hip fractures may involve the femoral neck or occur between the trochanteric processes (Fig. 3). Femoral neck, or cervical, fractures can be occult in the elderly, with little or no apparent trauma. The fracture line may be undetectable on initial radiographs, and bone scintigraphy may be required to establish the diagnosis. Scintigraphy additionally provides important information about vascular supply to the femoral head.

Intertrochanteric fractures usually result from a fall. The intertrochanteric region of the proximal femur contains about 50% trabecular bone, as compared to the femoral neck, which is about 25% trabecular bone (16).

Of interest is the fact that patients with intertrochanteric fractures are much more likely to have a recurrent fracture of the same type in the opposite hip (17,18). Likewise, recurrent femoral neck fractures are also more likely in patients with prior femoral neck

A   **B**

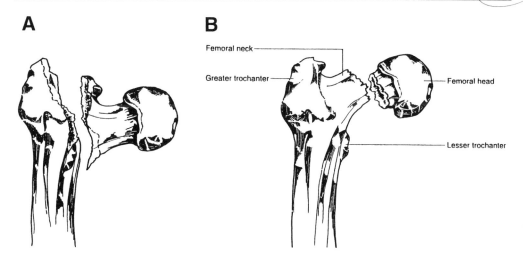

Fig. 3. **(A)** Intertrochanteric fracture, and **(B)** femoral neck fracture.

fractures on the opposite side *(17,18)*. There may also be different risk factors operative in the two types of hip fractures. *(19)*. Other nonspine fractures considered osteoporotic are listed in Table 2.

7.2. Vertebral Fractures

Although vertebral fractures are the most common of all osteoporotic fractures, their study has been hampered by the lack of consensus regarding the definition of vertebral fracture. Unlike nonspine fractures, where there is usually a distinct split or cleft in the bone, spine fractures are represented by a continuous range of vertebral deformations.

Vertebral radiographs are the primary diagnostic tool. Because a large proportion of vertebral fractures are asymptomatic and/or did not come to medical attention, self-reporting is not sufficiently accurate *(20)*. Height loss can result from vertebral fractures, but can also occur from other causes, rendering it nonspecific.

The interpretation of radiographs has traditionally been visual. Vertebral fractures have been classified as crush, wedge, and end plate (Fig. 4). More recently, quantitative vertebral morphometry has been employed as shown in Fig. 4.

7.2.1. INCIDENCE VERTEBRAL FRACTURES

The diagnosis of incidence vertebral fractures can be less problematic than the diagnosis of pre-existing fractures, particularly if a prior radiograph is available. Substantial vertebral height reductions usually represent a fracture, but there is some measurement error involved. Some studies have defined a new fracture as a ≥15% reduction in any one of the three measured heights (Ha, Hm, Hp). In order to reduce false positives, other investigators propose a more stringent criterion of ≥20%. For nonclinical, research purposes, a change exceeding 3 SDs of the mean of differences for that vertebral level has been proposed *(21)*. Although the best radiographic definition is not established, when there are questionable, new fractures in clinical practice, bone scintigraphy is usually employed to resolve the diagnosis. A new vertebral fracture will show diffusely increased

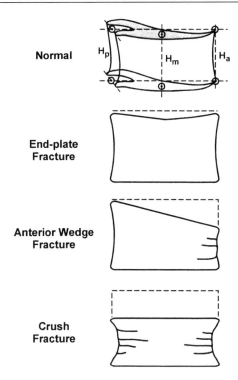

Fig. 4. Vertebral morphometry measurements are typically based on placement of six (6) points that define the anterior (H_a), middle (H_m), and posterior (H_p) heights of the vertebral body. Crush, wedge, and end-plate fractures are illustrated.

activity for approx 6 mo after the fracture occurs (Fig. 5). On occasion, bone scintigraphy will be positive prior to the appearance of radiographic collapse.

7.2.2. Prevalence Vertebral Fractures

There are more suggested definitions of prevalence vertebral fractures than there are vertebral bodies. The National Osteoporosis Foundation (NOF) convened a working group in 1994 to review criteria for definition of a prevalence vertebral fracture *(21)*. Since bone scintigraphy is useful only for the diagnosis of recent vertebral fractures, diagnosis of old fractures is based on radiographic and morphometric criteria. Also, since vertebral deformities can result from other processes, including congenital, degenerative, and malignant diseases, these etiologies must be excluded by visual interpretation of the radiograph.

The two basic approaches involve (1) comparison of vertebral dimensions or ratios within the same individual, and (2) comparison of an individual's vertebral dimensions to population-based normal ranges.

Although the population-based approach has advantages, it is not usually practical for clinical application. There are potential differences between ethnic groups and sexes, in addition to age cohorts. If an appropriate reference population is available, the fracture definition is based on comparison with normal values of means and standard deviations for each vertebral level. The NOF suggests that in studies involving community populations, prevalence vertebral fractures be defined as a reduction of 3 SDs or more below the

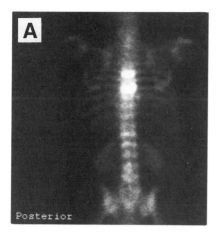
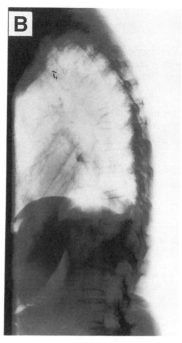

Fig. 5. (A) The ^{99}mTc-MDP scan reveals intensely increased activity in the T5 and T7 vertebral bodies, indicative of a recent fracture. The old fractures have healed and show no increased activity; **(B)** the spine radiograph reveals multiple thoracic and lumbar fractures, but the age of the fractures cannot be determined.

normal dimensions for that particular vertebral level. Less stringent criteria (i.e., –2 SDs) result in too many false positives, whereas a more stringent criterion of –4 SDs results in reduced sensitivity. The best criterion depends on the use; for higher sensitivity in clinical settings, a less stringent criterion (combined with visual interpretation) may be preferred. For studies involving groups or populations, a more stringent criterion, with fewer false positives, may be preferable.

In the absence of population-based normal ranges, the clinician can define vertebral deformities by several methods:

1. Ratios of vertebral dimensions within or between vertebrae (22,23);
2. Normalization of vertebral heights by dividing all other dimensions by the corresponding dimensions of T4 or T5 (24); and
3. Calculation of average vertebral size, and statistical confidence limits, for the individual (25).

8. SUMMARY

Low bone mass predicts fractures. Fractures also independently predict fractures. Individuals with both low bone mass and existing fractures have markedly elevated risks for future fractures. The clinical implications are several. First, the primary goal of interventional efforts should be the prevention of the first fracture. Second, patients who present with acute, nonviolent fractures, even though the fracture itself may have low morbidity (e.g., rib fractures), should have bone density routinely measured, and if osteoporosis is confirmed, appropriate intervention instituted. Finally, because fractures themselves provide important prognostic information, fracture histories should be carefully explored; vertebral fracture diagnosis should be radiographically investigated in older patients, particularly in those with low bone density.

REFERENCES

1. Consensus development conference. Diagnosis, prophylaxis, and treatment of osteoporosis. *Am J Med* 1993; 94: 646–650.
2. Wasnich RD, Ross PD, Heilbrun LK, Vogel JM. Prediction of postmenopausal fracture risk with bone mineral measurements. *Am J Obstet Gynecol* 1985; 153: 745–751.
3. Wasnich RD, Ross PD, McLean CJ, et al. A comparison of single versus multi-site BMC measurements for assessment of spine fracture probability. *J Nucl Med* 1989; 30: 1166–1171.
4. Hui SL, Slemenda CW, Johnston CC Jr. Baseline measurement of bone mass predicts fracture in white women. *Ann Intern Med* 1989; 111: 355–361.
5. Cummings SR, Black D, Nevitt MC, et al. Appendicular densitometry and age predict hip fracture in women. *JAMA* 1990; 263: 665–668.
6. Ross PD, Davis JW, Epstein RS, Wasnich RD. Pre-existing fractures and bone mass predict vertebral fracture incidence in women. *Ann Intern Med* 1991; 114: 919–923.
7. Melton LJ III. How many women have osteoporosis now? *J Bone Miner Res* 1995; 10: 175–177.
8. Seeley DG, Browner WS, Nevitt MC, et al. Which fractures are associated with low appendicular bone mass in elderly women? *Ann Intern Med* 1991; 115: 837–842.
9. Cooper AM, Greenfield D, Eastell R. Bone mineral density in women with previous ankle fracture. *J Bone Miner Res* 1995; 10(Suppl. 1): S265.
10. Kanis JA, Melton LJ, Christiansen C, et al. The diagnosis of osteoporosis. *J Bone Miner Res* 1994; 9: 1137–1141.
11. Black D, Cummings S, Melton LJ. Appendicular bone mineral and a women's lifetime risk of hip fracture. *J Bone Miner Res* 1992; 7: 639–646.
12. Wasnich RD, Ross PD, Vogel JM, Davis JW. *Osteoporosis. Critique and Practicum.* Honolulu: Banyan, 1989.
13. Gardsell P, Johnell O, Nilsson BE, Nilsson JA. The predictive value of fracture, disease and falling tendency due to fragility fractures in women. *Calcif Tissue Res* 1989; 45: 327–330.
14. Ross PD, Fujiwara S, Huang C, et al. Vertebral fracture prevalence in women in Hiroshima compared to Caucasians or Japanese in the U.S. *Int J Epidemiol* 1995; 24: 1–7.
15. Wasnich RD, Davis JW, Ross PD. Spine fracture risk is predicted by non-spine fractures. *Osteoporosis Int* 1994; 4: 1–5.
16. Riggs BL, Wahner HW, Seeman E, Offord KP, Dunn WL, Mazess RB, Johnson KA, Melton LJ. Changes in bone mineral density of the proximal femur and spine with aging: differences between the postmenopausal and senile osteoporosis syndromes. *J Clin Invest* 1982; 70: 716–723.
17. Dretakis E, Kritsikis N, Economou K, Christodoulou N. Bilateral and noncontemporary fractures of the proximal femur. *Acta Orthop Scan* 1981; 52: 227–229.
18. Melton LJ III, Ilstrup DM, Beckenbaugh RD, Riggs BL. Hip fracture recurrence: a population-based study. *Clin Orthop* 1982; 167: 131–138.
19. Fox KM, Cummings SR, Threets RD, et al. Intertrochanteric and femoral neck fractures have different risk factors. *J Bone Miner Res* 1995; 10(Suppl. 1): S170.
20. Cooper C, Atkinson EJ, O'Fallon WM, Melton LJ. Incidence of clinically diagnosed vertebral fractures: a population-based study in Rochester, Minnesota, 1985–1989. *J Bone Miner Res* 1992; 7: 221–227.
21. Assessing vertebral fractures. National Osteoporosis Foundation Working Group on vertebral fractures. *J Bone Miner Res* 1995; 10: 518–523.
22. Melton LJ. Epidemiology of vertebral fractures. In: Christiansen C, Johansen JS, Riis, BJ, eds. *Osteoporosis.* Denmark: Kobenhavn K, 1987, pp. 33–37.
23. Smith-Bindman R, Cummings SR, Steiger P, Genant HK. A comparison of morphometric definitions of vertebral fracture. *J Bone Miner Res* 1991; 6: 25–34.
24. Minne HW, Leidig G, Wüster Chr. A newly developed spine deformity index (SDI) to quantitate vertebral crush fractures in patients with osteoporosis. *Bone Miner* 1988; 3: 335–349.
25. Ross PD, Yhee YK, He YF, et al. A new method for vertebral fracture diagnosis. *J Bone Miner Res* 1993; 8: 167–174.

8 Bone Densitometry Techniques in Modern Medicine

Sydney Lou Bonnick, MD, FACP

Contents

The field of bone densitometry has grown rapidly, particularly in the last 15 years. A variety of techniques are now available from which the physician may choose. Beyond the simple consideration of geographic accessibility, the choice of technique may be determined by the intent of the measurement. Some techniques, because of the skeletal sites to which they can be applied, or because of their accuracy and reproducibility or both are better suited for certain types of measurements.

Bone density measurements can be broadly divided into two types: assessments of fracture risk or quantification of bone mineral content or density (BMC or BMD). Assessments of fracture risk can be further divided into global fracture risk assessments or site-specific fracture risk assessments. The quantification of bone density may be required to confirm osteopenia or osteoporosis suspected from the appearance of the skeleton on plain skeletal radiography, to confirm sufficient osteopenia to accept a diagnosis of fragility fracture, to detect the effects of disease processes on specific regions of the skeleton, or to detect changes in the bone mass or density over time from disease processes or therapeutic interventions. Once the intent of the desired measurement has been determined, the physician can decide which site or sites should be measured, and the degree to which the accuracy and precision of the various techniques will affect the interpretation of the test. Only then can the physician decide which technique to employ.

Plain skeletal radiographs when viewed by the unaided eye have never been useful for assessing bone density. Demineralization becomes visually apparent only after 40% or more of the bone density has been lost *(1)*. Beyond that general statement, no quantification of the bone density can be made. Plain radiographs have been used to perform qualitative

From: *Osteoporosis: Diagnostic and Therapeutic Principles*
Edited by: C. J. Rosen Humana Press Inc., Totowa, NJ

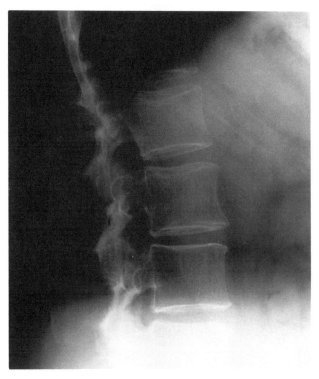

Fig. 1. Qualitative spinal morphometry. The vertebrae on this lateral lumbar spine film exhibit marked accentuation of the vertical trabecular pattern and thinning of the cortical shell. This is a Grade II spine.

and quantitative skeletal morphometry, which constituted some of the earliest attempts to assess bone density. Plain radiographs were also used to assess bone density based on the optical densities of the skeleton when compared to simultaneously X-rayed standards of known density. With the advent of the photon absorptiometric techniques, most of these early methods have fallen into disuse. Nevertheless, a brief review of these techniques should both enhance the appreciation of the capabilities of modern testing and provide a background for the understanding of modern technologies.

1. QUALITATIVE MORPHOMETRY
1.1. Qualitative Spinal Morphometry and the Singh Index
1.1.1. QUALITATIVE SPINAL MORPHOMETRY

Qualitative morphometric techniques for the assessment of bone density have been in limited use for over 50 years. Grading systems for the spine relied on the appearance of the trabecular patterns within the vertebral body and the appearance and thickness of the cortical shell (2).

Vertebra were graded from IV down to I as the vertical trabecular pattern became more pronounced with the loss of the horizontal trabeculae and the cortical shell became progressively thinned. The spine shown in Fig. 1 demonstrates a pronounced vertical trabecular pattern. The cortical shell appears as though it were outlined in white around the more radiotranslucent vertebral body. These vertebrae would be classified as Grade II.

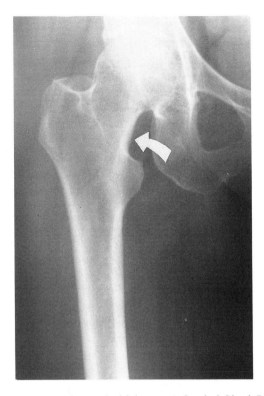

Fig. 2. The Singh Index and *calcar femorale* thickness. A Grade 2 Singh Index would be assessed here indicating the presence of osteoporosis. The arrow points to the *calcar femorale*, which measured 4 mm in thickness. Values <5 mm are associated with hip fracture.

1.1.2. THE SINGH INDEX

The Singh Index is a qualitative morphometric technique that was similarly based on trabecular patterns, but based on those seen in the proximal femur *(3)*. Singh and others had noted that there appeared to be a predictable pattern to the disappearance of the five groups of trabeculae in the proximal femur in osteoporosis. Based on this order of disappearance, radiographs of the proximal femur could be graded 1–6 with lower values indicating a greater loss of the trabecular patterns normally seen in the proximal femur. Studies evaluating prevalent fractures demonstrated a good association between Singh Index values of 3 or less with the presence of fractures of either the hip, spine, or wrist. Figure 2 shows a proximal femur with a Singh Index of 2. Only the trabecular pattern known as the principal compressive group, which extends from the medical cortex of the shaft to the upper portion of the head of the femur, remains. This patient was known to have had osteoporotic spine fractures as well as a contra lateral proximal femur fracture. Subsequent attempts to demonstrate a strong correlation with Singh Index values and bone density of the proximal femur measured by dual-photon absorptiometry (DPA) have not been successful *(4)*.

These qualitative morphometric techniques are highly subjective. In general, the best approach required the creation of a set of reference radiographs of the various grades to which all other radiographs could be compared.

2. QUANTITATIVE MORPHOMETRIC TECHNIQUES

2.1. Calcar Femorale *Thickness, Radiogrammetry and the Radiologic Osteoporosis Score*

2.1.1. CALCAR FEMORALE THICKNESS

A little-known quantitative morphometric technique involves the measurement of the thickness of the *calcar femorale*. The *calcar femorale* is the band of cortical bone immediately above the lesser trochanter in the proximal femur. In normal subjects, this thickness is >5 mm. In femoral fracture cases, it is generally <5 mm in thickness *(5)*. The arrow, seen in Fig. 2, is pointing to the *calcar femorale*. This patient had previously suffered a femoral neck fracture. The thickness of the calcar femorale measured 4 mm.

2.1.2. RADIOGRAMMETRY

Radiogrammetry is the measurement of the dimensions of the bones using skeletal radiographs. Metacarpal radiogrammetry has been in use for over 30 years. The cortical width of the metacarpal was measured in one of two ways. Using a plain radiograph of the hand and fine calipers or transparent ruler, the total width and medullary width of the metacarpals of the index, long, and ring fingers were measured at the midpoint of the metacarpal. The cortical width was calculated by subtracting the medullary width from the total width. Alternatively, the cortical width could be measured directly. A variety of different calculations were then made, such as the metacarpal index and the hand score. The metacarpal index (MI) is the cortical width divided by the total width. The hand score (HS), which is also known as the percent cortical thickness, is the MI expressed as a percentage. Measurements on the middle three metacarpals of both hands were also made and used to calculate the six metacarpal hand score (6HS). Other quantities derived from these measurements included the percent cortical area (%CA), the cortical area (CA), and the cortical area to surface area ratio (CA/SA). The main limitation in all of these measurements is that they were based on the false assumption that the point at which these measurements were made on the metacarpal was a perfect hollow cylinder. Nevertheless, using these measurements and a knowledge of the gravimetric density of bone, the bone density, bone ash, and bone calcium could be calculated. The correlation between such measurements and ashed bone is good, ranging from 0.79 to 0.85 *(6,7)*. The reproducibility of metacarpal morphometry is quite variable depending on the measurement used.* The measurement of total width is very reproducible. The measurement of medullary width or the direct measurement of cortical width is less reproducible, because the delineation between the cortical bone and medullary canal is not as distinct as the delineation between the cortical bone and soft tissue. Reproducibility has been variously reported as excellent to poor, but in expert hands, it is possible to achieve a reproducibility of 1.9% *(8)*.

Although metacarpal radiogrammetry is an old technique and somewhat tedious to perform, it remains a viable means of assessing bone density in the metacarpals. Metacarpal radiogrammetry demonstrates a reasonably good correlation to bone density at other skeletal sites measured with photon absorptiometric techniques *(9)*. The tech-

---

*Techniques are often compared on the basis of accuracy and reproducibility. Both are usually described with percent coefficients of variation (%CV). The %CV is the standard deviation divided by the mean of replicate measurements expressed as a percentage. The lower the %CV, the better the accuracy or reproducibility.

nique is very safe, since the biologically significant radiation dose from a hand X ray is extremely low at only 1 mrem.

Radiogrammetry can also be performed at other sites, such as the phalanx, distal radius, and femur *(10–12)*. Combined measurements of the cortical widths of the distal radius and the second metacarpal have been shown to be highly correlated with bone density in the spine as measured by DPA *(10)*.

2.1.3. THE RADIOLOGIC OSTEOPOROSIS SCORE

The radiologic osteoporosis score combined aspects of both quantitative and qualitative morphometry *(12)*. Developed by Barnett and Nordin, this scoring system utilized radiogrammetry of the femoral shaft and metacarpal, as well as an index of biconcavity of the lumbar vertebra. In calculating what Barnett and Nordin called a peripheral score, the cortical thickness of the femoral shaft divided by the diameter of the shaft and expressed as a percentage was added to a similar measurement of the metacarpal. A score of 88 or less was considered to indicate peripheral osteoporosis. The biconcavity index was calculated by dividing the middle height of usually the third lumbar vertebra by its anterior height and expressing this value as a percentage. A biconcavity index of 80 or less indicated spinal osteoporosis. Combining both the peripheral score and biconcavity index resulted in the total radiologic osteoporosis score, which was considered to indicate osteoporosis if the value was 168 or less.

3. RADIOGRAPHIC PHOTODENSITOMETRY

Much of the development of the modern techniques of single-photon absorptiometry (SPA) and DPA and dual-energy X-ray absorptiometry (DXA) actually came from early work on the X-ray-based method of photodensitometry. In photodensitometry, broad beam X-ray exposures of radiographs were obtained, and the density of the skeletal image was quantified using a scanning photodensitometer. The effects of variations in technique, such as exposure settings, beam energy, and film development, were partially compensated by the simultaneous exposure of a step wedge of known densities on the film. An aluminum wedge was most often used, but other materials, such as ivory, were also employed *(11)*. This technique could only be applied to areas of the skeleton in which the soft tissue coverage was <5 cm, such as the hand, forearm, and os calcis, because of technical limitations created by scattered radiation in thicker parts of the body and "beam hardening" or the preferential attenuation of the softer energies of the polychromatic X-ray beam as it passed through the body. It was also used in cadaver studies of the proximal femur *(14)*. Such studies noted the predictive power for hip fracture of the density of the region in the proximal femur known as Ward's triangle ** long before the prospective studies of Cummings et al., using the modern technique of DXA in 1993. The accuracy of such measurements was fairly good with a 5% error. The correlation between metacarpal photodensitometry and ashed bone was high at 0.88 *(6)*. This is a slightly better correlation than seen with metacarpal radiogrammetry. The reproducibility of photodensitometry was relatively poor, however, with a reproducibility ranging from 5 to 15% *(16)*. In this regard, the six metacarpal radiogrammetry hand score was

---

**Ward's triangle was first described by F. O. Ward in *Outlines of Human Osteology*, London: Henry Renshaw, 1838. It is a triangular region created by the intersection of three groups of trabeculae in the femoral neck.

superior *(2)*. Radiation dose to the hand was the same for metacarpal radiogrammetry and radiographic photodensitometry. In both cases, the biologically significant radiation dose was negligible.

Radiographic photodensitometry was developed and used extensively by Mack et al. *(17)*. Many of the original studies of the effects of weightlessness on the skeleton in the Apollo astronauts were performed by Mack and Vogt at Texas Woman's University *(18)*.

4. RADIOGRAPHIC ABSORPTIOMETRY (RA)

RA is the modern-day outgrowth of radiographic photodensitometry *(19,20)*. The ability to digitize high-resolution radiographic images and to perform computerized analysis of such images has largely eliminated the errors introduced by differences in radiographic exposure techniques and overlying soft tissue thickness. As performed in the US, RA of the hand involves taking two X-rays of the left hand using nonscreened film, each at slightly different exposures. The initial recommended settings are 50 kVp at 300 mA for 1 s and 60 kVp at 300 mA for 1 s. The exact settings will vary slightly with the equipment used and are adjusted so that the background optical density of each of the two hand films matches a sample film supplied by CompuMed, Manhattan Beach, CA. An aluminum alloy reference wedge, also supplied by CompuMed, is placed on the film prior to exposure, parallel to the middle phalanx of the index finger. The developed films are sent to CompuMed for analysis. The X-ray images are then captured electronically with a high-resolution video camera. The average density of the middle phalanxes of the index, long, and ring fingers is reported in RA units. Figure 3 illustrates the X-ray appearance of the hand and aluminum alloy reference wedge. Other manufacturers are employing updated radiographic absorptiometric techniques, such as the Bonalyzer by Teijin in Tokyo and the Osteoradiometer by NIM in Verona, Italy.

In cadaveric studies, the accuracy of RA for the assessment of bone mineral content of the middle phalanxes is very good *(21)*. The correlation between the RA values and the ashed weight in the phalanxes was excellent with $r = 0.983$. The accuracy was 4.8%. The authors of this study did note that increasing thicknesses of soft tissue, which might be seen in very obese subjects, could potentially result in an underestimation of RA values. The short-term reproducibility of these measurements was also excellent at 0.6%.

The ability to predict bone density at other skeletal sites from hand radiographic absorptiometry is as good as that seen with other techniques such as SPA, DPA, DXA, or quantitative computed tomography (QCT) of the spine. This does not mean that RA hand values can be used to predict accurately bone density at other skeletal sites. Although the correlations between the different sites as measured by the various techniques are correctly said to be statistically significant, the correlations are too weak to allow clinically useful predictions of bone mass or density at one site from measurement at another.

The utility of modern-day radiographic absorptiometry in predicting either a global or site-specific fracture risk remains to be established. A recent analysis of 1579 hand radiographs obtained with the older technique of photodensitometry during the National Health and Nutrition Examination Survey I (1971–1975) suggested its potential utility in this regard. During a median followup of 14 yr, which extended through 1987, 49 osteoporotic hip fractures occurred. Based on radiographic photodensitometry of the second phalanx of the small finger of the left hand, the age-adjusted relative risk for hip fracture was 1.6 *(23)*. This is a modern analysis of films acquired using the older technique

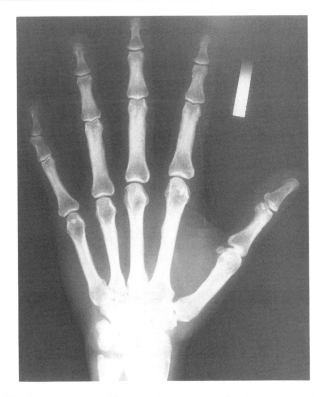

Fig. 3. Radiographic absorptiometry. The aluminum step wedge is seen, positioned adjacent and parallel to the middle phalanx of the index finger.

of photon absorptiometry and not truly representative of radiographic absorptiometry as it is performed today. Nevertheless, it suggests that modern-day RA may be similarly useful. A technique, such as RA, has the obvious advantages of being easy to perform and of widespread geographic accessibility, since standard X-ray equipment is used. The costs of RA include the costs of the X-ray film, the aluminum alloy reference wedge, which is reusable, the performance of two hand films, postage to CompuMed in California, and analysis costs from CompuMed. In general, these total costs will approach or equal the average cost of bone density testing with SPA, DPA, or DXA.

5. THE PHOTON ABSORPTIOMETRY TECHNIQUES

In radiology, attenuation refers to a reduction in the number and energy of photons in an X-ray beam. This is referred to as a reduction in the beam's intensity. To a large extent, the attenuation of X rays is determined by tissue density. A difference in tissue densities is responsible for creating the images seen on an X ray. The denser the tissue, the more electrons it contains. The number of electrons in the tissue determines the ability of the tissue either to attenuate or transmit the photons in the X-ray beam. The differences in the pattern of transmitted or attenuated photons create the contrast necessary to discern images on the X ray. If all the photons were attenuated (or none were transmitted), no image would be seen because the film would be totally white. If all of the photons were transmitted (or none were attenuated), no image would be seen because the film would

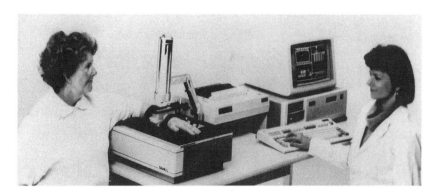

Fig. 4. SPA of the radius. Photo courtesy of Lunar Corp.

be totally black. The difference in the attenuation of the X-ray photon energy by different tissues is responsible for the contrast on an X ray, which enables us to see the images. If the degree of attenuation could be quantified, it would be possible to assess quantitatively the tissue density as well. This is the premise behind photon absorptiometry and the measurement of bone density.

5.1. Single-Photon Absorptiometry (SPA)

Writing in the journal *Science* in 1963, Cameron and Sorenson described a new method for determining bone density in vivo by passing a monochromatic or single-energy photon beam through bone and soft tissue *(24)*. The amount of mineral in the path transversed by the beam could be quantitated based on the difference between the beam intensity before and after passage through the region of interest. In the earliest SPA units, the results of multiple scan passes at a single location, usually the mid-radius, were averaged *(25)*. In later units, scan passes at equally spaced intervals along the bone were utilized, such that the mass of mineral per unit of bone length could be calculated. A scintillation detector was used to quantitate the photon energy after attenuation by the bone and soft tissue in the scan path. The photon source and the detector are both highly "collimated," which means that the size and shape of the beam are restricted. Both move in tandem across the region of interest on the bone, coupled by a mechanical motor drive system. Iodine-125 at 27.3 keV or americium-241 at 59.6 keV was originally used to generate the single-energy photon beam, although most SPA units subsequently developed in the US employed only [125]I.

The physical calculations for SPA determinations of bone mineral are valid only when there is uniform thickness of the bone and soft tissue in the scan path. In order to create this kind of uniform thickness artificially, the limb to be studied had to be submerged in a water bath or surrounded by a tissue-equivalent material. As a practical matter, this limited SPA to measurements of the distal appendicular skeleton, such as the radius and, later, the os calcis. Figure 4 illustrates a patient undergoing an SPA study of the midradius. Although difficult to see in the photograph, the area of interest in the forearm is wrapped with a tissue-equivalent gel-filled bag to produce the necessary uniform thickness. After the photon attenuation is quantified, the determination of the amount of bone mineral is based on a comparison to the photon attenuation seen with a calibration standard derived from dried defatted human ashed bone of known weight.

Table 1
The Relative Percentages
of Cortical and Trabecular Bone at Various Skeletal Sites[a]

Region of interest	% of Trabecular bone	% of Cortical bone
AP spine (DPA/DXA)	66	34
AP spine (QCT)	100	
Lateral spine (DXA)[b]	++++	
Femoral neck	25	75
Ward's area [b]	++++	
Trochanteric region	50	50
Os calcis	95	5
Midradius	1	99
Distal radius	20	80
Ultradistal 8-mm radius	25	75
Ultradistal 5-mm radius	40	60
Phalanges	40	60
Total body	20	80

[a]The exact composition of some of these skeletal sites is controversial. These are considered clinically useful characterizations of the percentages of cortical and trabecular bone.
[b]This site is highly trabecular, but the exact composition is not defined in the literature.

Several sites on the radius can be evaluated with SPA. Commonly used sites are the 33% site, the 50% site, the 10% sites and the 5- and 8-mm sites. The sites designated as a percentage are named based on the location of the site on the radius in relationship to the overall length of the ulna. In other words, the 50% site on the radius is located at a site on the radius that is directly across from the site on the ulna, which marks 50% of the overall ulnar length, not 50% of the overall radial length. The 5- and 8-mm sites are located on the radius at the point where the separation distance between the radius and ulna is 5 or 8 mm, respectively. The 33 and 50% sites are often referred to as midradial sites, whereas the 10% is considered a distal site. The 5- and 8-mm sites and a third site where the ulna and radius conjoin are considered "ultradistal" sites. The difference between these sites is in the relative percentages of cortical and trabecular bone found at the site. Table 1 summarizes the percentages of cortical and trabecular bone at a variety of skeletal sites that can be assessed with current densitometry techniques.

SPA is both accurate and reproducible, although these parameters will vary slightly with the site studied. For SPA measurements of the midradius, the accuracy has been reported as ranging from 3 to 5% and reproducibility as ranging from 1 to 2% (24,26–28). In expert hands, the reproducibility of midradial measurements should approach 1%. Early measurements of the distal and ultradistal radius did not demonstrate the same high degree of reproducibility primarily because of the marked changes in composition of the bone with very small changes in location along the distal and ultradistal radius. With newer instruments which employ computer enhanced localization routines and rectilinear scanning, SPA measurements of the distal and ultradistal radius should approach a reproducibility of 1% (29). Accuracy of measurements at the os calcis with SPA has been reported to be <3% and reproducibility as 3% or less (27). The skin radiation dose for both the radius and os calcis is 5–10 mrem (27,28). The biologically important radiation dose, the absorbed dose equivalent, is negligible. Results are reported as either BMC in grams or as bone mineral content per unit length (BMC/L) in g/cm. The time required to perform such studies is approx 10 min. The cost for SPA studies of the appendicular skeleton ranges from US $35.00 to US $125.00 *(28,30)*.

The ability to predict the risk of appendicular fractures with single-photon absorptiometric measurements of the radius is well established *(31–33)*. SPA measurements of the radius also appear to be good predictors of fracture risk of the spine and good predictors of global fracture risk *(31,34,35)*.

5.2. Dual-Photon Absorptiometry (DPA)

The basic principle involved in DPA for the measurement of bone density is the same as for SPA: the ability to quantitate the degree of attenuation of a photon energy beam after passage through bone and soft tissue. In dual-photon systems, however, an isotope that emits photon energy at two distinct photoelectric peaks or two isotopes, each emitting photon energy at separate and distinct photoelectric peaks, are used. When the beam is passed through a region of the body containing both bone and soft tissue, attenuation of the photon beam will occur at both energy peaks. If one energy peak is preferentially attenuated by bone, however, the contributions of soft tissue in beam attenuation can be mathematically subtracted *(36)*. As in SPA, the remaining contributions of beam attenuation from bone can be quantified and then compared to standards created from ashed bone. The ability to separate bone from soft tissue in this manner finally allowed quantification of the bone density in those areas of the skeleton that were surrounded by large or irregular soft tissue masses, notably the spine and proximal femur. DPA can also be used to determine the total body bone density. The development of DPA and its application to the spine, proximal femur, and total body is attributed to a number of investigators: B. O. Roos, G. W. Reed, R. B. Mazess, C. R. Wilson, M. Madsen, W. Peppler, B. L. Riggs, W. L. Dunn, and H. W. Wahner *(37–42)*.

The isotope most commonly employed in DPA is gadolinium-153, which naturally emits photon energy at two photoelectric peaks, 44 and 100 keV. It is at the photoelectric peak of 44 keV that bone preferentially attenuates the photon energy. The attenuated photon beams are detected by a NaI scintillation detector and quantified after passage through pulse-height analyzers set at 44 and 100 keV. The shielded holder for the [153]Gd source, which is collimated and equipped with a shutter that is operated by a computer, moves in tandem with the NaI detector in a rectilinear scan path over the region of interest. A point-by-point calculation of bone density in the scan path can be made. Figure 5 is the intensity-modulated image of the spine created with an early DPA device. Figure 6 demonstrates the intensity-modulated images of the same spine created with a later DPA device and newer pencil-beam and fan-array dual-energy X-ray absorptiometers.

Bone density studies of the lumbar spine are performed with the photon energy beam passing in a posterior to anterior direction. Because of the direction of the beam, the vertebral body and the posterior elements are included in the scan path. The transverse processes are eliminated. This results in a combined measurement of cortical and trabecular bone, which includes the more trabecular vertebral body surrounded by its cortical shell and the highly cortical posterior elements. The results are reported as an areal density in g of mineral/cm^2. The BMD of the proximal femur is also an areal density that is acquired with the beam passing in a posterior to anterior direction. Figure 7 shows an early dual-photon absorptiometer with the patient positioned for a study of the lumbar spine.

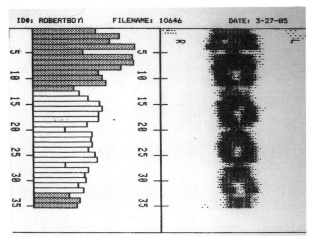

Fig. 5. The intensity-modulated image of the spine created with an early DPA device.

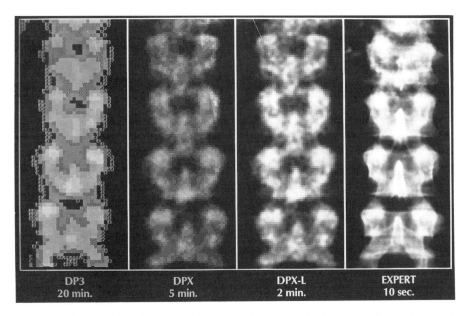

Fig. 6. An intensity-modulated image of the spine of the same patient created with four different devices. From left to right, a late DPA device, early DXA pencil-beam device, late DXA pencil-beam device, and a fan-array DXA device. Photo courtesy of Lunar Corp.

DPA studies of the spine require approx 30 min to complete. Studies of the proximal femur take 30–45 minutes to perform. Total body bone density studies with DPA require 1 h. Skin radiation dose is low during spine or proximal femur studies at 15 mrem. Accuracy of DPA measurements of the spine ranges from 3 to 6% and for the proximal femur, from 3 to 4% *(43)*. Reproducibility for measurements of spine bone density is 2–4% and around 4% for the femoral neck. The cost of a DPA study of the spine or proximal femur ranges from US $125 to US $200 and US $75 to US $125, respectively *(27,30)*.

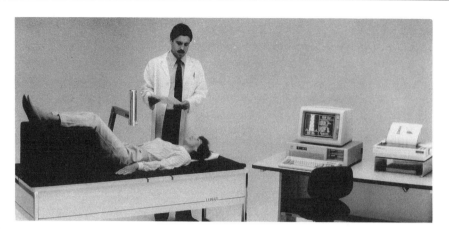

Fig. 7. DPA of the spine. Photo courtesy of Lunar Corp.

DPA was considered a major advance from SPA because it allowed the quantification of bone density in the spine and proximal femur. DPA does have several limitations, however. Machine maintenance is expensive. The ^{153}Gd source must be replaced yearly at a cost of $5000.00 or more. It has also been noted that as the radioactive source decays, values obtained with DPA increase by as much as 0.6%/mo *(44)*. With replacement of the source, values may fall by as much as 6.2%. Although mathematical formulas have been developed to compensate for this effect of source decay, it remains a cause for concern, affecting both accuracy and reproducibility. The overall reproducibility of 2–4% for DPA measurements of the spine and proximal femur limited its application for serial measurements of bone density. Two measurements performed with a technique that has a precision of 2% will yield a difference that is accurate at a 95% confidence level within ±5.5%. If the reproducibility is only 4%, the resulting difference is accurate to within ±11.1% *(45)*. Even at an 80% confidence level, these numbers fall to only ±3.6% and ±7.3%, respectively. This creates a margin of error that is too great to be clinically useful in following changes in bone density over time with only two measurements. Although these confidence intervals can be narrowed by performing multiple measurements within a given period of time, this increases the costs associated with the testing, which similarly serves to reduce its clinical utility in this regard.

As a practical matter, all spine bone density studies in which the photon beam passes in an AP or PA direction will be unable to separate the more highly trabecular vertebral body from its more cortical posterior elements. Calcifications in the overlying soft tissue or abdominal aorta will attenuate such a beam, falsely elevating the bone density values. Arthritic changes in the posterior elements of the spine will also affect the measurement *(46)*.

The ability to make site-specific predictions of fracture risk of the spine and proximal femur or global fracture risk predictions with dual photon absorptiometry has been established in prospective trials.

5.3. Dual-Energy X-Ray Absorptiometry (DXA)

The underlying principles of DXA are the same as those of DPA. With DXA, however, the radioactive isotope source of photon energy has been replaced by an X-ray tube. There are several advantages of X-ray sources over radioactive isotopes. There is no source decay, which would otherwise require costly replacement of the radioactive source. Similarly, there is no concern of a drift in patient values owing to source decay. The greater source intensity or "photon flux" produced by the X-ray tube and the smaller focal spot allows for better beam collimation which results in less dose overlap between scan lines and greater image resolution. Scan times are faster and precision is improved.

Because X-ray tubes produce a beam that spans a wide range of photon energies, the beam must be narrowed in some fashion in order to produce the two distinct photoelectric peaks necessary to separate bone from soft tissue. The major manufacturers of dual-energy X-ray absorptiometers in the US have chosen to do this in one of two ways. Lunar Corp. of Madison, WI and Norland Corp. of Fort Atkinson, WI use rare earth K-edge filters to produce two distinct photoelectric peaks. Hologic, Inc. of Waltham, MA uses a pulsed power source to the X-ray tube to create the same effect.

K-edge filters produce an X-ray beam with a high number of photons in a specific range. The energy range that is desired is the energy range that is just above the K-absorption edge of the tissue in question. The K-edge is the binding energy of the K-shell electron. This energy level varies from tissue to tissue. The importance of the K-edge is that at photon energies just above this level, the transmission of photons through the tissue in question drops dramatically. That is, the photons are maximally attenuated at this energy level *(47)*. Therefore, to separate bone from soft tissue in a quantifiable fashion, the energy of the photon beam should be just above the K-edge of bone or soft tissue for maximum attenuation. Lunar Corp. uses a cerium filter that has a K-shell absorption edge at 40 keV. A cerium-filtered X-ray spectrum at 80 kV will contain two photoelectric peaks at about 40 and 70 keV. The samarium K-edge filter employed by Norland Corp. has a K-shell absorption edge of 46.8 keV. The samarium-filtered X-ray beam at 100 kV produces a low-energy peak at 46.8 keV. In the Norland system, the high-energy peak is variable because the system employs selectable levels of filtration, but the photons are limited to <100 keV by the 100 kV employed. The K-edge of both cerium and samarium results in a low-energy peak, which approximates the 44-keV low-energy peak of gadolinium-153 used in most dual-photon systems.

The Hologic dual-energy X-ray absorptiometer utilizes a different system to produce the two photoelectric peaks necessary to separate bone from soft tissue. Instead of employing K-edge filtering of the X-ray beam, Hologic employs alternating pulses at 70 and 140 kV to the X-ray source.

Most regions of the skeleton are accessible with DXA. Studies can be made of the spine in both an anterior–posterior[†] and lateral direction. Although access to the lumbar spine in the lateral projection is limited by rib overlap of L1 and L2 and pelvic overlap of L4, the lateral projection offers the ability to eliminate the confounding effects of dystrophic calcification on densities measured in the AP direction *(48)*. It also eliminates the highly cortical posterior elements, which contribute as much as 47% of the density measured in the AP direction *(49)*. The proximal femur, radius, os calcis, and total body can also be evaluated with DXA. Scan times are dramatically shorter with DXA when compared to

---

[†]Although spine bone density studies with DXA are often referred to as AP spine studies, the beam actually passes in a posterior to anterior direction. Such studies are correctly characterized as PA spine studies, but it has become an accepted convention to refer to them as AP spine bone density studies. One of the new fan-array DXA scanners, the Lunar Expert, does perform AP spine studies.

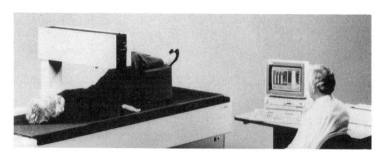

Fig. 8. The Lunar DPX, a DXA pencil-beam absorptiometer. Photo courtesy of Lunar Corp.

DPA. Early DXA units required approx 4 min for studies of the AP spine or proximal femur. Total body studies required 20 min in the medium scan mode and only 10 min in the fast scan mode. Later DXA units scan even faster, with studies of the AP spine or proximal femur requiring only 2 min to perform.

The values obtained with DXA studies of the skeleton are highly correlated with values from earlier studies performed with DPA and, consequently, its accuracy is considered comparable to that of DPA *(50–53)*. DXA values are consistently lower than values obtained with DPA. There are also differences in the values obtained with DXA equipment from the three major manufacturers. Values obtained with either a Hologic or Norland DXA unit are consistently lower than those obtained with a Lunar DXA·unit, although all are highly correlated with each other *(54–56)*. Comparison studies using all three manufacturers' equipment have resulted in formulas that allow for conversion of the values between the manufacturers, but the margin of error in such conversions is too large to make such comparisons clinically useful. The development of a universal standard to which the machines could be calibrated or a "standardized BMD" should eliminate this problem in the future.

Radiation exposure with dual-energy X-ray equipment is extremely low for all scan types. Expressed as skin dose, radiation exposure during an AP spine or proximal femur study is only 2 mrem. The biologically important absorbed dose equivalent is only 1 mrem *(57)*.

Perhaps the most significant advance seen with DXA is the marked improvement in reproducibility. Expressed as a coefficient of variation, short-term reproducibility in normal subjects has been reported as low as 0.9% for the AP lumbar spine and 1.4% for the femoral neck *(53)*. Reproducibility studies over the course of 1 yr have reported values of 1% for the lumbar spine and 1.7%–2.3% for the femoral neck *(53)*.

DXA has been used in prospective studies to predict fracture risk. In one of the largest studies of its kind, DXA studies of the proximal femur were demonstrated to have the greatest predictive ability for hip fracture compared to measurements at other sites with SPA or DPA *(15)*.

Figures 8, 9, and 10 illustrate DXA units from the three major manufacturers in the US. These units are considered first-generation DXA units or "pencil-beam" scanners. The next generation of DXA scanners are called "fan-array" scanners. The difference between these two types of scanners is illustrated in Figs. 11 and 12. Pencil-beam scanners employ a collimated X-ray beam, which moves in tandem in a rectilinear pattern with a single detector, or in the case of the Norland unit, two sequential detectors. Fan-array scanners

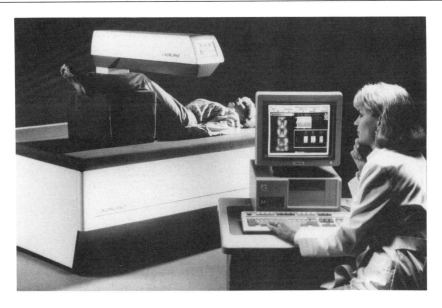

Fig. 9. The Norland XR-26, a DXA pencil-beam absorptiometer. Photo courtesy of Norland Corp.

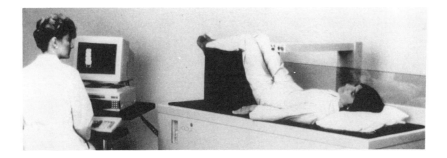

Fig. 10. The Hologic QDR 1000, a DXA pencil-beam absorptiometer. Photo courtesy of Hologic, Inc.

Pencil -Beam, Rectilinear Scanners

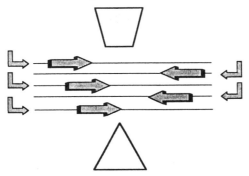

Fig. 11. Pencil-beam DXA absorptiometers. The single-detector and collimated X-ray beam move in tandem in a rectilinear scan path.

Fan-Array Scanners

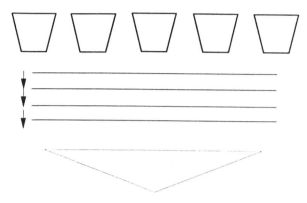

Fig. 12. Fan-array DXA absorptiometers. An array of detectors obviates the need for a rectilinear scan path.

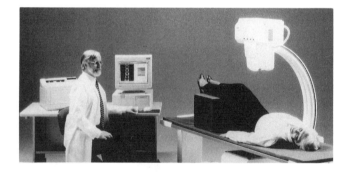

Fig. 13. The Lunar Expert, a fan-array DXA device. Photo courtesy of Lunar Corp.

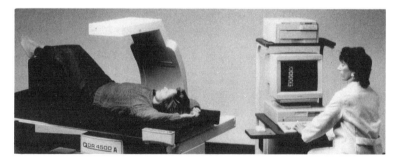

Fig. 14. The Hologic QDR 4500, a fan-array DXA device. Photo courtesy of Hologic, Inc.

employ an array of detectors, which obviates the need for a rectilinear scan path. Scan times are reduced to as low as 30 s for a study of the spine in the AP direction. Figure 13 is the Lunar fan-array scanner, the Expert, and Fig. 14 is the Hologic fan-array scanner, the QDR-4500. Image resolution is also enhanced with the fan-array scanners. Images of

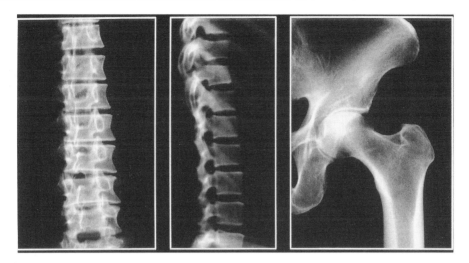

Fig. 15. Fan-array DXA Images. Photo courtesy of Lunar Corp.

radiographic or near-radiographic quality can be obtained as shown in Fig. 15. This has created a new application for bone densitometry scanning called morphometric X-ray absorptiometry or MXA. With MXA, images of the spine obtained in the lateral projection can be used for computer analysis of the vertebral dimensions and diagnosis of vertebral fracture. It is also conceivable that MXA software will be developed to measure hip axis length from studies of the proximal femur. Hip axis length has been shown to be an independent predictor of hip fracture risk *(58)*.

DXA is progressively replacing older DPA units in most clinical sites. The improved scan times, improved image resolution, lower radiation dose, greater precision, greater flexibility in application to a variety of skeletal sites, and lower cost of operation give DXA clear advantages over DPA.

5.4. Single-Energy X-ray Absorptiometry (SXA)

SXA is the X-ray based counterpart of SPA, much as DXA is the X-ray based counterpart of DPA. SXA units are being used to measure bone density in the distal radius and ulna and os calcis. Although the distal peripheral skeleton can be measured with DXA as well as SPA, SXA units have the advantage of not requiring radioactive isotopes, which reduces the cost of operating the equipment and should contribute to more reliable long-term performance. The accuracy and precision of SXA appears to be comparable to SPA *(59)*.

5.5. Quantitative Computed Tomography (QCT)

Although QCT is a photon absorptiometric technique like SPA, SXA, DPA, and DXA, it is unique in that it provides a three-dimensional quantitative image, which makes possible a direct measurement of density and a spatial separation of trabecular from cortical bone. In 1976, Ruegsegger et al. developed a dedicated peripheral quantitative CT scanner using ^{125}I for measurements of the radius *(60)*. Cann and Genant are credited with adapting commercially available CT scanners for the quantitative assessment of spinal bone density *(61,62)*. It is this approach that has received the most wide-spread use in the US, although dedicated CT units for the measurement of the peripheral skeleton, or pQCT units, are beginning to appear in clinical centers.

QCT studies of the spine utilize a reference standard or phantom that is scanned simultaneously with the patient. The phantom, which contains varying concentrations of K_2HPO_4, is placed underneath the patient during the study . A scout view is required for localization, and then an 8–10 mm thick slice is measured through the center of two or more vertebral bodies, which are generally selected from T12 to L3 *(63)*. A region of interest within the anterior portion of the vertebral body is analyzed for bone density and is reported as mg/cm³ K_2HPO_4 equivalents. This region of interest is carefully placed to avoid the cortical shell of the vertebral body such that a pure three-dimensional trabecular density is reported unlike the two-dimensional areal mixed cortical and trabecular densities reported with AP studies of the spine utilizing DPA or DXA. Figure 16 shows a QCT study of the spine.

A study of the spine with QCT requires about 30 min *(30)*. The skin radiation dose is generally 100–300 mrem. This overestimates the biologically important absorbed dose equivalent, because only a small portion of marrow is irradiated during a QCT study of the spine *(57)*. The absorbed dose equivalent is generally in the range of only 30 mrem, although this is still 30 times greater than the dose delivered with an AP spine study with DXA. The localizer scan, which precedes the actual QCT study, will add an additional 30 mrem to the absorbed dose equivalent. Nevertheless, these values are still quite acceptable in the context of natural background radiation of approx 200 mrem/mo. CT units that, by their design, are unable to utilize low-kVp settings for QCT studies, may deliver skin and absorbed doses 3–10 times higher.

The accuracy of QCT for measurements of spine BMD is affected by the presence of marrow fat *(63–65)*. Marrow fat increases with age, resulting in an increasingly large error in the accuracy of spine QCT measurements in older patients. The accuracy of QCT is reported to range from 5 to 15%, depending upon the age of the patient and percentage of marrow fat. The presence of marrow fat results in an underestimation of bone density in the young of about 20 mg/cc and as much as 30 mg/cc in the elderly *(63)*. The error introduced by marrow fat can be partially corrected by applying data on vertebral marrow fat with aging originally developed by Dunnill et al *(66)*. In an attempt to eliminate the error introduced by marrow fat, dual-energy QCT or DEQCT was developed by Genant and Boyd *(67)*. This method clearly reduced the accuracy error introduced by the presence of marrow fat to as low as 1.4% in cadaveric studies *(64,65)*. In vivo, the accuracy error with DEQCT is 3–6% *(30,63)*. The drawbacks of DEQCT are that the radiation dose is increased approx 10-fold compared to regular or single-energy QCT (SEQCT) and the precision is not as good. The precision of SEQCT for vertebral measurements in expert hands is 1–3% and for DEQCT, 3–5% *(63,68)*. Expertise in either SEQCT or DEQCT is, in the opinion of most, severely limited. The cost of a QCT spinal bone density measurement is around US $150 *(30)*.

The ability to measure bone density in the proximal femur with QCT is also limited. Using both dedicated QCT machines and standard CT units, investigators have attempted to utilize QCT for measurements of the proximal femur *(69,70)*. This capability remains restricted to a few research centers.

QCT of the spine has been used in studies of prevalent osteoporotic fractures, and it is clear that such measurements can distinguish osteoporotic individuals from normal individuals as well or even better than DPA *(71–74)*. Fractures are rare with values above

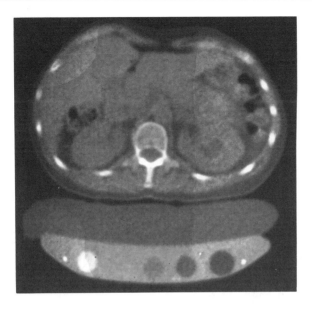

Fig. 16. QCT of the spine. The K_2HPO_4 phantom is seen underneath the patient. Photo courtesy of Dr. David Sartoris.

110 mg/cc and extremely common below 60 mg/cc *(75)*. Because QCT measures only trabecular bone, which is more metabolically active than cortical bone, rates of change in disease states observed with QCT spine measurements tend to be greater than those observed with AP spine studies performed with DPA or DXA *(61,76)*. This greater magnitude of change partially offsets the effects of the poorer precision seen with QCT compared to DXA. The correlations between spine bone density measurements with QCT and skeletal sites measured with other techniques are statistically significant, but too weak to allow accurate prediction of bone density at another site from measurement of the spine with QCT *(22,73,74)*.

Peripheral QCT or pQCT is becoming more widely available. These are small, dedicated units that are utilized primarily for the measurement of bone density in the forearm.

6. THE CHOICE OF TECHNIQUE

6.1. To Quantitate the Bone Mass or Density

While it is understood that not all techniques are readily available in all locales, additional logic can be applied to the choice of technique to be used in clinical practice. In certain circumstances, the clinician is primarily interested in quantitating the bone mass or density as opposed to assessing fracture risk. This situation might arise in circumstances in which demineralization is suggested on plain skeletal radiography or in which an apparent fragility fracture has occurred, and the clinician wishes to confirm the impression of osteopenia. In such cases, it is most appropriate to measure the site in question. As noted earlier, one cannot measure one skeletal site and predict bone density at another skeletal site with any technique with a degree of accuracy that would make such predictions clinically useful. The choice of technique, then, is based on the ability to measure the site in question with a high degree of accuracy. For example, if on plain films, demineralization of the spine is suspected, QCT, DPA, or DXA could be utilized to quantitate the bone density in the spine. Although the accuracy of QCT is affected by the presence of marrow fat in older individuals, the accuracy of AP spine studies with DPA or DXA may be affected by the presence of dystrophic calcification in the scan path. If it is known from plain films that dystrophic calcification is unlikely, DPA or DXA is an appropriate choice. If dystrophic calcification is present, QCT would be preferable. If an assessment of bone density in the proximal femur is desired, only DPA and DXA are generally available for this purpose. Studies of the radius or os calcis can be performed accurately with either SPA, DXA, SXA, or pQCT. As a practical matter, total body bone density assessments are restricted to DXA.

There are also circumstances in which a physician may be looking for the effects of a disease process on the skeleton and may wish to quantitate the bone mass or density in the region of the skeleton that may be affected. Certain disease processes will have a predilection for regions of the skeleton or types of bone. For example, primary hyperparathyroidism may cause a preferential loss of cortical bone. In such a case, a skeletal site that is primarily cortical bone should be measured. An SPA, SXA, or DXA study of the midradius would suffice for this assessment, as would a DPA or DXA study of the femoral neck. Cushing's disease or corticosteroid-induced osteoporosis will quickly devastate the trabecular bone of the axial skeleton. A bone density measurement of the spine with QCT, DPA, or DXA would be appropriate here.

If a bone density measurement is being performed in order to follow the effects of a disease process or therapeutic intervention over time, the choice of technique is determined by the technique that will measure the site that is expected to be affected with the greatest precision. For measurements of the spine, this would be DXA. For measurements of the proximal femur, again DXA would be the appropriate choice. For measurements of the midradius, SPA and DXA are equally excellent.

6.2. To Assess Fracture Risk

In assessing fracture risk, the clinician must decide if a site-specific or global fracture risk is desired. If a site-specific fracture risk assessment is indicated, then the technique that will measure the site in question with the greatest accuracy should be chosen. For global fracture risk assessments, measurements of the radius, spine, and proximal femur all have value, such that the physician can choose virtually any of the available techniques that will measure those sites.

REFERENCES

1. Johnston CC, Epstein S. Clinical, biochemical, radiographic, epidemiologic, and economic features of osteoporosis. *Orthop Clin North Am* 1981; 12: 559–569.
2. Aitken M. *Osteoporosis in Clinical Practice.* Bristol: John Wright & Sons, 1984, pp. 1–146.
3. Singh J, Nagrath AR, Maini PS. Changes in trabecular pattern of the upper end of the femur as an index of osteoporosis. *J Bone Joint Surg Am* 1970; 52-A: 457–467.
4. Bohr H, Schadt O. Bone mineral content of femoral bone and lumbar spine measured in women with fracture of the femoral neck by dual photon absorptiometry. *Clin Ortho* 1983; 179: 240–245.
5. Nordin BEC. Osteoporosis with particular reference to the menopause. In: Avioli LV, ed. *The Osteoporotic Syndrome*, New York: Grune & Stratton, 1983, pp. 13–44.
6. Shimmins J, Anderson JB, Smith DA, et al. The accuracy and reproducibility of bone mineral measurements "in vivo." (a) The measurement of metacarpal mineralisation using and X-ray generator. *Clin Radiol* 1972; 23: 42–46.

7. Exton-Smith AN, Millard PH, Payne PR, Wheeler EF. Method for measuring quantity of bone. *Lancet* 1969; 2: 1153–1154.

8. Dequeker J. Precision of the radiogrammetric evaluation of bone mass at the metacarpal bones. In: Dequeker J, Johnston CC, eds. *Non-invasive Bone Measurements: Methodological Problems*, Oxford: IRL, 1982: 27–32.

9. Aitken JM, Smith CB, Horton PW, et al. The interrelationships between bone mineral at different skeletal sites in male and female cadavera. *J Bone Joint Surg Br* 1974; 56B: 370–375.

10. Meema HE, Meindok H. Advantages of peripheral radiogrametry over dual-photon absorptiometry of the spine in the assessment of prevalence of osteoporotic vertebral fractures in women. *J Bone Min Res* 1992; 7: 897–903.

11. Bywaters EGL. The measurement of bone opacity. *Clin Sci* 1948; 6: 281–287.

12. Barnett E, Nordin BEC. Radiologic assessment of bone density. 1.-The clinical and radiological problem of thin bones. *Br J Radiol* 1961; 34: 683–692.

13. Mack PB, Brown WN, Trapp HD. The quantitative evaluation of bone density. *Am J Roentgenol Rad Ther* 1949; 61: 808–825.

14. Vose GP, Mack PB. Roentgenologic assessment of femoral neck density as related to fracturing. *Am J Roentgenol Rad Ther Nucl Med* 1963; 89: 1296–1301.

15. Cummings SR, Black DM, Nevitt MC, et al. Bone density at various sites for prediction of hip fractures. *Lancet* 1993; 341: 72–75.

16. Mazess RB. Noninvasive methods for quantitating trabecular bone. In: Avioli LV, ed. *The Osteoporotic Syndrome*, New York: Grune & Stratton, 1983: 85–114.

17. Mack PB, O'Brien AT, Smith JM, Bauman AW. A method for estimating degree of mineralization of bones from tracings of roentgenograms. *Science* 1939; 89: 467

18. Mack PB, Vogt FB. Roentgenographic bone density changes in astronauts during representative Apollo space flight. *Am J Roentgenol Rad Ther Nucl Med* 1971; 113: 621–633.

19. Cosman F, Herrington B, Himmelstein S, Lindsay R. Radiographic absorptiometry: a simple method for determination of bone mass. *Osteoporos Int* 1991; 2: 34–38.

20. Yates AJ, Ross PD, Lydick E, Epstein RS. Radiographic absorptiometry in the diagnosis of osteoporosis. *Am J Med* 1995; 98: 41S–47S.

21. Yang S, Hagiwara S, Engelke K, et al. Radiographic absorptiometry for bone mineral measurement of the phalanges: precision and accuracy study. *Radiology* 1994; 192: 857–859.

22. Kleerekoper M, Nelson DA, Flynn MJ, Pawluszka AS, Jacobsen G, Peterson EL. Comparison of radiographic absorptiometry with dual-energy X-ray absorptiometry and quantitative computed tomography in normal older white and black women. *J Bone Miner Res* 1994; 9: 1745–1749.

23. Yates AJ, Ross PD, Lydick E, Epstein RS. Radiographic absorptiometry in the diagnosis of osteoporosis. *Am J Med* 1995; 98: 415–475.

24. Cameron JR, Sorenson G. Measurements of bone mineral in vivo: an improved method. *Science* 1963; 142: 230–232.

25. Vogel JM. Application principles and technical considerations in SPA. In: Genant HK, ed. *Osteoporosis Update 1987*, San Francisco: University of California Printing Services, 1987: 219–231.

26. Johnston CC. Noninvasive methods for quantitating appendicular bone mass. In: Avioli LV, ed. *The Osteoporotic Syndrome*, New York: Grune & Stratton, 1983, pp. 73–84.

27. Barden HS, Mazess RB. Bone densitometry of the appendicular and axial skeleton. *Top Geriatric Rehabil* 1989; 4: 1–12.

28. Kimmel PL. Radiologic methods to evaluate bone mineral content. *Ann Intern Med* 1984; 100: 908–911.

29. Steiger P, Genant HK. The current implementation of single-photon absorptiometry in commercially available instruments. In: Genant HK, ed. *Osteoporosis Update 1987*, San Francisco: University of California Printing Services, 1987, pp. 233–240.

30. Chesnut CH. Noninvasive methods for bone mass measurement. In: Avioli L, ed. *The Osteoporotic Syndrome*, 3rd ed, New York: Wiley-Liss, 1993, pp. 77–87.

31. Gardsell P, Johnell O, Nilsson BE. The predictive value of bone loss for fragility fractures in women: a longitudinal study over 15 years. *Calcif Tissue Int* 1991; 49: 90–94.

32. Hui SL, Slemenda CW, Johnston CC. Baseline measurement of bone mass predicts fracture white women. *Ann Intern Med* 1989; 111: 355–361.

33. Ross PD, Davis JW, Vogel JM, Wasnich RD. A critical review of bone mass and the risk of fractures in osteoporosis. *Calcif Tissue Int* 1990; 46: 149–161.

34. Melton LJ, Atkinson EJ, O'Fallon WM, Wahner HW, Riggs BL. Long-term fracture prediction by bone mineral assessed at different skeletal sites. *J Bone Min Res* 1993; 8: 1227–1233.

35. Black DM, Cummings SR, Genant HK, Nevitt MC, Palermo L, Browner W. Axial and appendicular bone density predict fractures in older women. *J Bone Min Res* 1992; 7: 633–638.

36. Nord RH. Technical considerations in DPA. In: Genant HK, ed. Osteoporosis Update 1987, San Francisco: University of California Printing Services, 1987, pp. 203–212.

37. Dunn WL, Wahner HW, Riggs BL. Measurement of bone mineral content in human vertebrae and hip by dual photon absorptiometry. *Radiology* 1980; 136: 485–487.

38. Reed GW. The assessment of bone mineralization from the relative transmission of ^{241}Am and ^{137}Cs radiations. *Phys Med Biol* 1966; 11: 174

39. Roos B, Skoldborn H. Dual photon absorptiometry in lumbar vertebrae. I. Theory and method. *Acta Radiol Ther Phys Biol* 1974; 13: 266–290.

40. Mazess RB, Ort M, Judy P. Absorptiometric bone mineral determination using Gd. In: Cameron JR, ed. *Proceedings of Bone Measurements Conference*, US Atomic Energy Commission, 1970, pp. 308–312.

41. Wilson CR, Madsen M. Dichromatic absorptiometry of vertebral bone mineral content. *Invest Radiol* 1977; 12: 180–184.

42. Madsen M, Peppler W, Mazess RB. Vertebral and total body bone mineral content by dual photon absorptiometry. *Calcif Tissue Res* 1976; 2: 361–364.

43. Wahner HW, Dunn WL, Mazess RB, et al. Dual-photon Gd-153 absorptiometry of bone. *Radiology* 1985; 156: 203–206.

44. Lindsay R, Fey C, Haboubi A. Dual photon absorptiometric measurements of bone mineral density increase with source life. *Calcif Tissue Int* 1987; 41: 293–294.

45. Cummings SR, Black DB. Should perimenopausal women be screened for osteoporosis? *Ann Intern Med* 1986; 104: 817–823.

46. Drinka PJ, DeSmet AA, Bauwens SF, Rogot A. The effect of overlying calcification on lumbar bone densitometry. *Calcif Tissue Int* 1992; 50: 507–510.

47. Curry TS, Dowdey JE, Murry RC, eds. Attenuation. In: *Christensen's Physics of Diagnostic Radiology*. Philadelphia: Lea & Febiger, 1990, pp. 70–86.

48. Rupich RC, Griffin MG, Pacifici R, Avioli LV, Susman N. Lateral dual-energy radiography: artifact error from rib and pelvic bone. *J Bone Min Res* 1992; 7: 97–101.

49. Louis O, Van Den Winkel P, Covens P, Schoutens A, Osteaux M. Dual-energy X-ray absorptiometry of lumbar vertebrae: relative contribution of body and posterior elements and accuracy in relation with neutron activation analysis. *Bone* 1992; 13: 317–320.

50. Lees B, Stevenson JC. An evaluation of dual-energy X-ray absorptiometry and comparison with dual-photon absorptiometry. *Osteoporosis Int* 1992; 2: 146–152.

51. Kelly TL, Slovik DM, Schoenfeld DA, Neer RM. Quantitative digital radiography versus dual photon absorptiometry of the lumbar spine. *J Clin Endocrinol Metab* 1988; 76: 839–844.

52. Holbrook TL, Barrett-Connor E, Klauber M, Sartoris D. A population-based comparison of quantitative dual-energy X-ray absorptiometry with dual-photon absorptiometry of the spine and hip. *Calcif Tissue Int* 1991; 49: 305–307.

53. Pouilles JM, Tremollieres F, Todorovsky N, Ribot C. Precision and sensitivity of dual-energy X-ray absorptiometry in spinal osteoporosis. *J Bone Miner Res* 1991; 6: 997–1002.

54. Laskey MA, Crisp AJ, Cole TJ, Compston JE. Comparison of the effect of different reference data on Lunar DPX and Hologic QDR-1000 dual-energy X-ray absorptiometers. *Br J Radiol* 1992; 65: 1124–1129.

55. Pocock NA, Sambrook PN, Nguyen T, Kelly P, Freund J, Eisman J. Assessment of spinal and femoral bone density by dual X-ray absorptiometry: comparison of lunar and hologic instruments. *J Bone Min Res* 1992; 7: 1081–1084.

56. Lai KC, Goodsitt MM, Murano R, Chesnut CC. A comparison of two dual-energy X-ray absorptiometry systems for spinal bone mineral measurement. *Calcif Tissue Int* 1992; 50: 203–208.

57. Kalender WA. Effective dose values in bone mineral measurements by photon absorptiometry and computed tomography. *Osteoporos Int* 1992; 2: 82–87.

58. Faulkner KG, Cummings SR, Black D, Palermo L, Gluer C, Genant HK. Simple measurement of femoral geometry predicts hip fracture: the study of osteoporotic fractures. *J Bone Min Res* 1993; 8: 1211–1217.

59. Kelly TL, Crane G, Baran DT. Single x-ray absorptiometry of the forearm: precision, correlation, and reference data. *Calcif Tissue Int* 1994; 54: 212–218.

60. Ruegsegger P, Elsasser U, Anliker M, Gnehm H, Kind H, Prader A. Quantification of bone mineralisation using computed tomography. *Radiology* 1976; 121: 93–97.

61. Genant HK, Cann CE, Ettinger B, Gordan GS. Quantitative computed tomography of vertebral spongiosa: a sensitive method for detecting early bone loss after oophorectomy. *Ann Intern Med* 1982; 97: 699–705.

62. Cann CE, Genant HK. Precise measurement of vertebral mineral content using computed tomography. *J Comput Assist Tomogr* 1980; 4: 493–500.

63. Genant HK, Block JE, Steiger P, Gluer C. Quantitative computed tomography in the assessment of osteoporosis. In: Genant HK, ed. *Osteoporosis Update 1987*, San Francisco: University of California Printing Services, 1987, pp. 49–72.

64. Laval-Jeantet AM, Roger B, Bouysse S, Bergot C, Mazess RB. Influence of vertebral fat content on quantitative CT density. *Radiology* 1986; 159: 463–466.

65. Reinbold W, Adler CP, Kalender WA, Lente R. Accuracy of vertebral mineral determination by dual-energy quantitative computed tomography. *Skeletal Radiol* 1991; 20: 25–29.

66. Dunnill MS, Anderson JA, Whitehead R. Quantitative histological studies on age changes in bone. *J Pathol Bacteriol* 1967; 94: 274–291.

67. Genant HK, Boyd D. Quantitative bone mineral analysis using dual energy computed tomography. *Invest Radiol* 1977; 12: 545–551.

68. Cann CE. Quantitative computed tomography for bone mineral analysis: technical considerations. In: Genant HK, ed. *Osteoporosis Update 1987*, San Francisco: University of California Printing Services, 1987, pp. 131–144.

69. Sartoris DJ, Andre M, Resnick C, Resnick D. Trabecular bone density in the proximal femur: quantitative CT assessment. *Radiology* 1986; 160: 707–712.

70. Reiser UJ, Genant HK. Determination of bone mineral content in the femoral neck by quantitative computed tomography. 70th Scientific Assembly and Annual Meeting of the Radiological Society of North America, Washington, DC, 1984.

71. Gallagher C, Golgar D, Mahoney P, McGill J. Measurement of spine density in normal and osteoporotic subjects using computed tomography: relationship of spine density to fracture threshold and fracture index. *J Comput Assist Tomogr* 1985; 9: 634–635.

72. Raymakers JA, Hoekstra O, Van Putten J, Kerkhoff H, Duursma SA. Osteoporosis fracture prevalence and bone mineral mass measured with CT and DPA. *Skeletal Radiol* 1986; 15: 191–197.

73. Reinbold WD, Reiser UJ, Harris ST, Ettinger B, Genant HK. Measurement of bone mineral content in early postmenopausal and postmenopausal osteoporotic women. A comparison of methods. *Radiology* 1986; 160: 469–478.

74. Sambrook PN, Bartlett C, Evans R, Hesp R, Katz D, Reeve J. Measurement of lumbar spine bone mineral: a comparison of dual photon absorptiometry and computed tomography. *Br J Radiol* 1985; 58: 621–624.

75. Genant HK, Ettinger B, Harris ST, Block JE, Steiger P. Quantitative computed tomography in assessment of osteoporosis. In: Riggs BL, Melton LJ, eds. *Osteoporosis: Etiology, Diagnosis and Management*, New York: Raven, 1988, pp. 221–249.

76. Richardson ML, Genant HK, Cann CE, et al. Assessment of metabolic bone disease by quantitative computed tomography. *Clin Orth Rel Res* 1985; 195: 224–238.

9

Clinical Interpretation
and Utility of Bone Densitometry

Paul D. Miller, MD, FACP

Low bone mass is currently recognized to be the most important predictor of future fracture risk *(1)*. Its predictive value is as good as the predictive value of high cholesterol or high blood pressure for myocardial infarction or stroke *(1)*. It is now recognized that it is extremely important to diagnose osteoporosis before a fragility fracture occurs, just: as it is important to diagnose high blood pressure or high cholesterol in asymptomatic patients before strokes or heart attacks occur. This change in the clinical concept of osteoporosis diagnosis to the identification of asymptomatic patients prior to the occurrence of a fragility fracture is new, but important for all clinicians to understand. The diagnosis of osteoporosis before a fracture occurs requires a change in the definition of osteoporosis. Previously, the diagnosis of osteoporosis required the presence of a fragility fracture. The new definition in nonfractured patients is based on levels of bone mass reduction.

There are two major scientific justifications for making the diagnosis of osteoporosis before a fracture occurs based on bone mass reduction. First, the relationship between declining bone mass and increasing fracture risk is exponential (Fig. 1). For each standard deviation (SD) the bone mineral density (BMD) declines from the mean young normal BMD, the current relative fracture risk increases 1.5–2.5 times *(1–7)*. Hence, early identification of asymptomatic nonfractured patients, with smaller reductions in bone mass is important, since these patients are unaware of continued bone loss, which places them at increased risk of fracture. Second, once the first fragility fracture occurs, the risk for a second fracture increases enormously in patients with low bone mass. This increased risk has been shown to be as high as 25 times greater in some studies *(1)*. Conceptually, waiting for the first fracture to occur is analogous to diagnosing and treating hypertensive patients only after a stroke has occurred. Therefore, prevention of the first fragility fracture should be the clinician's goal. Making a prefracture diagnosis of osteopenia (low bone mass) or osteoporosis is conceptually important both for predicting current fracture risk and the remaining lifetime fracture probability. The current fracture risk is defined as the relative risk of a fragility fracture occurring within the subsequent 5 yr, and has been determined predominantly in elderly women *(1–7)*. The remaining life-time fracture probability (RLFP) is defined as the risk of fracture occurring during a woman's lifetime when bone mass has been determined at any age. RLFP is determined by a woman's current bone mass, current age, projected rate of bone loss, and anticipated life-

From: *Osteoporosis: Diagnostic and Therapeutic Principles*
Edited by: C. J. Rosen Humana Press Inc., Totowa, NJ

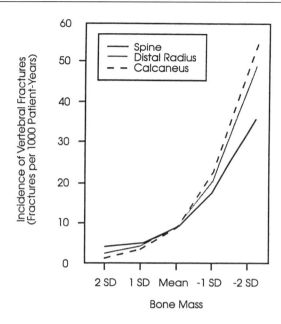

Fig. 1. Exponential relationship between decreasing bone mass (mean ± standard deviation [SD]; mean age, 63.7 yr) and increasing incidence of vertebral fractures. Adapted from ref. *22* with permission.

span *(8–10)*. These latter two variables are unknown in an individual patient, but can be defined using known ranges of bone loss rates and life expectancy. Nomograms can be used to estimate an individual patient's RLFP. The RLFP is greater in a younger woman than in an older woman with equal levels of bone loss, since the younger woman's life-span is longer and hence, time of exposure to low bone mass is longer. Thus, the younger woman is exposed to low bone mass and continual bone loss for a longer period of time with subsequent greater RLFP if no intervention is prescribed. Hence, detection of osteopenia or osteoporosis, based on levels of bone mass alone, has important implications for women of all ages.

The diagnostic thresholds to define osteopenia (low bone mass) and osteoporosis in nonfractured patients have recently been agreed on by international panels of the World Health Organization (WHO) and the International Society for Clinical Densitometry (SCD) *(11,12)*. Low bone mass or osteopenia is defined as any BMD between 1.0 and 2.5 SD below the mean BMD of young normal adult Caucasian women. Osteoporosis is defined as BMD more than 2.5 SD below the mean young normal value. The diagnostic threshold for osteoporosis is defined at this level, since over 95% of fragility fractures occur in patients with BMD more than 2.5 SD below the mean young normal bone mass. It is important to identify patients with osteopenia (BMD 1.0–2.5 SD below young normals), because they have both a greater current and life-time risk for fragility fractures as compared to patients with normal bone mass. If these patients remain unrecognized and untreated, and bone mass continues to decline, then they have a much greater risk of fracture as their age increases. It has been suggested that these definitions of osteopenia and osteoporosis may overdiagnose this disease, since by the age of 85 yr, nearly 85% of Caucasian women will fulfill these criteria, particularly if multiple skeletal sites are measured. However, justification for this diagnostic criteria rests with the knowledge that

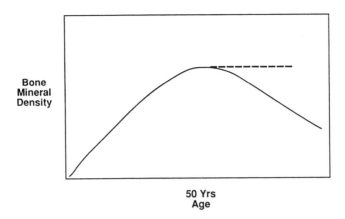

Fig. 2. Bone mass declines with aging after the menopause in an untreated woman (——). Ideally, this loss in bone mass could be preventable with current therapies and measurement techniques (---)

if left undetected and untreated, nearly 50% of all 50-yr-old Caucasian women will have an osteoporotic-related fracture in their life-time with one out of six women developing hip fractures. This high prevalence of osteoporosis-related fractures will not be reduced unless high-risk individuals are detected and some intervention takes place.

New techniques for bone mass measurement are accurate, precise, and objective. Routine radiographs are insensitive and subjective. However, they do provide valuable information. For example, the presence of a single fragility fracture of a vertebrae increases the relative risk of a second fracture five times, independent of bone mass. The risk of future fracture increases exponentially as the number of previous fragility fractures increases *(6,7,13)*.

The skeletal site of bone mass measurement and the technique to be used for screening a patient for osteoporosis should be decided by a clinician knowledgeable about the strengths and limitations of the skeletal site and the techniques. A few clinical caveats are important. First, in the female Caucasian population under the age of 65 yr, osteoporosis (BMD more than 2.5 SD below young normal values) is more often detected by measurements performed at the spine and/or the spine and hip measurements than at the wrist. This may be related to the higher metabolic turnover rate of cancellous bone, which is more readily measured at the spine, compared to cortical bone, which is the predominant bone type at the wrist *(14)*. Second, in the perimenopausal population, there is discordance in bone mass measured at different skeletal sites in an individual patient. Bone mass may be normal at the spine, but low at the hip or vice-versa *(15,16)*. Hence, measuring at least two skeletal sites (spine and hip) is usually advisable for the first diagnostic determination. In fact, the more skeletal sites measured, the greater are the chances of a diagnosis of low bone mass or osteoporosis being made *(7,17)*. It is possible that in untreated perimenopausal patients, monitoring bone loss at two skeletal sites might be also considered, since the rate of bone loss in an individual untreated patient might also be discordant. The determination of whether more than one skeletal site should be measured serially in a patient once therapy has been started is not clear. However, discordance in response to pharmacological therapy has been suggested in patients receiving estrogen and tamoxifen *(18,19)*.

In the elderly population, the PA-spine bone mass is often falsely elevated by osteophytes, and hence, the diagnosis of osteoporosis may be missed. This false elevation of the PA-spine may also be observed in younger rheumatology patients with axial arthropathies. In clinical states where low bone mass should be present (e.g., elderly women without estrogen replacement or patients with prevalent fragility fractures), but is not found using PA-spine measurements, then measuring a second skeletal site is necessary. In these cases, measurement of the lateral spine, which is predominantly cancellous bone, by lateral spine DXA, or measuring the center of the vertebral body, which is also predominantly cancellous bone, by QCT techniques may be very useful. It has been suggested that since such a large proportion of very elderly patients have false elevations of the PA-spine measurements owing to osteophytes, the hip measurement be substituted as the primary sites for DXA in this population for the determination of low bone mass (20). Hip measurements, in fact, might be more diagnostic in the elderly population (21); however, once a diagnosis is made, serial hip measurements (femoral neck and/or trochanter) change very slowly over time, both in response to pharmacological intervention and during normal aging. Additionally, the precision of DXA at the hip site is not as good as the precision of DXA at the PA-spine sites. Therefore, larger changes in bone mass are required at the hip before clinically significant changes owing to aging or intervention can be separated from changes related to errors in measurement (22–24). Hence, clinicians currently have a difficult decision in circumstances where the PA-spine measurement is falsely high and yet longitudinal monitoring is important for clinical decisions. There is currently no simple solution, since the long-term longitudinal precision of supine lateral DXA has yet to be established in the elderly population, and the longitudinal precision of QCT measurements is limited as well. If a QCT scanner is designated to perform only spine measurements and recalibration is performed prior to or during each use, then this technique may be precise enough to determine longitudinal changes in the spine. However, in most common hospital settings, this designated QCT application is the exception.

Clinicians interpreting bone mass measurements should be cognizant of the precision errors of the bone mass technology they use in order to interpret changes properly when following patients longitudinally. For any biological test, a change in an individual patient should be at least 2.8 times the precision error of the measurement (i.e., coefficient of variation) before a change can be considered to be real rather than within the variability of the test (22). In this case, for example, since the precision error of the PA-spine by DXA is 1.5–2.0%, then more than a 5.6% change at this skeletal site by this technology should be seen before a change is considered real rather than apparent. Hence, clinicians should not necessarily consider that bone loss is occurring or a change in therapy is needed when changes by any technique fall within the measurement error. Alternatively, a small change should not be totally discounted, since it might suggest a trend that needs to be monitored with future measurements.

In contrast to the detection and diagnosis of low bone mass, any skeletal site may be used for fracture prediction in the elderly population (3,5,25). In this population, any skeletal site is equally predictive of fracture at any other skeletal site. The measurement of BMD at the hip is slightly more predictive of a hip fracture than measurement of BMD at any other skeletal site to predict hip fracture (5,21). One may question why it is important to distinguish between the detection of low bone mass (which may be dependent on the technique used and skeletal site measured in the population under 65 yr old) and the prediction of fracture (which may not be dependent on the technique used or site measured in the population over 65 yr old). In the early menopausal patient, decisions regarding estrogen replacement or other preventive interventions are often made if low bone mass is found in order to preserve bone mass and are decisions that are independent of current fracture prediction decisions. Furthermore, since bone mass may be discordant in this population, two skeletal sites should be measured, especially if the initial site has a normal BMD, in order to make these clinical decisions.

In counseling patients about their fracture risk based on a bone mass measurement result, there are two distinct fracture risk assessments to consider: the current relative risk and the RLFP. Current fracture risk (e.g., the relative risk of a fracture occurring in the 5 yr following the bone mass measurement) has, with one exception, only been determined in longitudinal data in women with a mean age of 65 yr. Hence, it currently is not correct to equate the current fracture risk of a 50-yr-old to that of a 70-yr-old woman with equal levels of reduced bone mass. The younger woman's current fracture risk is likely to be lower, since age is an independent risk factor for fractures, independent of bone mass. The RLFP, however, for the younger woman with no treatment intervention is likely to be greater than for the older woman since the younger woman has many more years of exposure to low bone mass. The RLFP can be calculated from the woman's age, current level of BMD, rates of bone loss, and life-span in order to provide an absolute life-time fracture probability number that can enhance clinical decisions.

Specially trained clinicians should be involved, at some level, in the interpretation of bone mass measurements if the measurement is to have its most useful impact on patient care. The measurement of bone mass is not as simple to perform or interpret as a blood pressure measurement. Daily phantom calibration and quality control are required to prevent equipment drift and large measurement errors. Ongoing education is necessary for these trained clinicians and their technicians, since the technology of bone mass measurements is changing rapidly.

No one medical specialty should claim densitometry as its own unique area. Radiologists, endocrinologists, rheumatologists, gynecologists, and many others have substantial professional reasons to perform bone densitometry and include it as a part of their patient care. It is important, however, that continuing education and certification be maintained among these various professionals to assure the highest standards of professionalism.

The most useful type of information that can be provided to a physician requesting a bone mass measurement is one that allows that physician to understand what the test means in an individual patient, in order for that physician to make relevant decisions. Currently, the computer printout provided by the bone mass measurement manufacturers is confusing to most physicians receiving bone densitometry reports. The age-matched Z-scores are often misleading for the older population, but do have value in the pediatric and adolescent population. A normal age-matched Z-score in an older adult with fragility fractures is often misinterpreted as indicating that the patient does not have osteoporosis. In these cases, an incorrect misdiagnosis is the result, since the diagnosis of osteoporosis has been erroneously made by assessing the patient's bone mass as it compares to age-matched controls. At the present time, bone mass decreases in most postmenopausal women not on estrogen as their age increases. Therefore, if osteoporosis were to be defined on the basis of age-matched data, then the prevalence of osteoporosis would not increase with age, and yet it does at this time. However, postmenopausal bone loss should not be an accepted process of aging. The goal of osteoporosis prevention is to maintain peak bone mass and prevent bone loss. If this is achieved, then age-matched Z-score would be essentially the same as young adult Z-scores and age-matched Z-scores would be eliminated. Hence, the data shown in Fig. 2 should ideally apply. Therefore, the bone mass of an individual adult patient of any age for osteoporosis diagnosis and fracture prediction should be compared to the normal peak bone mass of young adults (i.e., T-score or young adult Z-score). This level of bone mass should be ideally maintained throughout life, and bone loss owing to aging (i.e., the age-matched Z-scores) should not be allowed to occur. Also since the strength of a bone is largely dependent on its ideal absolute bone mineral content (BMC), both the diagnosis of osteoporosis and the relationships between low bone mass and future fracture risk are related to the young normal bone mass and **not** to age-matched bone mass. As mentioned, this is especially clear when a physician observes an elderly woman with fragility fractures who has a very low bone mass when compared to a young adult but a normal age-matched bone mass. A diagnosis of "normal" in this case would certainly be misleading and a disservice to the patient.

The interpretation of bone mass measurement should also include an assessment of the relationship of a particular bone mass measurement to valuable information obtained from the patient. This information can also help the physician make clinical decisions. For example, providing a brief narrative report to the physician requesting a bone mass measurement can provide specific suggestions for both diagnostic and intervention regimens based on a patient questionnaire, and can make that individual test more meaningful for both the patient and the physician. The depth and range of these recommendations is dependent on the knowledge and experience of the individual clinician interpreting the report. Offering diagnostic suggestions (i.e., further laboratory tests, radiology tests, bone biopsies, and so forth) or suggestions for intervention (i.e., ERT in an osteopenic patient, or other pharmacological treatments in a patient with prevalent fragility fractures who is not a candidate for ERT) can enhance the value of bone mass measurements for both the patient and the physician. Any diagnostic and intervention suggestions should be carefully considered and based on and correlated with the bone mass measurement result and the patient historical data. This type of clinical interpretation can be performed in a professional and competent fashion in a physician-supervised practice where the patient is referred only for the bone mass testing and is not necessarily examined by the physician.

The measurement of bone mass for clinical decisions should be performed at any age on any sex when it will influence this clinical decision. It is an objective measurement. This measurement is not a risk for our patients, and will also have cost savings and be cost-effective by the early diagnosis and treatment of osteoporosis before the hip fractures occur *(26–30)*. Furthermore, by reducing fractures, the quality of life for our patient will be enhanced. If performed and interpreted correctly, bone mass measurement is a very useful objective tool that can enhance clinical decision making.

REFERENCE

1. Wasnich RD. Fracture prediction with bone mass measurement. In: Genant HK, ed. *Osteoporosis Update.* Berkeley, CA: University Press; 1987:95–101.
2. Melton LJ III, Atkinson EG, O'Fallon WM, Wahner HW, Riggs BL. Long-term fracture risk prediction with bone mineral measurements made at various skeletal sites. *J Bone Miner Res* 1991; 6(S1): S136.
3. Ross PD, Davis JW, Epstein RS, Wasnich RD. Pre-existing fractures and bone mass predict vertebral fracture incidence in women. *Ann Intern Med* 1991; 114: 919–923.

4. Hui SL, Slemenda CW, Johnston CC Jr. Age and bone mass as predictors of fracture in a prospective study. *J Clin Invest* 1988; 81: 1804–1809.
5. Cummings SR, Black DM, Nevitt MC, et al. Bone density at various sites for prediction of hip fractures. *Lancet* 1993; 341: 72–75.
6. Ross PD, Genant HK, Davis JW, Miller PD, Wasnich RD. Predicting vertebral fracture incidence from prevalent fractures and bone density among non-black, osteoporotic women. *Osteoporosis Int* 1993; 3: 120–126.
7. Wasnich RD, Ross PD, Davis JW, Vogel JM. A comparison of single and multi-site BMC measurements for assessment of spine fracture probability. *J Nucl Med* 1989; 30: 1166–1171.
8. Black DM, Cummings SR, Melton LJ III. Appendicular bone mineral and a women's lifetime risk of hip fracture. *J Bone Miner Res* 1992; 7: 639–646.
9. Melton LJ, Kan SH, Wahner HW, Riggs BL. Lifetime fracture risk: An approach to hip fracture risk assessment based on bone mineral density and age. *J Clin Epidemiol* 1988; 41: 985–994.
10. Wasnich RD, Ross PD, Vogel JM, Davis JW. *Osteoporosis. Critique and Practicum.* Honolulu, HI: Banyon; 1989: 133–136, 154–159.
11. Kanis JA, Melton LJ III, Christiansen C, Johnston CC, Khaltaev N. The diagnosis of osteoporosis. *J Bone Miner Res* 1994; 9: 1137–1141.
12. Miller PD. Guidelines for the clinical utilization of bone mass measurement in the adult population. *Calcif Tissue Int* 1995; 57: 251–252.
13. Wasnich RD, Davis JW, Ross PD. Spine fracture risk is predicted by non-spine fractures. *Osteoporosis Int* 1994; 4: 1–5.
14. Uebelhart D, Duboeuf F, Meunier PJ, Delmas PD. Lateral dualphoton absorptiometry: A new technique to measure the bone mineral density at the lumbar spine. *J Bone Miner Res* 1990; 5: 525–531.
15. Pouilles JM, Tremollieres R, Ribot C. Spine and femur densitometry at the menopause: Are both sites necessary in the assessment of the risk of osteoporosis? *Calcif Tissue Int* 1993; 52: 344–347.
16. Lai D, Rencken M, Drinkwater B, Chesnut CH III. Site of bone density measurement may affect therapy decision. *Calcif Tissue Int* 1993; 53: 225–228.
17. Davis JW, Ross PD, Wasnich RD. Evidence for both generalized and regional low bone mass among elderly women. *J Bone Miner Res* 1994; 9: 305–309.
18. Stevenson JC, Cust MP, Ganger KF, Hillard TC, Lees B, Whitehead MI. Effects of transdermal versus oral hormone replacement therapy on bone density in spine and proximal femur in postmenopausal women. *Lancet* 1990; 335: 265–269.
19. Love RR, Mazess RB, Barden HS, Epstein S, et al. Effects of tamoxifen on bone mineral density in postmenopausal women with breast cancer. *N Engl J Med* 1992; 326: 852–856.
20. Black DM, Bauer DC, Lu Y, Tabor H. Genant HK, Cummings SR. Should BMD be measured at multiple sites to predict fracture risk in elderly women? *J Bone Miner Res* 1995; 10: S140.
21. Looker AL, Johnston CC Jr, Wahner HW, Dunn WL, Calvo MS, Harris TB, Heyse SP, Lindsay RL. Prevalence of low femoral bone density in older vs women from NHANES III. *J Bone Miner Res* 1995, 10: 796–802.
22. Christiansen C. Postmenopausal bone loss and the risk of osteoporosis. *Osteoporosis Int* 1994; 9(S1): S47–S51.
23. He Y-F, Ross PD, Davis JW, Epstein RS, Vogel JM, Wasnich RD. When should bone mass measurement be repeated? *Calcif Tissue Int* 1994; 55: 243–248.
24. Verheij LF, Blokland JAK, Papapoulos SE, Zwinderman AH, Pauwels EKJ. Optimization of follow-up measurements of bone mass. *J Nucl Med* 1992; 33: 1406–1410.
25. Melton LJ III, Atkinson EJ, O'Fallon WM, Wahner HW, Riggs BL. Long-term fracture prediction by bone mineral assessed at different skeletal sites. *J Bone Miner Res* 1993; 8: 1227–1233.
26. Norris RJ. Medical costs of osteoporosis. *Bone* 1992; 13: 511–516.
27. Wasnich RD, Hagino R, Ross PD. Osteoporosis: will the use of new technology increase or decrease health care costs? *Hawaii Med J* 1987; 46: 199–200.
28. Tosteson A, Rosenthal DI, Melton LJ, Weinstein MC. Cost effectiveness of screening perimenopausal White women for osteoporosis: bone densitometry and hormone replacement therapy. *Ann Intern Med* 1990; 113: 594–602.
29. Ross PD, Wasnich RD, Maclean CJ, et al. A model for estimating the potential costs and savings of osteoporosis prevention strategies. *Bone* 1988; 9: 337–347.
30. Jonsson B, Christiansen C, Johnell O, et al. Cost-effectiveness of fracture prevention in established osteoporosis. *Osteoporosis Int* 1995; 5: 136–142.

10

Quantitative Ultrasound

Daniel T. Baran, MD

CONTENTS

INTRODUCTION
ULTRASOUND MEASUREMENTS
QUANTITATIVE ULTRASOUND TO ASSESS BONE MASS
ULTRASOUND VALUES AS A PREDICTOR OF FRACTURE
SUMMARY
REFERENCES

1. INTRODUCTION

Recent estimates suggest that osteoporosis affects 30% of postmenopausal Caucasian women in the US *(1)*. Osteoporosis is defined as a bone mineral density (BMD) more than 2.5 SD below the young normal mean. An additional 54% of postmenopausal women have osteopenia, defined as a BMD more than 1 SD below young normal mean, but <2.5 SD below. Osteoporosis accounts for 1.2 million fractures annually with an estimated annual cost of $10 billion.

Models have been developed to predict bone mass based on risk factors *(2,3)*. Although these models were highly significant in predicting bone mass at a given skeletal site, neither identified more than 73% of women with low bone density. Prospective studies have demonstrated the association between a maternal history of fragility fracture and the individual risk of osteoporosis *(4)*. Therefore, family history of fracture, particularly maternal, appears to be a significant risk factor for osteoporosis in postmenopausal women. In general, however, the assessment of risk factor status does not appear to be an efficient tool for the identification of perimenopausal women with low bone mass *(5)*. The poor performance of the risk factor models may be explained by unmeasured genetic factors, which are important determinants of bone mass.

Assessment of bone mass remains indispensable to determine osteoporosis risk, since risk factors alone are not sufficient for accurate delineation of either low or normal bone density. It is clear that bone density is a very good predictor of fracture risk (6-10). As bone density decreases, fracture rate increases. Women with bone density in the lowest quartile have an 8.5-fold greater risk of hip fracture than those in the highest

From: *Osteoporosis: Diagnostic and Therapeutic Principles*
Edited by: C. J. Rosen Humana Press Inc., Totowa, NJ

quartile *(7)*. Interestingly, calcaneal density is nearly as good a predictor of hip fracture as is hip density *(7)*.

Methods used to measure BMD include single energy X-ray absorptiometry (SXA), dual-energy X-ray absorptiometry (DXA), and quantitative computed tomography (QCT). Each of these methods is accurate and precise in measuring bone mass. Although quantitation of bone mass is the best predictor of fracture risk, the above instruments are relatively costly, and most importantly, are not readily available to the average physician and/or patient. Such techniques as quantitative ultrasound, which are not costly and are radiation-free, could make assessment of bone mass more readily available. This would allow the targeting of those women with lowest bone mass and greatest fracture risk for intervention with preventive therapy.

2. ULTRASOUND MEASUREMENTS

Bone density is a predictor of fracture risk *(6–10)*. The increase in risk of fracture with decreasing bone density is greater than those reported for the risk of coronary artery disease with increasing cholesterol levels or blood pressure *(11)*. The increase in risk of fracture is similar to the increase in risk of stroke-related mortality in women with increasing blood pressure *(12)*. However, in addition to density, it is believed that structure, elasticity, and geometry of bone are important determinants of its strength. These are variables about which current densitometric-based methodology provides no information, but which may be important in determining fracture risk. It has been suggested that quantitative ultrasound measurements (velocity and attenuation of the sound wave) may provide additional information about bone quality apart from density.

Ultrasound instruments may measure the velocity of the sound wave through bone and/or the speed of sound from one transducer to another. Velocity of the sound wave through bone assesses the speed of the sound wave from one bone surface to the other. Hence, the value represents the time it takes the sound wave to pass through bone alone. The speed of sound is the time it takes for the sound wave to travel from one transducer to another. Thus, the speed of sound through all materials between the transducers, e.g., bone, fat, soft tissue, and water, will be included in the measured value. The greater the connectivity or complexity of a structure, the greater will be the velocity of the sound wave through the structure. Thus, normal bone will have higher velocity values than osteoporotic bone. Measurements of velocity of sound through bone provide an index of microhardness and elastic properties, a reflection of the capacity of bone to resist deformation *(13–15)*. The velocity of the sound wave through bone is also dependent on the mineral content *(16)*. When bone mineral is decreased by demineralization with nitric acid, there is a linear decrease in velocity *(16)*. The velocity of the sound wave through bone is also largely influenced by trabecular separation *(17)*. As the parallel and perpendicular components of trabecular separation increase, the velocity of the sound wave through the bone deceases *(17)*.

The ultrasonic attenuation depends on bone structure, which can be described by the spatial distribution and size of the individual trabeculae. The more complex a structure, the more the sound wave passing through it will be blocked or attenuated. Thus, normal bone will have higher attenuation values than osteoporotic bone. The spatial arrangement of a structure also affects sound wave attenuation. The trabecular orientation of a bone affects ultrasound attenuation, but not BMD *(18,19)*. Ultrasound attenuation is also influenced by both trabecular separation and connectivity *(17)*, and correlates closely with bone volume *(20)*. This may be an important determinant of fracture risk, since osteoporosis is characterized by a process that removes entire trabeculae, leaving those that remain more widely separated, but only slightly reduced in thickness *(21)*. The broadband ultrasound attenuation and bone density of human femoral neck specimens correlate with femoral neck hardness determined by incremental indent depth *(22)*. Contrary to findings in bone specimens containing cortical and trabecular bone, incremental indent depth for trabecular bone cubes correlates only with BMD, not ultrasound attenuation. This suggests that the correlation between indent depth and broad-band ultrasound attenuation depends upon the presence of cortical bone *(19)*.

Thus, velocity of the sound wave through bone and the attenuation of the sound wave are related to biomechanical properties of bone: elastic modulus, compressive strength, and hardness. These are material characteristics that describe mechanical properties of a tissue that are independent of geometry and architecture *(23)*. Stiffness, which is available as a measurement on certain ultrasound instruments, does not reflect a biomechanical property of bone. It is an algorithm derived from the attenuation and the speed of the sound wave through bone, and as such, is dependent on those two measurements.

3. QUANTITATIVE ULTRASOUND TO ASSESS BONE MASS

Clinical studies have employed quantitative ultrasound to assess bone mass in adult women *(20,24–47)*, in pediatric subjects *(48)*, and in patients with primary hyperparathyroidism *(49)*. Broad-band ultrasound attenuation is not affected by heel width *(50–52)*. In contrast, increases in heel width and fat thickness result in an underestimation of the speed of sound *(52)*, demonstrating the importance of measuring velocity of sound through bone rather than speed of sound from one transducer to another.

Because ultrasound assesses properties of bone in addition to density, such as elasticity and structure, it should be expected that ultrasound values at a skeletal site do not correlate exactly with densitometric evaluation of that site. Broad-band ultrasound attenuation (BUA) and velocity of the sound wave (VOS) at the calcaneus correlate with density of the calcaneus determined by single-photon absorptiometry (SPA), $r = 0.51$ and $r = 0.72$, respectively *(28)*. Using SXA of the calcaneus, the correlation between the densitometric value and BUA in 25 women is $r = 0.72$ *(30)*, while with DXA the correlations are similar, $r = 0.66$ to 0.8 *(33,34)*. In a study of 64 Caucasian women, BUA and VOS correlate with heel density determined by DXA, $r = 0.73$ and $r = 0.66$, respectively *(31)*. These studies correlating density with quantitative ultrasound values at the same site suggest that approx 45%–50% of the BUA and VOS values can be accounted for by density. Even BUA and VOS values appear to measure different properties in humans ($r = 0.74$), suggesting that only 55% of the two measurements reflect similar properties of bone *(31)*.

Both BUA *(20,24,26,27,32–34,37,41,44,46)* and VOS *(41,42,45,46)* decrease with age in women. The fall in BUA values after menopause parallels the fall in lumbar spine BMD (Versace M., personal communication). BUA normative values have been reported in three different populations of women using the same instrument. Damilakis et al. *(32)* studied 93 normal Greek women between the ages of 25 and 87; Palacios et al. *(34)* studied 111 normal Spanish women between the ages of 30 and 70; Salamone et al. *(44)* examined 259 normal Caucasian women between the ages of 45 and 76 yr. A woman was defined as normal based on the absence of back pain and fracture. In the three studies, BUA values were similar at any given age in these diverse populations *(32,33,44)*.

BUA values are significantly decreased in women with osteoporosis *(24,27,32,33,36)* and increase during a program of brisk walking (29). The postmenopausal fall in BUA *(53)* and VOS *(42)* is prevented by estrogen replacement therapy. BUA values have a sensitivity and specificity for osteoporosis that range between 65 and 85% when osteoporosis is defined by bone density values *(24,26,33,40)*.

4. ULTRASOUND VALUES AS A PREDICTOR OF FRACTURE

Bone density is a very good predictor of fracture risk *(6–10)*. Nevertheless, it is clear that many women whose bone density is age-appropriate suffer fractures *(54,55)*. Although studies have shown that approx 75 to 80% of the variance in the ultimate strength of bone is accounted for by bone density *(56)*, a variety of changes in the material composition or structural geometry of the skeleton can modify the effects of altered bone mineral content *(57)*. Thus, it should not be surprising that ultrasound, a technique that assesses bone quality as well as density, is a predictor of fracture. There is a strong correlation between ultrasonic properties of the calcaneus and the load required to fracture cadaveric proximal femurs *(58)*. Femoral neck density and trochanteric density are strongly associated with femoral failure load ($r^2 = 0.79$ and 0.81, respectively, $p < 0.001$). Calcaneal density ($r^2 = 0.63$, $p < 0.001$) and BUA ($r^2 = 0.51$, $p = 0.002$) are also significantly associated with the femoral failure load *(58)*.

Women with VOS values approx 2 SD below young normals have a sixfold higher likelihood of having one or more fractures than women with velocities above that level *(59)*. Femoral neck density is decreased by 23% in women who sustain hip fractures, whereas BUA is decreased by 41% in these women *(24)*. BUA is as good a discriminator between normal subjects and patients with osteoporotic vertebral fractures, as is bone density of the spine measured by dual-photon absorptiometry (DPA) *(26)*. In a prospective study of 1414 elderly women, those most at risk of sustaining hip fractures were those with low BUA *(60)*, suggesting that, although the technique does not correlate perfectly with densitometry, it may identify women at greatest risk for later sustaining hip fracture. In a retrospective study of 50 women with hip fractures and 50 control subjects, BUA was a better discriminator of hip fracture than DXA at either the hip or spine *(61)*. BUA and VOS also have been shown to discriminate hip and vertebral fracture as well as densitometry of the respective sites in a study of 336 women over age 60 *(62)*. In this retrospective study, the ultrasound values remained as independent predictors of hip fracture even after correction for bone density, age, and years since menopause. This finding supports the hypothesis that ultrasonic measurements contain useful information about bone strength not contained in bone density measurements *(62)*. Ultrasound velocity at the tibia also discriminates between women with and without vertebral fracture as effectively as densitometry of the spine *(63)*. In a retrospective study of 4685 women over the age of 69 who are participating in the Study of Osteoporotic Fractures, BUA was compared with bone density of the spine, hip, and calcaneus as a predictor of fracture risk *(64)*. BUA was strongly associated with risk of fracture with odds ratios that remained significant even after correction for BMD. Thus, quantitative ultrasound measures characteristics of bone strength that are in part independent of density and in themselves are risk factors for fracture *(64)*. In a retrospective study of 649 women, the relationship of calcaneal BUA with vertebral fracture risk is similar in magnitude to associations observed for density measurements of the calcaneus and spine *(65)*.

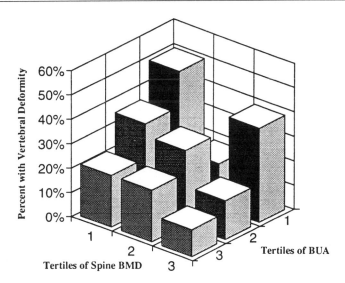

Fig. 1. The independent relation between BUA and vertebral fracture. Percentage with vertebral fracture by BUA and spine BMD. Tertiles labeled from lowest (1) to highest (3). reprinted from ref. *67* with permission of Blackwell Science, Inc.

Quantitative ultrasound values are better correlated to the type of hip fracture than DXA, discriminate subjects with hip and vertebral fracture equally well as DXA, and appear to provide an indication of fracture risk independent of BMD (Fig. 1) *(66,67)*. Ultrasound velocity is as good as single photon absorptiometry (SPA) in estimating odds of fracture *(68)*.

These studies *(59–68)* suggest that quantitative ultrasound is as good a predictor of fracture risk as BMD *(6–10)*. However, the studies have been retrospective *(59–68)* and may include unappreciated confounding variables. Two recent reports indicate that quantitative ultrasound can prospectively predict fracture risk. Incident vertebral deformities in 130 postmenopausal women were assessed over a 2-yr period. Women with ultrasound velocity values more than 1 SD below the mean for the group had a 3.3- to 4.6-fold greater likelihood of sustaining a vertebral fracture *(69)*. In a prospective study of 6,183 women followed for 1.4 yr, both low broad-band ultrasound attenuation and low BMD were associated with an increased risk of subsequent fracture, both nonspine and hip fractures *(70)*. However, the quantitative ultrasound values did not provide information about fracture independent of BMD *(70)*. This may be the result of the relatively small number of fractures, 250 nonspine including 38 hip fractures. Nevertheless, the combined retrospective *(59–68)* and prospective *(69,70)* studies indicate that quantitative ultrasound is as good a predictor of vertebral and hip fracture risk as bone densitometry and may provide additional information regarding bone quality.

5. SUMMARY

Decreased bone mass is the major risk factor for fracture. Osteoporosis-related fractures are responsible for increased morbidity and mortality, as well as increased health costs. The diagnosis of osteoporosis is often not made until a fracture occurs because of the lack of widespread availability of bone densitometry instruments. Quantitative ultrasound is a low-cost, radiation-free potential alternative to bone densitometry as a method to predict those individuals at greatest risk for subsequent fracture. Regardless of whether ultrasound provides information about bone that is independent of density, its ability to predict fracture risk will allow those patients to be targeted for preventive therapy.

REFERENCES

1. Melton LJ III. How many women have osteoporosis now? *J Bone Miner Res* 1995; 10: 175–177.
2. Ribot C, Pouilles JM, Bonnen M, et al. Assessment of the risk of postmenopausal osteoporosis using clinical factors. *Clin Endocrinol* 1992; 36: 225–228.
3. Slemenda CV, Hui SL, Longcope C, et al. Predictors of bone mass in perimenopausal women: a prospective study of clinical data using photon absorptiometry. *Ann Intern Med* 1990; 112: 96–101.
4. Fox EM, Cummings SR, Threets K. Family history and risk of osteoporotic fracture. *J Bone Miner Res* 1994; 95: S153.
5. Ribot C, Tremollieres F, Pouilles JM. Can we detect women with low bone mass using clinical risk factors? *Am J Med* 1995; 98(2A): 525–555.
6. Black DM, Cummings SR, Genant HK, et al. Axial and appendicular bone density predict fractures in older women. *J Bone Miner Res* 1992; 7: 633–638.
7. Cummings SR, Black DM, Nevitt MC, et al. Bone density at various sites for prediction of hip fractures. *Lancet* 1993; 341: 72–75.
8. Hui SL, Slemenda CW, Johnston CC. Baseline measurement of bone mass predicts fracture in white women. *Ann Intern Med* 1989; 111: 355–361.
9. Overgaard K, Hansen MA, Riis BJ, et al. Discriminatory ability of bone mass measurements (SPA and DXA) for fractures in elderly postmenopausal women. *Calcif Tissue Int* 1992; 50: 30–35.
10. Ross PD, Wasnich RD, Vogel JM. Detection of prefracture spinal osteoporosis using bone mineral absorptiometry. *J Bone Miner Res* 1988; 3: 1–11.
11. Neaton JD, Wentworth D. For the multiple risk factor intervention trial research group. Serum cholesterol, blood pressure, cigarette smoking and death from coronary artery disease: overall findings and differences by age for 316,099 white men. *Arch Intern Med* 1992; 152: 56–64.
12. Khaw K, Barrett-Connor E, Suarez L, et al. Predictors of stroke associated mortality in the elderly. *Stroke* 1984; 15: 244–88.
13. Abendschein W, Hyatt GW. Ultrasonics and selected physical properties of bone. *Clin Orthop* 1970; 69: 294–301.
14. Yoon HS, Katz JL. Ultrasonic wave propagation in human cortical bone. Measurements of elastic properties and microhardness. *J Biomech* 1976; 9: 459–464.
15. Ashman RB, Corin JD, Turner CH. Elastic properties of cancellous bone: measurement by an ultrasonic technique. *J Biomech* 1987; 20: 979–986.
16. Tavakoli MB, Evans JA. Dependence of the velocity and attenuation of ultrasound in bone on the mineral content. *Phys Med Biol* 1991; 36: 1529–1537.
17. Gluer CC, Wu CY, Jergas M, et al. Three quantitative ultrasound parameters reflect bone structure. *Calcif Tissue Int* 1994; 55: 46–52.
18. Gluer CC, Wu CY, Genant HK. Broadband ultrasound attenuation signals depend on trabecular orientation: an *in vitro* study. *Osteoporosis Int* 1993; 3: 185–191.
19. Duquette J, Lin J, Hoffman A, et al. Correlation between bone mineral density, broadband ultrasound attenuation, femoral neck strength, and bone orientation in bovine samples. *J Bone Miner Res* 1995; 10: S238.
20. Agren M, Karellas A, Leahey D, et al. Ultrasound attenuation of the calcaneus: a sensitive and specific discriminator of osteopenia in postmenopausal women. *Calcif Tissue Int* 1991; 48: 240–244.
21. Parfitt AM, Matthew CHE, Villanueva AR, et al. Relationships between surface, volume and thickness of iliac trabecular bone in aging and in osteoporosis. Implications for the microanatomic and cellular mechanisms of bone loss. *J Clin Invest* 1983; 72: 1396–1409.
22. Houde JP, Marchetti ME, Duquette J, et al. Correlation of bone mineral density and femoral neck hardness in bovine and human samples. *Calcif Tissue Int* 1995; 57: 201–205 .
23. Kaufman JJ, Einhorn TA. Ultrasound assessment of bone. *J Bone Miner Res* 1993; 8: 517–525.
24. Baran DT, Kelly AM, Karellas A, et al. Ultrasound attenuation of the os calcis in women with osteoporosis and hip fractures. *Calcif Tissue Int* 1988; 43: 138–142.

25. Rossman P, Zagzebski J, Mesina C, et al. Comparison of speed of sound and ultrasound attenuation in the os calcis to bone density of the radius, femur, and lumbar vertebrae. *Clin Phys Physiol Meas* 1989; 4: 353–360.

26. McCloskey EV, Murray SA, Miller C, et al. Broadband ultrasound attenuation in the os calcis: relationship to bone mineral at other skeletal sites. *Clin Sci* 1990; 78: 227–233.

27. Baran DT, McCarthy CK, Leahey D, et al. Broadband ultrasound attenuation of the calcaneus predicts lumbar and femoral neck density in Caucasian women: a preliminary study. *Osteoporosis Int* 1991; 1: 110–113.

28. Zagzebski JA, Rossman PJ, Mesina C, et al. Ultrasound transmission measurements through the os calcis. *Calcif Tissue Int* 1991; 49: 107–111.

29. Jones PRM, Hardman AE, Hudson A, et al. Influence of brisk walking on the broadband ultrasonic attenuation of the calcaneus in previously sedentary women Aged 30–61 Years. *Calcif Tissue Int* 1991; 49: 112–115.

30. Gluer CC, Vahlensieck M, Faulkner KG, et al. Site matched calcaneal measurements of broadband ultrasound attenuation and single X-ray absorptiometry: so they measure different skeletal properties? *J Bone Miner Res* 1992; 7: 1071–1079.

31. Waud CE, Lew R, Baran DT. The relationship between ultrasound and densitometric measurements of bone mass at the calcaneus in women. *Calcif Tissue Int* 1992; 51: 415–418.

32. Damilakis JE, Dretakis E, Gourtsoyiannis NC. Ultrasound attenuation of the calcaneus in the female population: normative data. *Calcif Tissue Int* 1992; 51: 180–183.

33. Roux C, Lemonnier E, Kolta S, et al. Broadband ultrasound attenuation of the calcaneus and bone density measurements. *Rev Rheumat* 1993; 60: 771–780.

34. Palacios S, Menendez C, Calderon J, et al. Spine and femur density and broadband ultrasound attenuation of the calcaneus in normal Spanish women. *Calcif Tissue Int* 1993; 52: 99–102.

35. Wapniarz M, Lehmann R, Banik N, et al. Apparent velocity of ultrasound at the patella in comparison to bone mineral density at the lumbar spine in normal males and females. *Bone Miner* 1993; 23: 243–252.

36. Lees B, Stevenson JC. Preliminary evaluation of a new ultrasound bone densitometer. *Calcif Tissue Int* 1993; 53: 149–152.

37. Herd RJM, Blake GM, Ramalingam T, et al. Measurements of postmenopausal bone loss with a new contact ultrasound system. *Calcif Tissue Int* 1993; 53: 153–157.

38. Miller CG, Herd RJM, Ramalingam T, et al. Ultrasonic velocity measurements through the calcaneus: which velocity should be measured. *Osteoporosis Int* 1993; 3: 31–35.

39. Massie A, Reid DM, Porter RW. Screening for osteoporosis: comparison between dual energy X-ray absorptiometry and broadband ultrasound attenuation in 1,000 premenopausal women. *Osteoporosis Int* 1993; 3: 107–110.

40. Young H, Howey S, Purdie DW, et al. Broadband ultrasound attenuation compared with dual energy X-ray absorptiometry in screening for postmenopausal low bone density. *Osteoporosis Int* 1993; 3: 160–164.

41. Schott AM, Hans D, Sornay-Rendu E, et al. Ultrasound measurements on os calcis: precision and age-related changes in a normal female population. *Osteoporosis Int* 1993; 3: 249–254.

42. Lehman R, Wapniarz M, Kvasnicka HM, et al. Velocity of ultrasound at the patella: influence of age, menopause, and estrogen replacement. *Osteoporosis Int* 1993; 3: 308–313.

43. Faulkner K, McClung MR, Coleman LJ, et al. Quantitative ultrasound of the heel: correlation with densitometric measurements at different skeletal sites. *Osteoporosis Int* 1994; 4: 42–47.

44. Salamone LM, Krall EA, Harris S, et al. Comparison of broadband ultrasound attenuation to single X-ray absorptiometry measurements at the calcaneus in postmenopausal women. *Calcif Tissue Int* 1994; 54: 87–90.

45. Miller CG, Herd RJM, Ramalingam T, et al. Ultrasonic velocity measurements through the calcaneus: which velocity should be measured. *Osteoporosis Int* 1993; 3: 31–35.

46. Van Daele PLA, Burger H, Algra D, et al. Age-associated changes in ultrasound measurements of the calcaneus in men and women. The Rotterdam study. *J Bone Miner Res* 1994; 9: 1751–1757.

47. Yamazaki K, Kushida K, Ohmara A, et al. Ultrasound bone densitometry of the os calcis in Japanese women. *Osteoporosis Int* 1994; 4: 220–225.

48. Jaworski M, Lebiedowski M, Lorenc RS, et al. Ultrasound bone measurement in pediatric subjects. *Calcif Tissue Int* 1995; 56: 368–371.

49. Minisola S, Rosso R, Scarda A, et al. Quantitative ultrasound assessment of bone in patients with primary hyperparathyroidism. *Calcif Tissue Int* 1995; 56: 526–528.

50. Blake GM, Herd RJM, Miller CG, et al. Should broadband ultrasonic attenuation be normalized for the width of the calcaneus. *Br J Radiol* 1994; 67: 1206–1209.

51. Wu CY, Gluer CC, Jerges M, et al. The impact of bone size on broadband ultrasound attenuation. *Bone* 1995; 16: 137–141.

52. Kotzki PO, Buyck D, Hans D, et al. Influence of fat on ultrasound measurements of the os calcis. *Calcif Tissue Int* 1994; 54: 91–95.

53. Houde JP, Marchetti M, Baran DT. Changes in broadband ultrasound attenuation of the calcaneus and bone density in early postmenopausal women. *Clin Res* 1994; 42: 210A.

54. Riggs BL, Wahner HW, Dunn WL, et al. Differential changes in bone mineral density of the appendicular and axial skeleton with aging: relationship to spinal osteoporosis. *J Clin Invest* 1981; 67: 328–35.

55. Riggs BL, Wahner HW, Seeman E, et al. Changes in bone mineral density of the proximal femur and spine with aging: differences between the postmenopausal and senile osteoporosis syndrome. *J Clin Invest* 1982; 70: 716–723.

56. Smith CB, Smith DA. Relations between age, mineral density, and mechanical properties of human femoral compacta. *Acta Orthop Scand* 1976; 47: 496–502.

57. Einhorn TA. Bone strength: the bottom line. *Calcif Tissue Int* 1992; 51: 333–339.

58. Bouxsein ML, Courtney AC, Hayes WC. Ultrasonic and densitometric properties of the calcaneus correlate with the strength of cadaveric femurs loaded in a full configuration. *Calcif Tissue Int* 1995; 56: 99–103.

59. Heaney RP, Avioli LV, Chesnut CC III, et al. Osteoporotic bone fragility detection by ultrasound transmission velocity. *JAMA* 1989; 261: 2986–2990.

60. Porter RW, Miller CG, Grainger D, et al. Prediction of hip fracture in elderly women: a prospective study. *Br Med J* 1990; 301: 638–641.

61. Stewart A, Reid DM, Porter RW. Broadband ultrasound attenuation and dual energy X-ray absorptiometry in patients with hip fractures: which technique discriminates fracture risk? *Calcif Tissue Int* 1994; 54: 466–469.

62. Turner CH, Peacock M, Timmerman L, et al. Calcaneal ultrasonic measurements discriminate hip fracture, but not vertebral fracture, independently of bone mass. *Osteoporosis Int* 1995; 5: 130–135.

63. Ogree J, McCloskey EV, Foster H, et al. Tibial Ultrasound velocity—a useful clinical measure of skeletal status. *J Bone Miner Res* 1994; 9: S156.

64. Gluer CC, Cummings SR, Bauer DC, et al. Associations between quantitative ultrasound and recent fractures. *J Bone Miner Res* 1994; 9: S153.

65. Vogel J, Huang C, Ross PD, et al. Broadband ultrasound attenuation (BUA) predicts risk of vertebral fractures. *J Bone Miner Res* 1994; 9: S154.

66. Schott AM, Weill-Engerer S, Hans D, et al. Ultrasound discriminates patients with hip fracture equally well as dual energy X-ray absorptiometry and independently of bone mineral density. *J Bone Miner Res* 1995; 10: 243–249.

67. Bauer DC, Gluer CC, Genant HK, et al. Quantitative ultrasound and vertebral fracture in postmenopausal women. *J Bone Miner Res* 1995; 10: 353–358.

68. Stegman MR, Heaney RP, Recker RR. Comparison of speed and sound ultrasound with single photon absorptiometry for determining fracture odds ratios. *J Bone Miner Res* 1995; 10: 346–352.

69. Heaney RP, Avioli LV, Chestnut CH III, et al. Ultrasound velocity through bone predicts incident vertebral deformity. *J Bone Miner Res* 1995; 10: 341–345.

70. Bauer DC, Gluer CC, Pressman AR, et al. Broadband ultrasonic attenuation and the risk of fracture: a prospective study. *J Bone Miner Res* 1995; 10: S175.

11

Biochemical Markers
of Bone Turnover

Clifford J. Rosen, MD

CONTENTS

INTRODUCTION
MARKERS OF BONE RESORPTION
CONCLUSIONS
REFERENCES

1. INTRODUCTION

Bone remodeling is a continuous and dynamic process of renewal, whereby a quantum of new bone is reformed following dissolution. As noted previously, this physiologic cycle serves to provide a constant source of calcium for homeostatic functions, while preserving the biomechanical properties of bone itself. During bone resorption, calcium and other matrix constituents are released into the bloodstream where they are metabolized or excreted. As bone formation proceeds, skeletal-specific proteins (enzymes or matrix components) can leach into the circulation in relatively high concentrations, permitting measurement by various techniques, including radioimmunoassay. Over the last decade several new assays for biochemical markers of bone remodeling have been developed (Table 1). These measurements have been shown to correlate with dynamic studies of bone histomorphometry and calcium kinetics. Therefore, these tests have the potential to become useful clinical tools in predicting bone loss and fractures.

Theoretically, knowing the dynamic state of the remodeling unit could provide critical information not obtainable from bone density studies. For example, an asymptomatic 52-yr-old postmenopausal woman presents to the office with a family history of osteoporosis and concern about possible use of estrogen. A lumbar spine bone density reveals that the patient is −0.5 SD below the mean for a 35-yr-old. At this point in time, it would be difficult for the clinician to predict her rate of bone loss or her future fracture risk without knowing an earlier (or latter) bone density. Even with this data, the question could be asked: Did this patient have a bone mineral density (BMD) + 1.0 SD from mean 3 yr ago, or has she always had a bone density near normal with minimal loss during her menopause? A single blood or urine test for one of these biochemical markers could provide

From: *Osteoporosis: Diagnostic and Therapeutic Principles*
Edited by: C. J. Rosen Humana Press Inc., Totowa, NJ

Table 1
Markers of Bone Turnover

Indices of bone formation	Indices of bone resorption
Total alkaline phosphatase (TAP)	Urinary calcium/creatine
skeletal alkaline phosphatase (SAP)	Urinary hydroxyproline
Serum osteocalcin (OC)	Urinary collagen crosslinks[a]
Procollagen I extension peptides (PICP)	deoxypyridinoline
	pyridinoline
	N-telopeptide crosslinks
	C-terminal crosslinks
	Serum Type I collagen crosslinks
	C-terminal crosslinks (ICTP)

[a]Collagen crosslinks can be assayed in urine and in serum by several different techniques. Total collagen crosslinks represent a chromatographic method of measuring both deoxy- and pyridinoline crosslinks. By chromatography, each component can also be determined. Free pyridinoline crosslinks (not bound to peptides) can be measured by ELISA; both N-terminal peptides and C-terminal peptides bound to the crosslinks can be measured by ELISA.

the clinician with an approximation of bone turnover, thereby alerting the provider to the need for some form of prophylactic therapy in this woman (e.g., estrogen, calcitonin, or a bisphosphonate). Furthermore, if the practitioner elects to treat this patient, a biochemical marker could demonstrate whether the drug was or was not successful in suppressing bone resorption. Finally, a single biochemical marker at one point in time might predict how this individual will respond to antiresorptive therapy in terms of bone density *(1)*. Hence, in this patient, clinical application of bone markers may provide potentially useful information.

Despite the theoretical scenario presented above, it is important to note that biochemical markers of bone turnover cannot make the diagnosis of osteoporosis. Still, markers do have a role in clinical medicine and can be used (as in the case) to measure bone remodeling indirectly. With rapid technological advances, it is likely that more markers will become available. Hence, within 5 yr, at least one biochemical marker will be accessible on multiphasic screening in a manner analagous to cholesterol or calcium. By choice or not, the provider will have to deal with interpretation of these markers. Therefore, understanding the strengths and limitations of these indices will become increasingly more important in the management of osteoporosis.

2. MARKERS OF BONE RESORPTION

2.1. Background

Bone is composed of a mineral or inorganic component (calcium hydroxyapatite) and an organic or protein matrix. The organic matrix is composed primarily of collagen, 97% of which is Type I collagen *(2)*. *De novo* synthesis of collagen, a three peptide chain held together in a helical structure (Fig. 1), is critical to subsequent bone formation, since it provides the lattice necessary for crystalization and mineralization. Type I collagen is secreted by osteoblasts as procollagen-containing peptide extensions *(3)*. During extracellular processing and just prior to mature fibril formation, amino- (N-) and carboxy- (C-) terminal extensions are cleaved and released into the circulation. The

Type I Bone Collagen

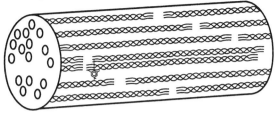

Fig. 1. Type I collagen is the predominant peptide within the bone matrix. It is a helical structure composed of three peptide strands held together through CCLs.

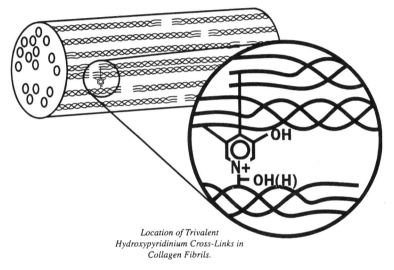

Location of Trivalent
Hydroxypyridinium Cross-Links in
Collagen Fibrils.

Fig. 2. The trivalent hydroxypyridiinium crosslinks (including deoxypyridinoline and pyridinoline) anchor Type I collagen peptides at the N-terminal and C-terminal ends.

C-terminal fragment remains intact, but the N-terminal fragment can be incorporated back into bone as a low-mol-wt fragment.

The final step in the extracellular processing of collagen is the crosslinking of the three collagen fibrils at both the C- and N-terminal portions (telopeptides) of the molecule (Fig. 2). This occurs at unique amino acids (hydroxylysine or lysine) in collagen. In bone and cartilage, hydroxylysine predominates. Hence, most crosslinks are pyridinoline (pyr) or hydroxypyridinoline (deoxypyridinoline, D-pyr) (*see* Fig. 2). D-pyr is found exclusively in bone and dentin while pyr is a crosslink component of skin, joint and cartilaginous tissues. In human bone, the ratio of pyr/D-pyr is approx 2:3 *(4)*. The breakdown of these crosslinks during the early stages of bone resorption guarantees their presence in the circulation bound to peptide fragments (C-telopeptides), whereas excretion in the urine represents a combination of free peptide ($\approx$30%) and bound pyridinolines (N-telopeptides) *(5)*. Pyridinolines are not metabolized but are excreted in a diurnal pattern with a peak at night and a nadir during the afternoon *(6)*. Hence, timed collections of pyridinolines may provide an integrated measure of bone turnover.

The most abundant noncollagen protein in bone (and the seventh most abundant protein in the body) is osteocalcin (also called bone Gla-protein). It is a 49 amino acid peptide with three glutamic acid residues and a strong affinity for hydroxyapatite (7). It is synthesized by osteoblasts, and is specific for bone and dentin. Its precise biologic function is unknown although it is a marker of the differentiated osteoblast. The vast majority of osteocalcin is deposited in bone by osteoblasts, although 1% is released into the circulation and can be measured by radioimmunoassay (8). During bone resorption, osteocalcin fragments can be detected in the serum and urine.

Total alkaline phosphatase is the most widely used marker of bone formation, even though it is the least specific and sensitive for most metabolic bone diseases (except Paget's disease of the bone). There are three isoenzymes of alkaline phosphatase, which differ according to posttranslational glycosylation. This processing allows the enzyme to attach to cell membranes and vesicles (9). The principal substrates for alkaline phosphatase in bone are organic and inorganic phosphates and pyrophosphates, thus making its enzymatic activity critical for mineralization. Total serum alkaline phosphatase (TAP) represents the spillover from several tissues. Fifty percent of TAP is skeletal alkaline phosphatase (SAP) derived almost exclusively from osteoblastic synthesis.

Osteocalcin, alkaline phosphatase, collagen, collagen crosslinks (CCLs), and hydroxyproline are the basic remodeling proteins that commercial assays can currently measure in either serum or urine (see Table 1). Each will be examined in the following sections under bone resorption markers or bone formation indices.

2.2. Markers of Bone Resorption

2.2.1. Urinary Calcium/Creatinine

Twenty-four-hour urine collections for calcium and creatinine have been used to extrapolate the status of bone remodeling activity in various metabolic bone conditions. As noted in Chapter 2, Albright reported increased urinary calcium excretion in postmenopausal women, suggesting negative calcium balance during menopause (10). Since then, this test has been widely used and modified by a simultaneous assay for urinary creatinine. However, use of the ratio of urinary calcium to creatinine is plagued by low specifity and sensitivity. Numerous factors can affect calcium excretion (dietary calcium, PTH, vitamin D status, salt intake, and so on). Furthermore, there is a large intrasubject coefficient of variation (up to 50%). Finally, 24-h urinary collections are particularly cumbersome even in the most experienced hands. Hence, even though urinary calcium is the cheapest of the biochemical markers, this test has low sensitivity, lacks specificity and is a very poor predictor of bone loss.

2.2.2. Urinary Hydroxyproline

After collagen synthesis by osteoblasts, the amino acid proline is hydroxylated and incorporated into bone matrix where it contributes to collagen fibril stability. About 13% of collagen contains hydroxyproline (11). During collagen breakdown (i.e., bone resorption), hydroxyproline is released into the circulation both free and bound to polypeptides. The free and peptide-bound constituents are filtered in the urine; free hyroxyproline is completely reabsorbed and metabolized in the liver, whereas peptide fragments remain in the urine. Unfortunately, a significant proportion of urinary hydroxyproline originates from the breakdown of nonskeletal collagen (12). Furthermore, dietary hydroxyproline is absorbed readily and is present in several food sources, including gelatins. Urinary measurements are made by high-performance liquid chromatography (HPLC) or calo-rimetry, and are usually expressed as a ratio of hydroxyproline to creatinine clearance. Owing to complex metabolic pathways, and the lack of specificity, urinary hydroxypro-line correlates poorly with bone resorption assessed by calcium kinetics or bone histomorphometry *(13)*.

In summary, hydroxyproline excretion is a sensitive marker of increased bone turn-over, but its specificity is poor. Furthermore, special dietary instructions are an absolute necessity. In general, newer biochemical markers with enhanced specificity have sup-planted hydroxyproline as an indicator of bone turnover.

2.2.3. URINARY CCLS

Pyridinoline CCLs represent one of the final steps in the maturation and stabilization of collagen within the bone matrix. As noted previously, these crosslinking amino acids are generated extracellularly and provide stability for the helical fibrils of Type I col-lagen. CCLs are rapidly dissolved during bone resorption, are relatively specific for bone, are not influenced by diet, and are not metabolized in the circulation. Therefore, these compounds have been considered the best markers of bone turnover. Furthermore, mea-surement of pyridinoline CCL excretion correlates closely with histomorphometric determinants of bone resorption in women with osteoporosis *(14)*.

In the past 5 yr, clinical experience with pyridinoline CCLs has grown, especially in states of high bone turnover (Paget's disease of bone, thyrotoxicosis, hyperpara-thyroidism). CCL excretion has been shown to correlate with histomorphometric evi-dence of increased bone resorption in these disorders *(15–17)*. Recent studies have focused on pyridinoline CCL excretion in osteoporosis in order: (1) to determine the precise rate of bone loss in a postmenopausal woman; and (2) to assess an individual's response to antiresorptive therapy. Technological modifications have recently improved the speed and accuracy of measuring pyridinoline CCLs. A brief (nontechnical) discussion of these different methodologies follows.

Pyridinoline CCLs are released into the circulation during bone resorption and are excreted as both free pyridinolines (deoxypyridinoline and pyridinoline) and pyridino-lines bound to bone specific C- or N- terminal ends of Type I collagen (Figs. 1 and 2). There are several different ways to measure pyridinoline CCLs. The most sensitive and accurate methodology for urinary pyridinoline CCL excretion is high performance liquid chromatography (HPLC) which permits quantitation of total CCLs into D-pyr and pyr *(18)*. In addition to the expense, there are several other disadvantages that prevent wide-spread clinical utility of HPLC. First, only a few laboratories have the capability to determine D-pyr and pyr by this methodology. Second, the assay involves a rather labo-rious multistep procedure of acid hydrolysis, extraction, and then HPLC. In addition, CCL recovery by HPLC may be incomplete. Finally, the extent of intrasubject variability has not been studied.

In the past 3 yr, there have been considerable advances in the development of simpler, more precise measures of pyridinoline CCLs both in the urine and serum These tests rely on ELISA (enzyme-linked substrate assays: N-telopeptide and free pyridinoline) or RIA technology (serum type I collagen crosslinked C-telopeptide, ICTP). The N-telopeptide urinary assay uses a monoclonal antibody (MAb) to the intermolecular crosslink domain on the N-terminal region of the Type I collagen molecule, thereby measuring the pyridinoline link and a portion of the collagen protein (*see* Fig. 2) *(19)*. Free pyridinoline crosslinks are measured in the urine by an ELISA assay, which preferentially detects free CCLs rather than those bound to N-terminal fragments of collagen (20). Serum ICTP is assayed by RIA, and it employs antisera directed against the C-terminal region (C-telopeptide) of the peptide bound to pyridinoline crosslinks. These compounds are released directly into the serum during bone resorption (21).

For each of these resorption markers, studies have been conducted to determine their sensitivity and specificity for detecting bone loss and predicting responsiveness to anti-resorptive therapy. Although evidence that these markers can predict future fractures is lacking, the ease of these measures should permit critical data to be forthcoming relatively shortly. Fig. 3 illustrates the value of each of these tests in detecting accelerated bone turnover among 85 postmenopausal osteoporotic women (22). In these women four of the five indices of bone turnover (not ICTP) were well above levels of normal premenopausal women (33–171% above normal; $p < 0.001$). In addition to measuring changes in bone turnover, D-pyr by HPLC and N-telopeptide by ELISA were both able to predict accurately spinal bone loss over 15 mo (22). Thus, these data suggest that several markers of bone turnover could be useful adjuncts for detecting bone loss in postmenopausal women.

In addition to detecting accelerated bone loss, biochemical markers of bone remodeling may provide important patient-specific information about bone responsiveness to antiresorptive therapy. Several studies have confirmed that pyridinoline CCLs are suppressed by conventional therapies. In 12 older postmenopausal women, 6 wk of conjugated equine estrogen (0.625 mg/d) suppressed pyridinoline CCL excretion (by HPLC), free pyridinolines (ELISA), and N-telopeptides (by ELISA) by 30% (23). In this study, after discontinuation of estrogen, indices of bone resorption returned to pretreatment levels. In a separate study of 65 early postmenopausal women, 5, 20, and 40 mg of alendronate suppressed N-telopeptide excretion in a dose-dependent manner up to 60% of baseline (19). Finally, 10 mg of alendronate to 85 postmenopausal women for 15 mo reduced N-telopeptide and total pyridinoline excretion (HPLC) to premenopausal levels within 1 mo of therapy and predicted bone density changes over the ensuing 15 mo (see Fig. 4) (22).

These data reinforce the potential significance of biochemical markers in determining the extent of bone loss and responsiveness to treatment. However, longer clinical trials will be needed to assess how accurately pyridinoline CCLs predict long-term bone loss and fractures. Moreover, many questions remain unanswered. For example, there are no studies that have shown that women with high bone turnover have a higher fracture incidence. Second, urinary pyridinoline CCL determinations still have a relatively high coefficient of variation (10–40%) (19). Third, over the course of several years, postmenopausal women change their rate of bone loss in both directions (24). Finally, predictions based on CCL excretion about the rate of bone loss have been most extensively studied only in early and late postmenopausal women. Generalizations about pyridinoline CCLs in other populations are not yet supported by critical data.

In the meantime, commercially available pyridinoline CCL studies can provide a relatively precise and accurate indication of bone turnover in most postmenopausal women. In addition, these tests are accessible to primary care providers and are relatively inexpensive ($55–100/test) compared to serial bone mass measurements. Furthermore, pyridinoline CCL assays can be performed reliably on morning 2-h collections, thereby eliminating the need for cumbersome 24-h urinary collections. Their future clinical utility will depend on newer technologies that should lower the cost of these tests, increase accessibility, and hopefully permit fracture prediction.

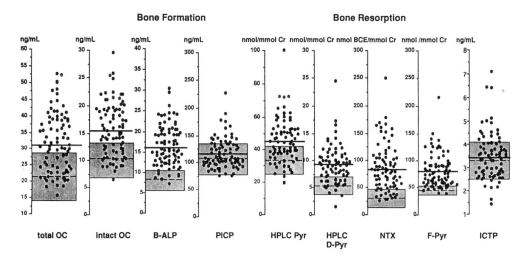

Fig. 3. Individual values for four markers of bone formation and five markers of bone resorption in 84 elderly osteoporotic women. For each marker, the solid line represents the mean of the patient population; the dotted line and the gray zone in the background are the mean and the normal range, respectively (±1 SD) for premenopausal controls. Reprinted from ref. *22* with permission.

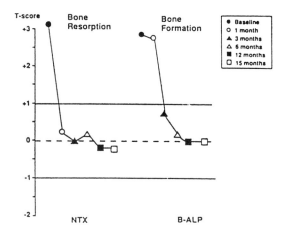

Fig. 4. Mean t-score values for N-telopeptide and bone alkaline phosphatase in elderly osteoporotic women at baseline and after 1, 3, 6, 12, and 15 mo of treatment with 10 mg/d of alendronate. T-scores are the number of SD from the mean of 46 premenopausal women. Reprinted from ref. *22* with permission.

2.3. Markers of Bone Formation

2.3.1. BACKGROUND

Biochemical markers of bone formation have been utilized for many yr in the management of metabolic bone diseases. For example, TAP remains one of the most sensitive and specific indicators of clinical activity in Paget's disease. However, Paget's disease is characterized by tremendous increases in bone remodeling activity. Osteoporosis, on the other hand, is not associated with the same degree of bone resorption. Therefore, other tests that reflect bone formation have been studied.

In general, markers of bone formation reflect increased osteoblastic function. In that context, during stages of osteoblast differentiation, collagen metabolites are expressed first, followed by osteocalcin, and then alkaline phosphatase. Therefore, it would be expected that the earliest markers of differentiation would be the most sensitive to changes in bone formation *(25)*. However, other factors contribute to the metabolism of these markers, making each somewhat unique in its ability to correlate with bone turnover activity. Furthermore, it should be remembered that in almost all cases of osteoporosis, bone formation remains at least partially coupled to bone resorption, even though resorption rates can far exceed formation. Therefore, during states of high turnover, markers of bone formation should be increased. In contrast, during treatment of osteoporosis with drugs that block bone resorption, bone formation is suppressed. Therefore, these markers may be potentially useful in detecting accelerated bone turnover (increases in serum markers) and response to therapy (decreases in serum markers).

Because bone formation markers are assayed in serum, their measurements tend to have better precision (i.e., the percent variation with repeated testing in the same individual), but lower sensitivity than urinary markers. Therefore, attempts have been made to combine urine and serum testing to determine the precise rate of bone turnover in a given individual. However, this model has not proven cost-effective nor has it been shown to predict fractures. In this chapter, I will focus only on individual measures of bone formation.

2.2.2. ALKALINE PHOSPHATASE

TAP activity comprises the sum of skeletal, intestinal, and hepatic components, and therefore lacks specificity for mild abnormalities in bone remodeling. Fifty percent of TAP is derived from osteoblastic production; hence, increased TAP can be noted in some patients with osteoporosis. The most common causes for a mildly elevated TAP are:

1. Recent fracture;
2. Coexisting osteomalacia;
3. Numerous medications, including anticonvulsants; and
4. Metastatic disease to bone. These disorders limit the clinical utility of TAP, except in the diagnosis and treatment of Paget's disease.

Since SAP and hepatic alkaline phosphatase (HAP) are derived from a single gene, attempts have been made to enhance the specifity and sensitivity of TAP by examining fractions of circulating alkaline phosphatase. Electrophoresis, heat inactivation, lectin precipitation, and MAb with RIA have been used in assays for SAP. However, none of the above, except the RIA, have produced results which greatly enhance sensitivity and specificity. Two groups of investigators previously demonstrated that SAP levels (by RIA) clearly distinguish osteoporotic from normal postmenopausal women *(26,27)*. More recently Garnero et al. reported twofold higher SAP levels among late postmenopausal women than premenopausal controls (*see* Figs. 3 and 4) *(22)*. Furthermore, SAP was found to be the best discriminator among bone formation markers between older osteoporotics and younger controls, and could predict the rate of bone loss and response to alendronate in 85 women treated for 15 mo *(22)*.

Bone formation markers may be important in monitoring the response to treatment with anabolic agents that stimulate new bone. Fluoride therapy increases TAP and SAP, and these markers predict favorable responses (in terms of BMD) to this treatment *(28)*. hPTH *(1–38)* administered to postmenopausal osteoporotic patients also produces a significant rise in TAP *(29)*. On the other hand, SAP levels do not increase during either rhGH or rhIGF-I therapy in elderly women *(30)*.

In conclusion, SAP has the potential to become a clinically relevant marker for bone turnover in postmenopausal women. Further studies will be required to assess its predictive value in fractures and its response to antiresorptive therapy. In addition, the cost and application of these tests in clinical practice require further study. However, it is clear that SAP represents an improvement over TAP in both sensitivity and specificity.

2.2.3. OSTEOCALCIN

Osteocalcin is a bone-specific protein produced by osteoblasts late in the differentiation scenario *(25)*. Its function is unknown, although it is produced in both carboxylated and decarboxylated forms, serum levels increase with age, and osteocalcin synthesis is modulated by vitamin D *(31)*. Serum osteocalcin is not stable if left at room temperature for several hours or with repetitive defrosts. Furthermore, there is significant diurnal variation (up to 25%) between peak and trough levels. Some osteocalcin cam be released from bone directly into the circulation during bone resorption.

Osteocalcin has traditionally been measured by RIA, although recently sandwich immunoradiometric and ELISA assays have become commercially available through kits or in reference laboratories *(32)*. Osteocalcin levels are increased during states of accelerated bone remodeling, such as hyperparathyroidism, hyperthyroidism, Paget's disease of bone, and acromegaly. These levels also correspond with histomorphometric changes in these disorders *(33)*. Serum levels of osteocalcin are suppressed during chronic treatment with glucocorticoids, estrogens, and bis-phosphonates.

In idiopathic postmenopausal osteoporosis, serum osteocalcin levels are either normal or elevated. In general, the higher the osteocalcin, the greater the remodeling frequency and the lower the bone density *(34,35)*. Among 52 postmenopausal osteoporotic women, Charles et al. reported a significant correlation between osteocalcin and bone mineralization rates *(36)*. Several groups have now demonstrated that osteocalcin levels are markedly increased in elders compared to premenopausal women *(22,39)*. This is consistent with histomorphometric evidence of increased bone turnover during aging. Recently, Szulc et al. reported that decarboxylated osteocalcin (in contrast to fully carboxylated osteocalcin) was a good predictor of hip fracture in elderly women *(37)*. Changes in carboxylation of osteocalcin are thought to be related to alterations in vitamin K within the skeleton, although the functional significance of these alterations is unknown *(38)*.

Civitelli et al. were the first to report that high levels of osteocalcin prior to treatment with calcitonin predicted an enhanced bone density response to antiresorptive therapy *(1)*. Although many physicians treating metabolic bone diseases select women for antiresorptive therapy based on these data, confirmation with other therapeutic agents has not been forthcoming. However, at least one subsequent study has shown that in elders, changes in osteocalcin during 3 mo can predict bone density responses to alendronate over 12 mo of therapy *(22)*. Hence, there may be value in doing serial osteocalcin levels to assess long-term effects of antiresorptive therapy.

Once again, as with all the bone formation indices, more studies will be needed before this marker can be used reliably to predict future fracture or rate of bone loss in postmenopausal women. Furthermore, the cost of serum osteocalcin remains relatively prohibitive ($80–150/assay). Therefore, its role in the assessment and management of osteoporotic patients remains to be determined.

2.3.4. PROCOLLAGEN I EXTENSION PEPTIDES (PICPS)

Collagen is synthesized as procollagen-containing peptide extensions in both the C- and N-terminal ends. These are cleaved from the rest of the molecule before its incorporation into collagen fibrils. Procollagen peptides are produced in equimolar ratios to collagen and then are released into the circulation, where they are metabolized in the liver after a relatively short half-life *(40)*. Immunologically different propeptides are produced in various tissues, but the contribution to serum PICP from collagen other than type I is relatively small. A commercially available RIA can detect these peptide fragments in serum *(41)*. PICPs are synthesized by osteoblasts and exhibit fairly significant diurnal variation. Although these peptides are relatively specific for bone formation some N-terminal peptide fragments make their way into the circulation after bone resorption. Hence, the commercial assays employ antibodies to the C-terminal end of the PICP.

Since the development of the radioinamunoassay for PICP is new, definitive statements about its predictive value in osteoporosis must await further studies. It is known that PICP levels correlate with histological indices of bone formation and calcium kinetic studies *(36,42)*. However, the onset of menopause is associated with only a mild increase in serum PICP, and this rise does not predict subsequent bone loss *(43)*. Likewise, Charles et al. could not show differences in PICP levels between osteoporotics and normal controls *(36)*. Hence, in 1996, PICP does not appear to have an advantage over other bone formation markers and may, in fact, be less sensitive. Further longitudinal studies will be required to assess the value of this biochemical marker in osteoporosis.

3. CONCLUSIONS

Biochemical markers of bone turnover cannot make the diagnosis of osteoporosis. However, development of more sensitive and specific tests that reflect bone remodeling have proven useful in predicting an individual's rate of bone loss and response to therapeutic interventions. At the present time, there remain several variables that limit universal application of these markers to clinical practice. These include:

1. Cost: Most of the newer assays are around $100/sample, although urinary N-telopeptide at one reference laboratory is approx $50. In the managed care environment of the mid- and late 1990s, it is unlikely that these tests will find widespread use, unless they can be used to predict fractures or the risk of osteoporosis. Since a similar amount of money can buy a patient a single-site bone density measurement, which can accurately predict fracture risk, it seems certain that biochemical markers will not replace bone densitometry. Furthermore, a combination of assays may improve sensitivity and specificity, but would increase costs. Paradigms that predict future loss or fracture rate need to be developed, since these tests are being considered for reimbursement by most third-party payers.
2. The clinical significance of biochemical markers: Until greater information is available about the reliability of these markers in clinical practice, many practitioners may not understand the strengths and limitations inherent in these studies. Paradoxically, endocrinologists and rheumatologists have used some of these markers for years. However, little data exist about their practical utility or cost-effectiveness. Certainly, greater educational efforts will be needed for all providers before these tests are widely used. Until then, it remains to be seen whether these biochemical markers will be employed routinely for management decisions in osteoporotic patients.
3. Intrinsic variability of the tests: For physicians who manage osteoporotic patients, bone densitometry is valued as a highly precise clinical tool (precision errors of 0.5–4.0%) However, in the vast armamentarium of clinical medicine, no laboratory test can approach

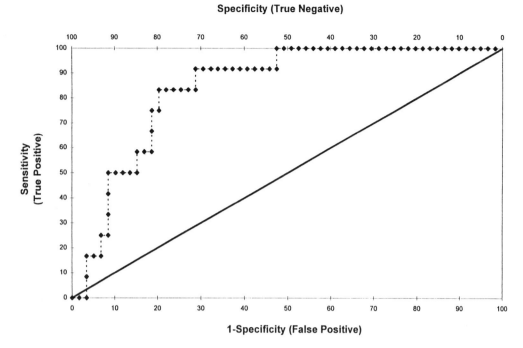

Fig. 5. A ROC analysis was used to determine the sensitivity and specificity of percent change in N-telopeptide excretion 3 mo after hormone replacement therapy for change in BMD of the spine at 1 yr. The change in bone resorption at 3 mo determines the probability of change in spine BMD from baseline to 1 yr with a 84% sensitivity and 80% specificity. Reprinted from ref. *44* with permission.

that level of precision. Indeed, most biochemical markers of bone turnover have relatively reasonable precision errors (10–40%), but pale in comparison to densitometry. Hence, expectations about these studies must be tempered by the realization that they represent a single blood or urine test in a complex individual. Furthermore, biochemical markers have inherent variability because they reflect bone remodeling, a process that is very sensitive to seasonal change, circadian rhythms, ethnicity, menstrual cycles, and dietary changes. Therefore, prediction of bone mass by biochemical markers awaits further studies.

Having stated those concerns, however, it seems likely that biochemical markers of bone resorption and formation can play an important role in the day-to-day management of patients with osteoporosis. For example, in the hypothetical patient presented earlier who had a spine bone density –0.5 SD below the mean and was worried about hormone replacement, a biochemical marker, such as urinary N-telopeptide, might provide the clinician with enough information to urge therapeutic intervention. Moreover, if 10–15% of postmenopausal women are nonresponders to HRT, then an N-telopeptide measurement could demonstrate this relatively quickly, rather than waiting for an annual bone density measurement. In that same vein, a recent multicenter study suggests that the N-telopeptide response to estrogen therapy in postmenopausal women could provide the clinician with a firm prediction of future BMD changes in that patient *(44)*. In that trial of 248 postmenopausal women, the percent change in N-telopeptide excretion after 3 mo of HRT was a very strong predictor of 1-yr spine BMD *(44)*. Receiver–operator characteristic analysis (ROC) for that trial is shown in Fig. 5. These data further support the notion that a >30% decrease in N-telopeptide excretion three mo after initiation of HRT is 91–95% sensitive of a maintenance or gain in spine BMD.

In summary, there is a role for biochemical markers of bone turnover in the patient with osteoporosis. Like everything in clinical medicine, the practitioner must understand the strengths and limitations of these assays prior to their utilization in order to derive the greatest benefit for his/her patient.

REFERENCES

1. Civitelli R, Gonelli S, Sacchei F. Bone turnover in postmenopausal osteoporosis. Effect of calcitonin treatment. *J. Clin Invest* 1988; 82: 1268–1274.
2. Herring GM. The organic matrix of bone. In: Bourne GH, ed. *The Biochemistry and Physiology of Bone*, vol. I. New York: Academic, 1972, pp. 127–189.
3. Eriksen EF, Brixen K, Peder C. New markers of bone metabolism: clinical use in metabolic bone disease. *Eur J Endocrinol* 1995; 132: 251–263.
4. Eyre D. New Biomarkers of bone resorption. *J Clin Endocrinol Metab* 1992; 74: 470.
5. Bienkowski RS, Cowan MJ, McDonald JA, Crystal RC. Degradation of newly synthesized collagen. *J Biol Chem* 1978; 253: 4356–4363.
6. Schlemmer A, Hassager C, Jensen SB, Christiansen C. Marked diurnal variation in urinary excretion of pyridinium cross-links in premenopausal women. *J Clin Endocrinol Metab* 1992; 74: 476–480.
7. Poser JW, Esch PS, Ling NC, Price PA. Isolation and sequence of the vitamin K dependent protein from human bone. *J Biol Chem* 1980; 225: 5685–5691.
8. Lian JB. Osteocalcin: biochemical considerations and clinical applications. *Clin Orthop* 1988; 226: 267–283.
9. Hamilton BA, Mcphee JI, Hawrylak K, Stinson RA. Alkaline phosphatase releasing activity in human tissues. *Clin Chim Acta* 1990; 186: 249–254.
10. Albright F. Postmenopausal osteoporosis. *JAMA* 1941; 116: 2465–2474.
11. Kivirikko K, Laitinen O, Prockop DJ. Modifications of a specific assay for hydroxyproline in urine. *Anal Biochem* 1967; 19: 249–255.
12. Bienkowski RS, Cowan MJ, McDonadd JA, Crystal RG. Degradation of newly synthesized collagen. *J Biol Chem* 1978; 253: 4356–4363.
13. Delmas PD. Biochemical markers of bone turnover for the clinical assessment of metabolic bone disease. *Endocrinol Metab Clin North Am* 1990; 19: 1–18.
14. Delmas PD, Schlemmer A, Gineyts E, Riis B. Christiansen C. Urinary excretion of pyridinoline cross-links correlates with bone turnover measured on iliac crest biopsy in patients with vertebral osteoporosis. *J Bone Miner Res* 1991; 6: 639–644.
15. Harvey RD, McHardy KC, Reid IW. Measurement of bone collagen degradation in hyperthyroidism and during thyroxine replacement therapy using pyridinium cross-links as specific urinary markers. *J Clin Endocrinol Metab* 1991; 72: 1189–1194.
16. Uebelhart D, Gineyts E, Chapuy MC, Delmas PD. Urinary excretion of pyridinium cross links: a new marker of bone resorption in metabolic bone disease. *Bone Miner* 1990; 8: 87–90.
17. Seibel MJ, Gartenberg F, Silverberu SJ, Ratcliffe A, Robins SP, Bilezikian JP. Urinary hydroxypyridinium cross links of collagen in primary hyperparathyroidism. *J Clin Endocrinol Metab* 1992; 74: 481–486.
18. Eyre DR, Koob TJ, Van Neww KPI. Quantitation of hydroxypyridinium cross-links in collagen by high performance liquid chromatography. *Anal Biochem* 1984; 137: 380–388.
19. Gertz BJ, Shao P, Hanson DA, Quan H, Harris ST, Genant HK, Chestnut SH, Eyre DR. Monitoring bone resorption in early postmenopausal women by an immunoassay for cross-linked collagen peptides in urine. *J Bone Miner Res* 1994; 9: 135–140.
20. Seyedin SM, Kung VT, Daniloff YN. Immunoassay for urinary pyridinoline: the new marker of bone resorption. *J Bone Miner Res* 8: 635–641.
21. Risteli J, Elomaa I, Niemi S, Novamo A, Risteli L. Radioimnlunoassay for the pyridinoline cross-linked carboxy-terminal telopeptide of type I collagen: a new marker of bone degradation. *Clin Chem* 1993; 39: 635–640.
22. Garnero P, Shih WJ, Gineyts E, Karpf DB, Delmas PD. Comparison of new biochemical markers of bone turnover in late postmenopausal osteoporotic women in response to alendronate treatment. *J Clin Endocrinol Metab* 1994;79: 1693–1670.

23. Prestwood KM, Pilbeam CC, Burleson JA, Woodiel FN, Delmas PD, Deftos LJ, Raisz LG. The short term effects of conjugated estrogen on bone turnover in older women. *J Clin Endocrinol Metab* 1994;79:366–371.

24. Hui SL, Slemenda CW, Johnston CC. The contribution of bone loss to postmenopausal osteoporosis. *Osteoporosis Int* 1990; 1: 30–34.

25. Stein GS, Lian JB. Molecular mechanisms mediating proliferation/differentiation interrelationships during progressive development of the osteoblast phenotype. *Endocrine Rev* 1993; 14: 424–444.

26. Farley JR, Chestnut CH, Baylink DJ. Improved method for quantitative determination in serum of alkaline phosphatase of skeletal origin. *Clin Chem* 1981; 27: 2002–2007.

27. Stepan J, Pacovsky V, Horn V, Sillinkova-Makova B. Relationship of the activity of the bone isoenzyme of serum alkaline phosphatase to urinary hydroxyproline excretion in metabolic and neoplastic bone diseases. Eur *J. Clin Invest* 1978; 8: 373–378.

28. Pouilles JM, Tremollieres F, Causse E, Louvet JP, Ribot C. Fluoride therapy in postmenopausal osteopenic women: effect on vertebral and femoral bone density and prediction of bone response. *Osteoporosis Int* 1991; 1: 103–109.

29. Hodsman AB, Fraher LJ, Ostbye T, Adachi J. Steer BM. An evaluation of several biochemical markers for bone formation and resorption in a protocol utilizing cyclical PTH and calcitonin therapy for osteoporosis. *J. Clin Invest* 1993; 91; 1138–1148.

30. Thompson J, Holloway L, Hoffman AR, Butterfield GE. Effects of rhGH and IGF-I on bone turnover in elderly women. *J Bone Miner Res* 1994; 9: S328.

31. Lian JB. Bone and serum concentrations of osteocalcin as a function of 1,25 dihydroxyvitamin D circulating levels in bone disorders in rats. *Endocrinology* 1987; 120: 2123–2126.

32. Tracy RP, Andrianorivio A, Riggs BL, Mann KG. Comparison of monoclonal and polyclonal antibody based immunoassays for osteocalcin. A study of sources of variation in assay results. *J Bone Miner Res* 1990; 5: 451–461.

33. Delmas PD, Malaval L, Arlot M, Meunier PJ. Serum bone gla-protein compared to histomorphometry in endocrine diseases. *Bone* 1985; 6: 329–341.

34. Delmas PD, Wahner HW, Mann KG, Riggs BL. Assessment of bone turnover in postmenopausal osteoporosis by measurement of bone gla protein. *J Lab Clin Med* 1983; 102: 470–476.

35. Brown JP, Malaval L, Chapuy MC, Delmas PD, Edouard C, Maunier PJ. Serum bone Gla protein: a specific marker for bone formation in postmenopausal osteoporosis. *Lancet* 1984; I: 1091–1093.

36. Charles P, Hasling C, Ristell L, Ristell J, Mosekilde L, Eriksen EF. Assessment of bone formation by biochemical markers in metabolic bone disease. *Calcif Tissue Int* 1992; 51: 406–411.

37. Szulc P, Chapuy MC, Meunier PJ, Delmas PD. Noncarboxylated serum osteocalcin is a predictor of the risk of hip fracture in elderly women. *Bone Miner* 1992; 17: S80, abstract #40.

38. Plantalech L, Guillaumont M, Vergnaud P, Leclercq M, Delmas PD. Impairment of gamma carboxylation of circulating osteocalcin in elderly women. *J Bone Miner Res* 1991; 6: 1211–1216.

39. Eastell R, Delmas PD, Hodgson SF, Ericksen EF, Mann KG, Riggs BL. Bone formation rate in older normal women: concurrent assessment with bone histomorphometry, calcium kinetics and biochemical markers. *J Clin Endocrinol Metab* 1988; 67: 741–748.

40. Hassager C, Risteli J, Risteli L, Jensen SB, Christiansen C. Diurnal variation in serum markers of type I collagen synthesis and degradation in healthy postmenopausal women. *J Bone Miner Res* 1992; 7: 1307–1311.

41. Melkko J, Niemi S, Risteli L, Risteli J. RIA of the carboxyterminal propeptide of the human type I procollagen. *Clin Chem* 1990; 36: 1328–1332.

42. Parfitt AM, Simon LS, Villantleva AR. Procollagen type I carboxyterminal extension peptide in serum as a marker of collagen biosynthesis in bone. Correlation with iliac bone formation rates and comparison with total alkaline phosphatase. *J Bone Miner Res* 1987; 2: 427–436.

43. Hassager C, Fabbri-Mabelli G, Christiansen C. The effect of the menopause and hormone replacement therapy on serum carboxyterminal propeptide of type I collagen. *Osteoporosis Int* 1993; 3: 50–52.

44. Campodavre L, Ulrich U, Bell N, Clark G, Drinkwater B, English S, Johnston CC, Notelovitz M, Rosen C, Mallinak N, Cain D, Fressland K, Chestnut C. Urinary N-telopeptide of type I collagen monitors bone resorption and may predict change in bone mass of the spine in response to HRT. *J Bone Miner Res* 1995; 10: S182.

IV THE TREATMENT OF OSTEOPOROSIS

12

An Introduction to Clinical Decision Making in Osteoporosis

Gordon H. Guyatt, MD, MSc, FRCPC

CONTENTS

The decision to offer patients a particular treatment is rarely straightforward. In the area of osteoporosis, the choices are particularly complex. In clinical trials of osteoporosis, the outcomes that are easy to measure are of questionable importance, and the important outcomes occur infrequently and often far in the future. In the prevention of osteoporosis, the patient faces years of changes in lifestyle and possible side effects of medication, for a distant and uncertain outcome. In this chapter, I will outline the issues we should consider when offering a treatment recommendation. The discussion follows closely an approach my colleagues and I have offered in another publication *(1)*.

1. DESCRIBING THE IMPACT OF A TREATMENT

One reason clinicians give medication is to prevent a specific adverse outcome, such as a hip fracture. The extent to which a treatment reduces the likelihood of such an adverse outcome can be presented in different ways. These include the relative risk, which is the ratio of the risk of the adverse events in treated patients to the risk of adverse events in the untreated patients; the relative risk reduction or (1 − relative risk) *(2)*; the absolute risk reduction, which is the difference in the absolute risk of the adverse outcome between treatment and control groups; and the number needed to treat, which is the inverse of the absolute risk reduction. The size of the treatment effect will play an important part in the decision to administer or withhold therapy.

From: *Osteoporosis: Diagnostic and Therapeutic Principles*
Edited by: C. J. Rosen   Humana Press Inc., Totowa, NJ

2. COLLECTING THE EVIDENCE

Traditionally, investigators presenting literature reviews have failed to specify how they selected their evidence, to appraise systematically the methodological quality of the evidence, or to present a quantitative summary of their results. This traditional approach contrasts with systematic overviews of the evidence. By "systematic," I mean overviews that meet the following five standards: the overview addresses a focused clinical question, uses appropriate criteria to select studies for inclusion, conducts a comprehensive search; appraises the validity of the individual studies, and applies appropriate statistical methods to summarizing the data *(3)*. Ideally, treatment recommendations should be made on the basis of systematic overviews. Treatment recommendations that are based on a literature review that meets these five criteria are stronger than those that do not.

3. STRENGTH OF EVIDENCE

Because randomized trials provide unique protection against bias, they yield stronger evidence about intervention efficacy than other study designs. Overviews of randomized trials, therefore, provide far stronger evidence about efficacy than do overviews of cohort and case-control studies (Table 1). The strength of evidence from an otherwise systematic overview of randomized trials will, however, depend on the consistency of the results from study to study. When different studies in the same overview yield very different estimates of intervention efficacy (a situation we refer to as "heterogeneity" of study results), one must question why. Possibilities include differences in the patients, the way the interventions were administered, the way the outcomes were measured, or the way the studies were conducted. An alternative to each of these explanations is that the simple "play of chance" is responsible for heterogeneity in study results. If investigators cannot explain large variation in study results, any inferences we make about treatment effect will be weaker. We therefore rank the strength of evidence from overviews of randomized trials according to the presence or absence of unexplained differences in results from study to study (Table 1), and overviews with significant and important heterogeneity (Level B) are ranked lower than those without significant and important heterogeneity (Level A).

Because the potential for bias is much greater in cohort and case-control studies than in randomized trials, recommendations from overviews combining studies with these latter designs will be much weaker (Table 1). Frequently, randomized trials yield smaller estimates of efficacy than do observational studies of the same treatments *(4,5)*. Thus, we classify observational studies as providing weaker evidence than randomized trials (Table 1).

4. CHOICE OF THE RIGHT OUTCOME

If we told a patient that a medication would increase her bone density but would do nothing else (not prevent fractures or reduce pain), she would be very unlikely to take the treatment, and she would be right. Although there is appreciable evidence of a moderate relationship between bone density and fracture, it does not follow that increasing bone density will reduce fracture rate or that the magnitude of any reduction in fracture rate that does occur will be clinically important. We are in the same situation with bone density and fractures as we were with hypertension and stroke or coronary artery

Table 1
Proposed Levels of Evidence for Treatment Recommendations in Osteoporosis

Strength of the study design
    Level A: RCTs, no clinically important or statistically significant heterogeneity
    Level B: RCTs, significant heterogeneity
    Level C: Observational studies
Strength of the outcome
    Level A: Important to patients (pain, functional limitation, fracture of long bones)
    Level B: Of questionable importance to patients (vertebral fractures)
    Level C: Important to patients only through relation to other variables (bone density)
Precision of the outcome
    Level A: Entire confidence interval below threshold number needed to treat
    Level B: Confidence interval overlaps threshold number needed to treat

disease 30 yr ago, or that we continue to be in with cholesterol and coronary disease. Thirty years ago, we knew of the strong association between hypertension and stroke, but we did not know whether reducing blood pressure would reduce the stroke rate. Establishing that effect required randomized trials focusing on stroke itself.

Even if we had randomized trials demonstrating that an intervention reduces vertebral fractures, this may not be important to patients. Only if this reduction in fractures is associated with decreased pain and deformity are patients likely to consider the intervention important for them. Treatment recommendations based on substitute end points are weaker than recommendations based on outcomes that are indisputably important to patients.

5. DECIDING WHAT CONSTITUTES AN IMPORTANT DIFFERENCE

Any decision about initiating a preventive or therapeutic regimen represents a trade-off between patient or public benefits, on the one hand, and toxicity, cost, and administrative burden to patients and providers, on the other. Clinicians do not, therefore, administer all efficacious treatments (efficacious in that they have a positive effect on some important outcome) to all potentially eligible patients.

For administration of preventative or treatment interventions for patients with osteoporosis, it is useful to think of a threshold effect, above which one would treat and below which one would not treat. One way of thinking about this threshold is in terms of the number of patients one would need to treat to prevent a single adverse outcome *(6,7)*. For instance, a 50-yr-old woman has a 15% lifetime risk of fracturing her hip, and the median age of the fracture is 79 *(8)*. Observational studies suggest that long-term estrogen therapy will reduce this risk by 25%. Thus, our best estimate is that 15 of 100 untreated women will have a hip fracture, whereas approx 11 treated women will have a hip fracture, a difference of 4 in 100. We must therefore treat 25 women for 30 yr to prevent a single fracture.

In considering whether it is worthwhile to treat 25 women for 30 yr with hormones to prevent one fracture, we identify two sorts of undesirable events. One is the clinical event that treatment is preventing (which we will call the target event, in this case, a hip fracture), and the other is the adverse effects attributable to treatment. These adverse effects include symptoms and associated impairment of quality of life, the side effects, the inconvenience, and the cost. Whether it is worth treating will depend on the relative values we place on preventing the target event and incurring the adverse effects of treatment. Treatment recommendations will be strengthened if they include each of the following steps:

1. Estimating the risk of adverse outcomes, which patients can expect if they are not treated;
2. The extent to which the risk can be reduced by the treatment (from which follows the number needed to treat);
3. All the adverse effects that follow from treatment, including inconvenience and cost; and
4. The values placed on avoiding the target event or avoiding the adverse effects.

6. THE THRESHOLD NUMBER NEEDED TO TREAT, AND THE PRECISION OF THE ESTIMATE OF THE TREATMENT EFFECT

Consideration of the adverse effects of therapy implies that there is a threshold number needed to treat above which it is no longer worthwhile treating. Most people would agree, for instance, that if we had to treat 1000 women for 30 yr with hormone replacement therapy to prevent a single fracture, it would not be worth it. A recommendation to treat will be strong if we are confident that the number needed to treat falls below the threshold value above which treatment is no longer worthwhile. Deciding on a threshold number needed to treat for use of hormone replacement therapy is challenging, for we would have to take into account possible effects on coronary artery disease and uterine cancer, side effects of the medication, and issues of convenience and acceptability.

Our confidence in the number needed to treat falling below the threshold value above which we would no longer treat will depend, in part:, on the precision of the estimate of treatment effect. We represent this precision by the confidence interval, the range within which the true treatment effect is likely to lie. Let us assume we decide that our threshold number needed to treat for hip fractures is 30: we are willing to administer 30 yr of estrogen therapy to no more than 30 women to prevent a single hip fracture—if more than 30 must be treated, we would withhold therapy. Although the point estimate of the relative risk reduction with hormone replacement therapy is 0.25, the 95% confidence interval ranges from 0.32 to 0.16 *(8)*. Given the risk of fracture without treatment of 15%, our best estimate of number needed to treat, 25 patients, suggests we should treat. However, if the true risk reduction is only 0.16, we would need to treat approx 40 women to prevent a hip fracture and would therefore recommend that treatment not be offered.

A recommendation to treat gains strength when the precision of the estimate of the treatment effect is such that the highest plausible number needed to treat is still lower than the threshold above which we would not treat. If the range of plausible number needed to treats exceeds this threshold, treatment recommendations lose strength (Table 1).

7. CONCLUSION

Considering each of the issues I have raised requires a great deal from those making recommendations. Ideally, the investigator will either find or conduct a rigorous overview of the literature, identify all the relevant benefits and adverse effects of the therapy, determine whether treatment is worthwhile by explicitly valuing the benefits and adverse effects, and decide whether the recommendation to treat or not to treat is robust. This last decision involves considering the study design of the investigations, the extent to which they considered outcomes of importance to patients, and the precision of our estimates of the treatment effect. Currently, very few recommendations about treatment meet all these criteria.

Although those recommending treatment policies may despair when they view the criteria I have proposed, they (and their readers!) must at least consider these issues. If a recommendation to treat is based on an unsystematic sampling of the literature, if it is based on observational studies, if the outcome prevented is a substitute end point, if all the adverse outcomes have not been considered and valued, and if the estimate of the treatment effect is imprecise, the reader is entitled to considerable scepticism about the recommendation. Thus, authors will assist their readers if, in considering the issues I have raised, they explicitly label the strength of the recommendations they put forth.

REFERENCES

1. Guyatt GH, Sackett DL, Sinclair J. Hayward RS, Cook DJ, Cook TW. A method for grading health care recommendations. *JAMA* 1995; 274: 1800–1804.
2. Sinclair JC, Bracken MB. Clinically useful measures of effect in binary analyses of randomized trials. *J Clin Epidemiol* 1994; 47: 881–889.
3. Oxman AD, Cook DJ, Guyatt GH for the Evidence-Based Medicine Working Group. Users' guides to the medical literature VI. How to use an overview. *JAMA* 1994; 272: 1367–1371.
4. Sacks HS, Chalmers TC, Smith H Jr. Sensitivity and specificity of clinical trials. Randomized versus historical assignment in controlled clinical trials. *Arch Intern Med* 1983; 143: 753–755.
5. Chalmers TC, Celano P, Sacks HS, Smith H Jr. Bias in treatment assignment in controlled clinical trials. *N Engl J Med* 1983; 309: 1358–1361.
6. Laupacis A, Sackett DL, Roberts RS. An assessment of clinically useful measures of the consequences of treatment. *N Engl J Med* 1988; 318: 1728–1733.
7. Guyatt GH, Sackett DL, Cook DJ and the Evidence-based Medicine Working Group. A users' guide to the medical literature. How to use an article about therapy or prevention. Part B. What are the results and will they help me in caring for my patients. *JAMA* 1994; 271: 59–63.
8. Grady D, Rubin SM, Petitti DB, et al. Hormone therapy to prevent disease and prolong life in postmenopausal women. *Ann Intern Med* 1992; 117: 1016–1037.

13

Calcium as a Primary Treatment and Prevention Modality for Osteoporosis

Robert Marcus, MD

CONTENTS

I. INTRODUCTION

The skeleton contains 99.5% of body calcium and provides a mineral reservoir to support plasma calcium concentrations at times of need. Since the intestine is the only site for calcium to enter the body, it seems obvious that dietary calcium intake should be a major determinant of skeletal acquisition and maintenance. However, the truth of this statement has been difficult to establish. Seemingly contradictory interpretations of the literature receive widespread publicity in the scientific and lay media regarding the proper role of dietary calcium, resulting in a substantial residue of misunderstanding and skepticism among physicians and other health professionals, as well as the community at large. In this chapter, I propose to clarify what is currently understood with respect to this issue. If successful, I hope to convince the reader that the importance of dietary calcium is linked to specific phases in the life cycle and that proper attention to calcium intake at specific times of life is, in fact, an effective strategy to improve bone health. This chapter will not deal with nutritional aspects of normal and low birthweight infancy because of the highly specialized nature of that topic.

Epidemiological data are mixed concerning relationships between calcium intake and either bone density or fracture incidence. The major constraint on such data is that it is

From: *Osteoporosis: Diagnostic and Therapeutic Principles*
Edited by: C. J. Rosen Humana Press Inc., Totowa, NJ

remarkably difficult to determine with accuracy exactly how much calcium a person habitually consumes. The tools used to assess nutrient intake, food frequency and dietary recall questionnaires, diet diaries, and the like are notoriously inaccurate. Correlations among them, even including test–retest comparisons of the same instrument, are fairly weak, requiring that surveys include hundreds or even thousands of individuals to demonstrate statistically meaningful relationships. Many published surveys do not even approach having adequate statistical power for this purpose. This is particularly the case when attempting to determine the relationship between calcium intake and bone acquisition during growth and development, a time when genetically determined factors already account for about 80% of the population variance in bone mass, leaving only a small component that could possibly be influenced by diet. Moreover, the nutrient composition tables on which these analyses rely are also frequently inaccurate. Substantial variation in calcium content of foodstuffs occurs in different geographical regions owing largely to differences in water hardness, and the published nutrient data bases may be in error by several hundred percent for given foods. Finally, absorption and utilization of calcium do not simply reflect crude mineral intake, but vary highly, depending on such factors as intrinsic absorption efficiency, vitamin D status, renal function, and other dietary constituents that may affect absorption and/or excretion, including protein, fiber, and sodium. None of these issues has been adequately addressed or controlled for in epidemiological studies.

On the other hand, it has been much easier to demonstrate prospectively that calcium supplementation protects bone mass. Most, if not all, randomized controlled trials, even of relatively small size, have been able to show differences in bone gain or loss over time between calcium- and placebo-treated subjects.

2. CALCIUM NUTRITURE
DURING ACQUISITION OF PEAK BONE MASS

Following the rapid accumulation of body mass during the years of infancy, there is a relatively gradual and linear acquisition of bone throughout the prepubertal years. With the onset of adolescent growth begins an acceleration in bone acquisition, so that about 60% of final adult bone mass is acquired by girls across the age span ~12–16 yr (with a 2-yr delay and prolongation in boys). In any individual case, the period of greatest acquisition is restricted to a 2–3 yr interval corresponding to the time of greatest growth velocity. During puberty itself, dramatic changes in reproductive hormone status, particularly estrogen, are the primary driving force for bone acquisition, both for boys and girls. At that time, an independent effect of dietary calcium is difficult to prove. However, an important study by Johnston et al. (1) clearly demonstrated an effect of calcium supplementation in children who had not yet entered puberty. In that study of twins, one member of each twin pair was given supplemental calcium, whereas the other pair received a placebo. Following 3 yr of intervention, there was a significant advantage in bone mineral density (BMD) acquired by the calcium-supplemented twin. When twins who had entered puberty were analyzed, no effect of calcium could be seen (Fig. 1). This elegant study eliminated many possible confounding factors related to physiologic and environmental variability by using twins, and the data seem compelling. The question that must be posed, however, is whether the bone density advantage in the supplemented children will persist. That is, when these children reach skeletal maturity, will there still

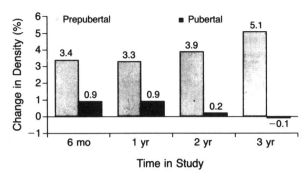

Fig. 1. Mean differences within twin pairs in the change in BMD of the radial midshaft among prepubertal and older children according to time in the study. Differences were significant among prepubertal children at 6 months and thereafter. Reproduced from ref. *1* with permission.

be an advantage to the supplemented group? Another study of calcium supplementation was carried out in late-adolescent women by Lloyd et al. *(2)*. In that 2-yr study, calcium supplementation led to a small, but statistically significant increase in bone mass compared to changes in a placebo group.

Although about 95% of final peak bone mass in women seems to be acquired by age 18, Recker et al. *(3)* have shown continued small increases in BMD until age 28. In that study, two factors emerged as important determinants of bone acquisition during the third decade, habitual physical activity and calcium intake. In fact, for dietary calcium, a progressive increase in bone acquisition was observed without any sign of attenuation even at a remarkably high level of 2000 mg/d (Table 1).

Thus, a reasonably strong case can be made for an important role for dietary calcium in the optimization of peak bone mass. Unfortunately, actual intakes of calcium by women in the US and many other countries are woefully inadequate. Figure 2 shows recent data from the Health and Nutrition Evaluation Survey (NHANES) *(4)*. It can be seen that, beginning at age 11, American girls fail on average to meet recommended intake levels and never improve thereafter. These data reflect the fact that milk and dairy product consumption by female Americans has decreased substantially over the past 40 yr.

3. CALCIUM NUTRITURE DURING YOUNG ADULT LIFE

After peak bone mass is achieved, measurable changes in BMD can be shown only inconsistently until about age 50 in either men or women. Measurements of trabecular bone mass by iliac crest biopsy or by quantitative computed tomography do show a gradual reduction over this age span, but this has generally not been detected by single- or dual-photon projection densitometry. Regardless of when bone loss actually begins, the young adult years are generally a time of robust physiological compensations. It is possible for healthy young adults to subject their bodies to substantial degrees of nutritional abuse without important consequences. The compensatory response to inadequate calcium intake includes hypersecretion of parathyroid hormone (PTH), which is followed by a cascade of PTH-dependent alterations in renal function aimed at conservation of calcium. These include increasing the efficiency of renal tubular calcium reabsorption and activating the 1α-hydroxylase enzyme that converts 25-hydroxyvitamin D (25-OH-D, the major circulating form of vitamin D), to its hormonal form, 1,25-dihydroxyvitamin

Table 1
Estimated Effect of Dietary Calcium on Percentage
of Change in Spinal BMD in the Third Decade[a]

Calcium intake, mg	% BMD change/decade
220	−1.05
700	+3.39
1000	+6.17
1400	+9.87
2106	+16.4

[a]Adapted from ref. (3) with permission.

D (1,25 [OH]$_2$D) (calcitriol). Calcitriol, in turn, promotes intestinal calcium absorption. In addition, PTH signals an increase in bone remodeling activity and delivery of skeletal mineral to the circulation. In young adults, these responses are generally prompt, and calcium balance is relatively quickly restored. At this time of life, it is very difficult to show any effect of calcium intake on rates of change in bone mass (5).

4. THE SIXTH DECADE AND THE EFFECT OF MENOPAUSE

In both men and women, onset of measurable bone loss can be easily and consistently shown after age 50. In men, this likely represents the accumulation over time of small deficits resulting from bone remodeling imbalance throughout adult life. In women, this same effect is magnified by an added component owing specifically to menopausal loss of endogenous estrogen.

In the US, the average age of menopause is ~51 yr. During this period of about 6 yr, the greatest component of bone loss is owing to estrogen loss and not to other factors. Therefore, it should be no surprise that calcium supplementation would be a relatively unimportant intervention for recently menopausal women. Nonetheless, in 1988, enormous confusion over the role of calcium was introduced by a paper published by Riis et al. (6). In that study, a group of Danish women within 2 yr of menopause was randomly assigned to take placebo, calcium, or estrogen for 2 yr. As predicted, the placebo group lost bone. The calcium group also lost bone, but, particularly in the cortical skeleton, this loss was significantly less than was seen for placebo. By contrast, the estrogen group maintained bone mass. The authors concluded that for this group of women, estrogen was a superior intervention to calcium. This study was widely reported in the lay press and has ultimately been seriously misrepresented to assert that calcium supplements are generally of no value.

Interpretation of the Riis study requires an understanding of two issues: who these women were and where they lived. As stated, these subjects were all within 2 yr of their last menstrual period. They were therefore in a time of accelerated bone loss owing to estrogen deficiency. It makes no more sense to use calcium to counteract this particular component of bone loss than it would to treat pernicious anemia with iron. Moreover, it must be mentioned that the dietary calcium of this Danish population averages 1100 mg/d, which is about double that of North American women (4) (Fig. 2). Therefore, it is actually remarkable that the calcium-treated subjects of Riis et al. (6) actually sustained less bone

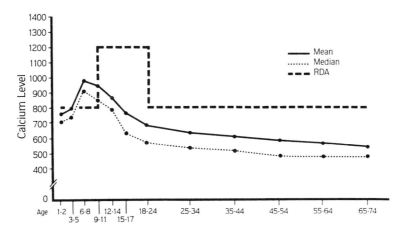

Fig. 2. Daily calcium intake (mg) for females in the US population, 1976–1980. Reproduced from ref. *7* with permission.

loss than the placebo group. The most plausible interpretation of that result is that even in this calcium-replete population, there still exists a subset of individuals with relatively low calcium intake who benefit from supplemental calcium.

5. THE LATER YEARS

After age 60, the compensatory mechanisms that serve young adults so well gradually diminish. The renal response to PTH gradually attenuates, as does the ability of skin to synthesize vitamin D. Intrinsic deficits in intestinal mucosal and renal function accumulate, and bone remodeling itself becomes more inefficient. Thus, it is no longer possible to adapt readily to reduced calcium intakes. Work from the laboratory of Heaney *(8)* and colleagues shows that elderly women who are not receiving replacement estrogen require about 1500 mg/d of calcium simply to achieve neutral calcium balance.

Several important clinical trials now demonstrate skeletal benefit from assuring adequate calcium intake to elderly men and women. In the US, Dawson-Hughes and colleagues *(9)* have shown that women who are beyond the first several years postmenopause achieve significant increases in BMD, particularly if their habitual calcium intake is low. Supportive results have been published in other small series from this country and abroad. Most impressive is an enormous French clinical trial from Chapuy et al. *(10)*. In this study, more than 3000 elderly French women, average age 84, who were living in sheltered residential communities, were assigned randomly to receive placebo or a daily supplement of calcium (1000 mg) plus vitamin D (800 IU). At 18 mo followup, there was a reduction in all nonvertebral fractures and specifically in hip fracture of about 30% in the active treatment group relative to placebo. This reduction was actually evident by 6 mo of study, and has continued unabated over 4 yr of continuous followup. At 4 yr, there was actually a significant reduction in overall mortality of about 15% (Pierre Meunier, personal communication). Thus, a simple and inexpensive supplement of calcium and vitamin D achieved greater antifracture efficacy in a brief time than has been reported for any pharmaceutical intervention yet described for treatment of osteoporosis!

6. CALCIUM AND THE LIFE CYCLE, A SUMMARY

1. During years of peak bone acquisition, calcium intake is limiting, yet underconsumption of this nutrient by women is widespread. In this age group, it is an enormous challenge to promote greater calcium intake. Whether this can be best achieved by nutrition education programs, by calcium fortification of foods that young women will eat, or by recommending the use of calcium supplements remains to be established.
2. Between ages 25 and 50 yr, little evidence supports a critical role for calcium as an influence on skeletal maintenance. Unfortunately, this is the age group at which the great preponderance of calcium advertising revenue is directed.
3. At menopause, the primary deficit is estrogen, and calcium alone simply does not make up for this lack. However, it appears that some component of bone loss at this time may be responsive to calcium intake. Whether very high calcium intakes can make up for estrogen lack has not been adequately studied.
4. Beyond age 65, based on current evidence, a recommendation for men and women to consume at least 1000 mg/d of calcium, either in the diet or with the addition of supplement, seems prudent. Moreover, women who are not taking hormone replacement therapy should have a total calcium intake of at least 1500 mg. This recommendation assumes that the individual does not suffer a condition that would contraindicate it, such as idiopathic hypercalciuria or untreated primary hyperparathyroidism.

7. PROMOTING CALCIUM INTAKE: FOOD VS SUPPLEMENTS

In the western diet, about 75% of calcium is obtained from milk or dairy products. Although it is possible to construct a strictly vegetarian diet that would provide calcium sufficiency, one should realize that it may take several cups of green vegetables to provide as much calcium as is present in a single 8-oz. glass of milk. One quart of milk contains about 1100 mg calcium, regardless of whether it is whole, reduced fat, skim, or chocolate milk. The calcium content of cheese varies widely. Aged natural cheeses, such as cheddar, may contain several hundred milligrams of calcium/100 g of cheese. On the other hand, cottage cheese, which enjoys a fine reputation as a healthy food, contains relatively little calcium, about 90 mg/100 g. This reflects the fact that cottage cheese is actually an acidified hydrolysate of whole milk, and that calcium, being readily soluble in an acid environment, is eluted in the whey.

Calcium absorption from dairy products is not adversely influenced by lactase deficiency. For individuals who become symptomatic with lactose ingestion, lactase tablets can be taken with milk, or lactase-fortified milk can be purchased. In addition, yogurt is a calcium-rich product in which the lactose has been hydrolyzed.

The bioavailability of calcium from dairy products and from most vegetables is comparable, averaging about 25–30%. An exception to this rule is spinach, which, for reasons that are still unclear, is very poorly absorbed (~2%). This is not related to the oxalate content of spinach, since other vegetables that contain similar amounts of oxalate are absorbed with much greater efficiency. Considerable amounts of calcium can also be obtained from soups cooked with bones, but the duration of cooking and the broth pH are important concerns that are difficult to standardize. Small fish served with the bones, such as anchovies and herring, are also fairly rich sources of calcium.

There is no absolutely compelling reason that calcium adequacy cannot be achieved by supplements as opposed to diet. However, there are some concerns that cause me to stress dietary modification as a first goal. Patients with osteoporosis have been shown to have marginal or inadequate intakes of multiple nutrients, not just of calcium. These, of course, are not satisfied by the simple administration of a calcium supplement. Single nutrient supplements can occasionally induce undesirable nutrient–nutrient interactions. For example, some evidence has been presented that supplemental calcium may impair absorption of iron. Finally, even though inducing a long-term dietary modification may be a challenge, there is no reason to believe that long-term compliance with nutrient supplements is any more successful, and I think (although without firm evidence to support my view) that if healthful dietary choices can be instituted by an educated consumer, long-term dietary adherence is likely to be maintained.

That being said, it is clear that many older adults are unwilling or unable to increase their dietary calcium intake to recommended levels, and for such people, use of calcium supplements is perfectly appropriate. Many calcium supplements are currently available at low cost. It is true that various studies show statistically significant advantages of one supplement over another. For example, the Dawson-Hughes studies indicate a better response to calcium-citrate-malate than to calcium carbonate. My own view of this issue is that since we are recommending a supplement for long-term, perhaps lifelong, consumption, the most important factor is that it be palatable and affordable to the individual patient, and that the number of pills to be taken should be minimized. In my personal experience, I have found calcium carbonate to be well suited to most patients. It is well tolerated, it contains 40% calcium by weight, which is more than most other salts, and it is available in tablets that each contain 500 mg or more calcium. Calcium carbonate can be well absorbed even by patients with achlorhydria, as long as it is taken with food. Difficulty in calcium absorption has been described with certain generic calcium carbonate preparations, but several reliably absorbed products are widely available.

Certain preparations offer "chelated" minerals, magnesium, manganese, and/or other micronutrients in addition to calcium. No credible evidence supports a clinical benefit to those preparations, and I see no value in them. In addition, I am singularly unimpressed with the so-called benefits of "natural" calcium hydroxyapatite preparations.

Calcium supplements are generally well tolerated. Some patients become constipated at high doses (~2000 mg/d). Patients frequently ask about the best time to take calcium supplements. My view is that whatever schedule will lead to long-term compliance should be encouraged, although there is a theoretical basis for taking part of the supplement just before bedtime. Dietary calcium has generally been completely assimilated by 6 h after a meal. From that time to the next meal, maintenance of circulating calcium may require hypersecretion of PTH and could lead to increased bone turnover. Nocturnal rises in blood levels of PTH, of urinary calcium excretion, and of biochemical markers of bone turnover have been frequently observed. Suppression of these changes by administering a bedtime oral calcium load seems reasonable. However, not all of the nocturnal surge in bone turnover reflects nutrient availability. Some of this effect could be owing to the nocturnal surge in adrenal steroid production or to several hours of recumbency.

8. IS THERE A NEED FOR SUPPLEMENTAL VITAMIN D?

Classical presentations of vitamin D-deficiency osteomalacia are associated with circulating 25-OH-D concentrations of 8 ng/mL or less. Therefore, published "normal" ranges for this marker of vitamin D nutritional status are frequently given as 10–50 ng/mL. Considerable evidence indicates that this so-called normal range is seriously flawed. In fact, it appears that 25-OH-D concentrations below ~25 ng/mL may be associated with hypersecretion of PTH, increased bone turnover, and increased bone loss in elderly people. I consider it a reasonable goal to maintain the 25-OH-D concentration above 25 ng/mL. In most regions of North America, there is a very high prevalence of vitamin D concentrations below this level among elderly people. This reflects not only the physiological inefficiencies that develop with age, but also the fact that, particularly at latitudes north of Saint Louis, the UV spectral content of sunlight does not stimulate vitamin D synthesis for much of the year. Therefore, in view of these considerations as well as the powerful impact of calcium/vitamin D on fracture incidence shown in the Chapuy study *(8)*, it seems reasonable to recommend modest vitamin D supplementation (400–800 IU/d) as a general prescription for older men and women. Certainly, many robust elderly who live in more temperate areas of the US do maintain vitamin D status without the need for supplements, so this intervention should be individualized. However, at the 800 IU dose level, even fully vitamin D-replete individuals would not be harmed by taking a supplement.

Prescribing 800 U of vitamin D is not as easy as it may sound. Very few single-nutrient preparations of vitamin D are actually marketed at the present time. Many health food stores sell 400 IU vitamin D capsules at a reasonable price. Some calcium supplements contain small amounts of vitamin D (usually ~125 U/tablet). However, marketing emphasis has certainly been placed on the more potent (and more expensive!) forms of the vitamin, 25-OH-D or $1,25(OH)_2D$ (calcitriol). For patients with reasonably normal renal function, I see no advantage to either of these potent agents, and particularly with calcitriol, the substantial risk for hypercalciuria and hypercalcemia complicates care by mandating regular laboratory surveillance.

REFERENCES

1. Johnston CC, Jr., Miller JZ, Slemenda CW, Reister TK, Hui S, Christian JC, Peacock M. Calcium supplementation and increases in bone mineral density in children. *N Engl J Med* 1992; 327: 82–87.
2. Lloyd T, Andon MB, Rollings N, Martel JK, Landis R, Demers LM, Eggli DF, Kieselhorst K, Kulin HE. Calcium supplementation and bone mineral density in adolescent girls. *JAMA* 1993; 270: 841–844.
3. Recker RR, Davies M, Hinders SM, Heaney RP, Stegman MR, Kimmel DB. Bone gain in young adult women. *JAMA* 1992; 268: 2403–2408.
4. Carroll MD, Abraham S, Dresser CM. Dietary Intake Source Data: United States, 1976–1980. Vital and Health Statistics. Series II, No. 231, DHHS Publ No. (PHS) 83–1681. National Center for Health Statistics. Public Health Service, Washington DC: US Government Printing Office, March 1983.
5. Riggs BL, Wahner HW, Melton LJ III, Richelson LS, Judd HL, O'Fallon M. Dietary calcium intake and rates of bone loss in women. *J Clin Invest* 1987; 80: 979–982.
6. Riis B, Thomsen K, Christiansen C. Does calcium supplementation prevent postmenopausal bone loss? A double-blind, controlled clinical study. *N Engl J Med* 1987; 316: 173–177.
7. National Dairy Council, *Dairy Council Digest* 1984; 55(1).
8. Heaney RP, Recker RR, Saville PD. Calcium balance and calcium requirements in middle-aged women. *Am J Clin Nutr* 1977; 30: 1603–1611.
9. Dawson-Hughes B, Dallal GE, Krall EA, Sadowksi L, Sahyoun N, Tannenbaum S. A controlled trial of the effect of calcium supplementation on bone density in postmenopausal women. *N Engl J Med* 1990; 323: 878–883.
10. Chapuy MC, Arlot ME, Duboeuf F, Brun J, Crouzet B, Arnaud S, Delmas PD, Meunier PJ. Vitamin D_3 and calcium to prevent hip fractures in elderly women. *N Engl J Med* 1992; 327: 1637–1642.

14

Use of Estrogen for Prevention and Treatment of Osteoporosis

Robert Marcus, MD

CONTENTS

INTRODUCTION
MENOPAUSAL CHANGES IN SKELETAL HOMEOSTASIS
SKELETAL EFFECTS OF ESTROGEN REPLACEMENT THERAPY
EFFECTS OF ESTROGEN ON FRACTURE
PRACTICAL ASPECTS OF ESTROGEN REPLACEMENT
HELPING THE PATIENT DECIDE WHETHER TO TAKE ESTROGEN
CONCLUSIONS, CONCERNS, AND FUTURE DIRECTIONS
REFERENCES

I. INTRODUCTION

Two decades of experience leave no doubt that sustained administration of estrogen to menopausal women conserves bone throughout the skeleton. Such conservation should theoretically protect against osteoporotic fracture, and, indeed, epidemiological studies support the view that long-term estrogen replacement does afford women such protection. On the other hand, uncertainty remains about many aspects of this issue. Questions persist regarding the therapeutic schedule itself: the type, dose, and mode of administration of estrogen that is optimal. Other questions concern the individuals who will receive estrogen: the age at which treatment begins, its duration, and the consequence of adding progestins to the treatment regimen. The level of uncertainty for these questions grows considerably when the end point is fracture protection rather than bone mass. In this chapter, I discuss the therapeutic use of estrogen to prevent or treat osteoporosis.

2. MENOPAUSAL CHANGES IN SKELETAL HOMEOSTASIS

2.1. Calcium Economy

Women entering menopause experience a daily calcium loss of about 60 mg, compared to premenopausal values of 20 mg (1). This change reflects an increase in bone-resorbing over forming activity brought about mainly by an increased activation of new bone remodeling units. It is attended by measurable changes in whole-body calcium

From: *Osteoporosis: Diagnostic and Therapeutic Principles*
Edited by: C. J. Rosen Humana Press Inc., Totowa, NJ

economy: decreased intestinal absorption efficiency and increased urinary excretion, which may be the result of suppressed parathyroid hormone (PTH) secretion. The magnitude of this change in calcium balance may appear trivial, but after a decade, it would account for about 13% of an original whole body calcium mass of 1000 g, equivalent to a standard deviation in bone mineral density (BMD), and would lead to a two to threefold increase in the risk for fracture (2–4). In contrast, women who received estrogen replacement as they entered menopause show calcium balance and rates of mineral turnover that were the same as those of premenopausal women (5). To accommodate the menopausal changes in calcium economy by dietary means alone, a rise in daily calcium intake from 1000 to about 1500 mg was necessary.

The following sequence of events offers a plausible model for these menopausal changes:

1. A reduction in circulating estrogen increases bone remodeling by promoting secretion by osteoblasts of skeletally active cytokines that, in turn, recruit osteoclast precursors;
2. Increased osteoclastic bone resorption increases plasma ionized calcium activity, consequently increasing the load of calcium filtered by the kidney and suppressing PTH secretion;
3. Reduced PTH concentrations decrease renal synthesis of $1,25(OH)_2D$, thereby decreasing the efficiency of intestinal calcium absorption. When estrogen is replenished, bone remodeling is suppressed, $1,25(OH)_2D$ levels rise (6,7), intestinal calcium absorption improves (6), and calcium balance is restored (1).

2.2. Bone Mass

After peak bone mass is achieved by about age 30 yr (8), it remains relatively stable until about age 50. This statement may not apply to all skeletal sites; for example, earlier bone loss from the hip may occur (9), and the notion that conservation of bone mass is absolute prior to menopause or (in men) age 50 remains a function of the sites measured, as well as being an artifact of the detection system.

The weight of evidence supports the concept that bone loss accelerates at menopause, and it appears that this acceleration begins when FSH levels increase in association with a reduction in circulating estradiol. Menopausal acceleration of bone loss affects the entire skeleton, but is particularly marked in trabecular bone, reflecting its higher prevalence of bone surfaces, where turnover occurs. The magnitude of this change represents a two- to threefold increase in turnover rate and results 5 yr later in a typical decrease in BMD of about 15%, or about 1 SD.

Considerable attention has been given to identifying women who are likely to be "fast losers," and therefore most likely to benefit from hormonal intervention. Although predictive formulas based on body fat mass, urinary calcium and hydroxyproline excretion, and serum alkaline phosphatase activity have been proposed (10), it remains uncertain whether a discrete subgroup actually exists or whether rates of bone loss at menopause are normally distributed.

2.3. The Later Menopausal Years

Several years following last menses, bone turnover decreases. Based on cross-sectional studies, it has been commonly stated that the annual decrease in BMD slows and even stabilizes after about age 70 yr. Recent studies indicate a need to revise this view. Biochemical evidence of increased bone turnover in estrogen-deplete women persists well

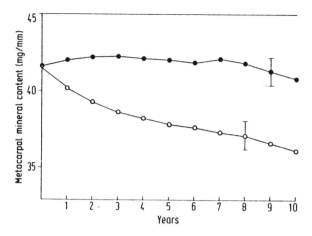

Fig. 1. Effect of estrogen on metacarpal BMC. Filled circles represent estrogen-treated women; open circles represent placebo treatment. Reproduced from ref. *14* with permission.

into the eighth decade *(11,12)*. Body weight has a major influence on postmenopausal bone loss, heavier subjects being relatively protected *(13)*, perhaps related to their higher degree of mechanical loading or to their higher circulating concentrations of estrone.

3. SKELETAL EFFECTS OF ESTROGEN REPLACEMENT THERAPY

3.1. Background

Enthusiastic claims for the skeletal benefits of exogenous estrogen have been made for at least 40 yr. Conjugated estrogens were approved for marketing in the US in 1942 under provisions of the Food, Drug, & Cosmetics Act of 1938. This product was approved initially because it had satisfied a requirement to be shown safe for its intended use in the treatment of menopausal symptoms, vaginitis, and amenorrhea. Following amendments to the Act in 1962, when it became necessary to show efficacy as well as safety, the Food and Drug Administration (FDA) announced a group of estrogen products to have satisfied this additional requirement for their original intentions and to be "probably effective" for selected cases of osteoporosis. In 1986, FDA upgraded the status of estrogen to "effective" for use in postmenopausal osteoporosis. At present, the following preparations and daily doses have received approval for osteoporosis:

1. Conjugated equine estrogens, 0.625 mg (Premarin®);
2. 17β-estradiol transdermal patches, 0.05 mg (Estraderm®)
3. Piperazine estrone sulfate tablets, 0.75 mg (Ogen®, 0.75 mg).

3.2. Effects of Estrogen on Bone

Initiation of estrogen replacement at the time of oophorectomy or within the first few years after natural menopause indisputably conserves bone mass. In 1976, Lindsay et al. *(14)* reported a clinical trial in which oophorectomized women had been randomly assigned to receive mestranol, average dose 24 mcg, or placebo. The placebo group progressively lost metacarpal bone, but bone mineral was maintained in the treatment group, a finding that persisted for 10 yr of followup *(15)* (Fig. 1). Similar results were achieved subsequently with other estrogen preparations, with other measurement tech-

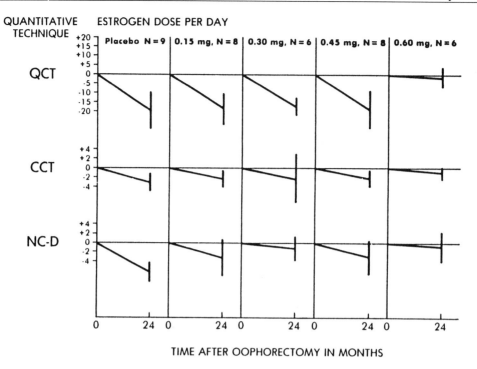

QUANTITATIVE   ESTROGEN DOSE PER DAY
TECHNIQUE

Fig. 2. Effect of estrogen on bone mass of recently oophorectomized women. Women were randomly assigned to placebo or to 1 of 4 doses of conjugated estrogen. Bone was assessed at entry and after 24 mo at multiple sites. QCT, lumbar spine trabecular bone mineral density (BMD) by quantitative computed tomography; CCT, combined cortical thickness from hand radiographs; NC-D, BMD of the mid-radius using single photon absorptiometry (Norland-Cameron densitometry). Reproduced from ref. *16* with permission.

niques, and at multiple skeletal sites *(16–19)*. Genant et al. *(16)* administered estrogen for 2 yr to women who had undergone oophorectomy within 2 mo of enrolling. Results showed a progressive reduction in lumbar spine BMD across a conjugated estrogen dose range of 0.15–0.6 mg/d, with maintenance of baseline BMD at only the 0.6-mg dose level (Fig. 2). In a 2-yr comparison against other agents thought likely to constrain bone loss, Christiansen et al. *(19)* reported that estrogen was significantly more effective than calcium vitamin D and its metabolites, thiazide diuretics, and fluoride.

The curvilinear nature of menopausal bone loss engendered the idea that once the accelerated phase of early menopause subsides, there is little to be gained by starting estrogen. Fairly strong evidence argues against this view. Early studies demonstrating the efficacy of estrogen consisted of mixed groups of patients with established osteoporosis, many in their 60s when hormone therapy was started. Beginning in 1978, a series of papers appeared that established conclusively that estrogen confers skeletal benefits even beyond the initial menopausal years. Recker et al. *(17)* reported the effects of placebo, cyclic conjugated equine estrogens (0.625 mg with 5 mg methyltestosterone), and calcium carbonate (1000 mg/d) in postmenopausal women, age 55–65 yr. Loss of forearm bone mass was observed in the control and calcium groups, but was not significant for the estrogen group.

Lindsay et al. *(20)* treated osteoporotic postmenopausal women who were on average more than 14 yr beyond menopause with conjugated equine estrogens. After 2 yr, vertebral bone mass increased significantly, with an upward trend at the proximal femur, whereas a calcium-treated control group lost bone from both sites. Quigley et al. *(21)* conducted a trial of estrogen in a large group of women whose age at entry was 51–80 yr. When results were stratified by age, significant protection of forearm bone mass was seen in all estrogen groups, without attenuation in the 71–80-yr-old group. Most recently, Holland et al. *(22)* demonstrated the efficacy of percutaneous estradiol implants on bone mass in older women. Thus, skeletal benefit can be achieved even when initiation of estrogen is delayed by more than a decade. There is insufficient specific information regarding fracture outcomes in women who start estrogen at an advanced age.

As opposed to skeletal maintenance that was observed in very early menopausal women, BMD responses of women who are several years beyond last menses generally follow a pattern that is predictable from an understanding of the hormone's role as an antiresorptive agent: a rise in bone mass over 12–18 mo, followed by a plateau. This pattern is most compatible with an estrogen-induced decrease in the "remodeling space," a transient deficit in bone that represents areas where resorption has taken place, but where the formation response has not yet started or remains in progress. The plateau indicates restoration of this remodeling transient to a new steady-state level. In the recently concluded 3-yr multicenter Postmenopausal Estrogen/Progestin Interventions Trial (PEPI) *(23)*, unopposed estrogen increased lumbar spine BMD in a curvilinear pattern, resulting in a 4–5% increase over 3 yr. A similar trajectory was, observed at the proximal femur, although the magnitude of response was only about 2% *(24)*. The reason that most studies of even recently menopausal women show this increased plateau trajectory rather than simple maintenance reflects the fact that, in contrast to Genant et al. *(25)*, who assessed women within 2 mo of oophorectomy, other studies have generally required women to be at least 12 mo away from last menses to validate that they were truly postmenopausal. This delay is more than adequate for bone turnover to increase and for an expansion of the remodeling space to have occurred.

Data from the Study of Osteoporotic Fractures (SOF), a prospective study of incident fractures in 9700 women who were at least 65 yr of age at entry *(3)*, establish that older estrogen-replete women do lose bone, although at a slow rate. The maintenance effect that seemed absolute in younger women is not absolute, probably because estrogen does not completely forestall age-related changes in intestinal, renal, and parathyroid function.

4. EFFECTS OF ESTROGEN ON FRACTURE

Data suggesting that estrogen protects against fragility-related fractures are relatively sparse compared to those showing effects on bone mass. In an early clinical trial, Nachtigall et al. *(25)* showed less vertebral deformity in women assigned to take conjugated equine estrogens than in placebo-treated women. This study was remarkable for two features: it was extremely small in size, and the estrogen dose, 2.5 mg/d of conjugated equine estrogens, was fourfold greater than that typically prescribed for menopausal hormone replacement. That study notwithstanding, most evidence supporting antifracture efficacy of estrogen comes from epidemiologic studies rather than clinical trials. The reason for this, of course, is the nontrivial nature of conducting prospective studies with adequate statistical power. Current industry-sponsored trials aimed at showing antifracture benefit have enrolled several thousand osteoporotic women for at least 3 yr of observation.

Epidemiological studies confirm a lower risk of fracture among women who have taken estrogen *(26–30)* and suggest a magnitude of protection of about 60%. Full realization of this benefit requires sustained hormone administration, probably for 5 yr or more *(27)*. Results from the Framingham study *(29)* indicate that at least 7 yr of estrogen may be needed to achieve protection against fracture, and, in addition, suggest that even this degree of exposure is not adequate to protect bone mass in women beyond 75 yr of age. In contrast, Kanis et al. *(28)* found a 30% reduction in hip fracture risk for estrogen users beyond 80 yr of age. The importance of continuing to take estrogen therapy is seen in the report of Cauley et al. *(30)* from SOF. After adjusting for many potential confounding factors, current estrogen use was associated with a 34% decreased risk for all nonspinal fractures. Current users who initiated estrogen within 5 yr of last menses had a 50% reduction in risk, but those women who had stopped estrogen experienced no fracture protection, even if they had at one time taken estrogen for more than 10 yr.

It is generally assumed that fracture protection directly reflects preservation of bone mass. Although this assumption is certainly compatible with the evidence, additional factors should be considered. In the SOF study *(30)*, estrogen users showed a reduced risk for all nonspinal fractures even after the data were adjusted for bone mass. Subjects in case-control or observational cohort studies did not randomly decide to take estrogen, and pretreatment characteristics of these women might themselves underlie a lower fracture risk. Women choosing to take estrogen may already exhibit higher than average commitment to healthful behaviors, such as patterns of diet, exercise, and use of alcohol or tobacco, that themselves reduce fracture risk. An important contribution to fracture risk, particularly hip fracture, is the tendency to fall. The great majority of hip fractures occur as the immediate consequence of a fall (*see* Chapter 19). The suggestion that long-term estrogen may influence the risk of falls is not unreasonable and requires investigation.

5. PRACTICAL ASPECTS OF ESTROGEN REPLACEMENT

5.1. When to Initiate Estrogen Replacement

Fears that irreversible bone loss might occur if estrogen is withheld until all menstrual periods cease have led some physicians to consider initiation of therapy prior to menopause. Since accelerated bone loss does not occur in perimenopausal women with low circulating FSH values, commencing estrogen in the early perimenopausal years will probably not be beneficial. Insufficient data preclude a definitive judgment about women with increased FSH concentrations who still have menstrual periods. Estrogen products used for menopausal indications do not provide effective contraception. If a physician wishes to prescribe estrogen for a woman who still has menses, oral contraceptive pills may be a superior choice.

5.2. Choice of Drug and Dose Requirement

The epidemiological studies discussed above establish a skeletal protective effect of oral estrogen. In the US, most estrogen-treated women during the past four decades have received a single drug, conjugated equine estrogens (Premarin®) at a single dose, 0.625 mg/d, without the use of progestins. This preparation consists of a mixture of 10 steroidal compounds, the most important of which are estrone and equilin sulfates. The fracture epidemiology thus depends heavily on this particular agent. Until recently, experience with other forms of estrogen has centered in Europe and the UK. Most, if not all, estrogens prescribed for menopausal women provide skeletal benefit. In addition to conjugated estrogens, these include 17β-estradiol, ethinyl estradiol, estrone sulfate, mestranol, and others.

Before discussing what is known about estrogen dosage and skeletal protection, a few general statements must be given that point out inadequacies of knowledge in this field. First, the number of studies that directly assess dosing requirements is very small and generally involve very few patients. For example, in the major study on which FDA approval of estrogen was based, only six women were assigned the 0.6-mg hormone dose at which BMD maintenance was observed *(16)*. Second, studies have generally been conducted to assess the dose of hormone necessary for a treatment group to show BMD conservation relative to a placebo group. They have rarely had adequate power to compare one dose of hormone with another. Further, it is very difficult, indeed, almost impossible, to determine anything beyond group responses. If dosing studies are to be an aid to effective therapy, one must know how many patients can be expected to respond (or not to respond) to any given dose. Finally, with few exceptions, conclusions regarding minimum effective dose reflect the experience at only one skeletal site.

Doses of estrogen sufficient to elevate plasma 17β-estradiol concentrations to about 70 pg/mL suppress bone remodeling and protect bone mass at the spine. In one study *(31)*, >25 μg/d of 17β-estradiol promoted bone gain, whereas <15 μg did not prevent loss. Ettinger et al. *(32)* conducted a dose-response test of micronized 17β-estradiol in women who had been menopausal for up to 5 yr. Women receiving 0.5, 1.0, and 2.0 mg of drug showed annual increases in lumbar spine BMD of 0.3, 1.8, and 2.5%, respectively. In an interesting twist to this study, after one year of followup, women were all placed on open-label 17β-estradiol at 1.0 mg/d and followed for another 18 mo. Those who had previously received placebo increased BMD by 4.3%/yr. Changes in women who had initially received active drug varied inversely according to the initial dose assignment. Women receiving the 2.0-mg dose during the first phase actually **lost** bone when the dose was reduced. Changes in BMD at the radius were in the same direction as those at the spine, but of lesser magnitude.

For conjugated equine estrogens, 0.625 mg/d is sufficient. Very few patients, <5%, so treated show significant bone loss from the spine or hip over 3 yr of followup. Some evidence suggests that spine BMD may be protected by as little as 0.3 mg of conjugated estrogens if patients also receive supplemental calcium *(33)*. However, not all skeletal regions respond with identical sensitivity to estrogen, and the adequacy of the latter approach for conserving hip BMD is not established. Differential sensitivity may also affect the response to different estrogens, particularly those with intrinsically lower potency, such as estrone or estriol. For example, 2-yr treatment with 0.625 mg/d of estrone sulfate conferred protection at the spine, but 1.25 mg was necessary to protect the proximal femur *(34)*.

Some consideration has been given to the possibility that much higher doses of estrogen might afford additional skeletal benefit. The basis for this supposition is evidence from animal studies that high doses of estrogen may have an osteotropic effect beyond the well-established antiresorptive action. Human evidence in favor of such an effect is scanty. Studd and Smith *(35)* carried out dose–response studies using percutaneous estradiol implants at doses ranging from 25 to 100 mg. At the highest doses, circulating estradiol levels around 200 pg/ml were achieved, and increases in BMD at both the spine and hip correlated significantly with dose.

Neither the side effect profile nor the impact of long-term high-dose estrogen on cardiovascular, breast, or other morbidity is known. At present, high-dose estrogen cannot routinely be recommended for patient management.

5.3. Route of Administration

The route of estrogen delivery appears not to be critical for skeletal response, since transdermal 17β-estradiol influences bone turnover and bone mass similarly to oral hormone (36).

Field et al. (37) conducted a 2-yr placebo-controlled trial of 127 women who had undergone oophorectomy from 6 wk to 2 yr before entry. Women in active treatment groups were assigned to either 25, 50, or 100 μg/d 17β-estradiol transdermal patches. By 2 yr, BMD of the lumbar spine decreased 6.4% in the placebo group and 3.0% in the women receiving 25 μg estradiol, but increased by 0.8 and 3.7% in the higher-dose groups. At the midradius, placebo women lost 4.9% and the lowest-dose estradiol group lost 1.8%, but the higher-dose active groups lost 0.8 and 1.1%, respectively. At both sites, changes in BMD for all active groups differed significantly from placebo. This study therefore supports a dose–responsive preservation of bone mass by transdermal estradiol, with a minimum dose for spine BMD conservation at ~50 μg.

In a 2-yr study of early postmenopausal women using 28-d cycles of estradiol cream supplemented by progesterone, Riis et al. (38) showed significant improvement in BMD at the spine, radius, and whole body compared to a placebo group. Although this study was carefully executed and the results convincing, dosing characteristics seem to me less consistent and predictable with creams than with oral or patch estrogen, and are therefore less desirable. Studd et al. (39) conducted a year-long trial of percutaneous estradiol implants in postmenopausal women. Implant doses of 25–75 mg consistently achieved plasma estradiol concentrations >70 pg/mL, and were all associated with significant improvement in BMD at multiple sites.

The favorable and equivalent skeletal response to both oral and other forms of estrogen delivery means for the prescribing physician that choice of estrogen preparation should probably be based on other considerations. In particular elevations in high density lipoprotein (HDL) cholesterol and reductions in low density lipoprotein (LDL) cholesterol have been observed primarily with oral estrogen. For women in whom achieving such changes is an important consideration (i.e., in women with higher risk for cardiovascular disease and in whom lipoprotein profiles are unfavorable), an oral estrogen would appear to be a superior choice. On a more practical basis, some women uniquely experience headaches, malaise, or other systemic side-effects with one particular form of estrogen, but can tolerate other preparations. The physician can take comfort in the knowledge that, at least with respect to the skeleton, the method of delivery is not a matter of consequence.

Other differences in metabolic response to oral and transcutaneous estrogen have been described, although their significance is not known. Oral therapy increases circulating concentrations of growth hormone and decreases blood levels of insulin-like growth factor I (IGF-I), whereas transdermal estrogen has been reported to increase IGF-I levels without changing those of GH (40). Since human osteoblasts possess receptors for and respond to both growth hormone and IGF-I (41,42), a clinically relevant consequence of this difference cannot be excluded.

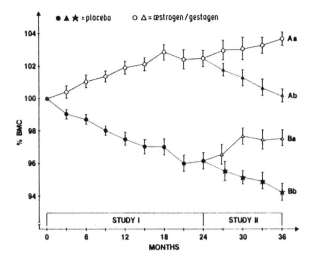

Fig. 3. Effect of estrogen withdrawal on forearm BMC. Subjects were treated initially with either estrogen/progestin (open circles) or placebo (filled circles) for 18 mo. They were then randomly assigned to continue hormone of placebo for an additional 12 mo. Subjects assigned initially to active treatment subsequently lost bone at a rate that was equivalent to that of the original placebo group. Reproduced from ref. *44* with permission.

5.4. Cessation of Estrogen Therapy

Uncertainty persists regarding the consequences of stopping estrogen. Lindsay et al. *(43)* observed an accelerated rate of bone loss in women who abruptly terminated estrogen replacement therapy. In a more complex protocol, Christiansen et al. *(44)* randomly assigned women to estrogen or placebo for 24 mo, at which time the estrogen group either switched to placebo or continued estrogen. The secondary placebo group lost bone over the next 12 mo at the same rate that was observed in subjects who had taken placebo from the beginning (Fig. 3). Thus, the authors found that bone is lost after termination of estrogen, but do not confirm the accelerated rate reported by Lindsay et al. *(43)*.

5.5. The Role of Progestins

Until very recently, the dominant form of estrogen therapy in the US was continuous unopposed estrogen. Concerns over protecting the uterus from hyperplasia and endometrial carcinoma have led to the creation of multiple schedules for interposing a progestin on a cyclic or continuous basis. Since progesterone antagonizes some of the actions of estrogen, it was important to determine whether antagonism occurred on bone. Short-term administration of the most commonly used progestin, medroxyprogesterone acetate (MPA), 10 mg/d, had no independent effect, nor did it blunt the effect of estrogen on circulating concentrations of calciotropic hormones, on urinary calcium excretion, or urinary hydroxyproline *(45)*. In the PEPI trial, no interaction of any of three progestin regimens on the beneficial effect of unopposed estrogen was observed, either on lumbar spine or on proximal femur BMD *(24)*. These regimens included cyclic MPA, 10 mg/d for 12 d each month, continuous MPA 2.5 mg/d, or micronized progesterone, 200 mg/d for 12 d each month. Progestins other than MPA, such as norethindrone, may interact with the testosterone receptor, and have anabolic effects on muscle and bone *(46)*.

Enthusiasm has been expressed for the use of MPA as sole therapy, without estrogen. This idea comes from data suggesting that endogenous progesterone secretion may be important for skeletal maintenance in women of reproductive age. Prior et al. *(47)* reported that young athletic women who experienced >1 anovulatory or short-luteal-phase cycle during a year of observation had increased rates of trabecular bone loss from the spine. In another study, the same group reported that treatment of such women with 10 mg MPA for 10 d each month was associated with a gain in spinal bone mass, whereas a placebo group lost bone *(48)*. Several problems surround these reports. Assessments of menstrual abnormality were done by a method that is fairly imprecise for assigning the day of ovulation. The 4% annual rate of bone loss in women with anovulatory cycles is far beyond that which is generally observed in populations of healthy young women, yet had a fairly high prevalence in that small study. Finally, attribution of the skeletal effect to deficiency of progesterone alone is not justified, since women with luteal-phase abnormalities often have abnormal follicular phase estrogen production as well.

On the other hand, Gallagher et al. *(49)* reported a clinical trial in postmenopausal women, in which one treatment arm was MPA, 20 mg/d. This group lost bone significantly from all sites. For the present, I remain unconvinced of a clinically meaningful osteotropic effect of nonandrogenic progestins. The data of Gallagher et al. *(49)* show clearly that bone mass decreases at multiple sites if women are treated with MPA alone. My greatest concern in this area is for younger women treated with long-acting MPA (Depo-Provera®) for contraception, since ovulation is interrupted, an estrogen-deficient state is induced, and bone loss is predictable.

5.6. The Effect of Tamoxifen, an Antiestrogen

One of the most problematic categories of patient to treat is the woman who has recovered or is recovering from breast cancer. Although clinical trials are currently under way to determine whether this policy is wrong, the standard of care in the US as of 1995 is **not** to offer estrogen to such women. This is a source of great apprehension on the part of patients, many of them young, who are postmenopausal or who have been rendered postmenopausal by their oncologic management. It appears that tamoxifen, an antiestrogen frequently used as adjuvant therapy for breast cancer, may provide a reasonable solution for many women. Tamoxifen is not a pure estrogen antagonist, but shows partial agonist activity on bone. Several reports indicate that postmenopausal women treated with tamoxifen mainain bone mass *(50–52)*. Additional work with this compound is required, particularly in younger women. It is also important to note that although tamoxifen may act like estrogen in postmenopausal women whose endogenous estrogen concentrations are very low, its use as preventive therapy (e.g., the current NIH-sponsored breast cancer prevention trial) by healthy young women with normal estrogen production may permit its estrogen antagonism to dominate, leading to bone loss.

6. HELPING THE PATIENT DECIDE WHETHER TO TAKE ESTROGEN

The decision whether or not to take estrogen is highly personal and must be based on an individualized assessment of multiple health factors. The essential minimal components of this analysis include an understanding of a patient's risks for ischemic heart disease, osteoporosis, and breast cancer, of her personal view of hormone replacement, and of any other factor in her personal health history that might bear on this decision, for example, the presence of menopausal symptoms, estrogen-related thromboembolic disorder, history of endometrial hyperplasia or cancer, or lupus erythematosis.

6.1. Ischemic Heart Disease

A large and increasing body of epidemiological evidence supports the conclusion that sustained use of estrogen confers about a 50% reduction in risk for coronary heart disease, and as much as a 40% reduction in all-cause mortality *(53–55)*. This literature presumes the standard estrogen regimen received by most postmenopausal American women over the past several decades, conjugated equine estrogens **without** added progestins. The protective effect is linked to the known ability of estrogen to increase plasma concentrations of HDL cholesterol, but this linkage may account for only about 50% of the total effects Other possible mechanisms include direct vascular actions of estrogen, i.e., on vascular smooth muscle tone, and direct effects on endothelial nitric oxide or endoperoxide pathways, as well as on more systemic metabolic pathways. The degree of protection by estrogen mirrors the number of risk factors already present. Thus, an obese, hypertensive smoker with low HDL cholesterol values will achieve greater benefit than a thin, athletic, normotensive nonsmoker who has a relatively high HDL cholesterol concentration.

6.2. Breast Cancer

Despite a truly voluminous literature on this topic, no definitive conclusion is currently possible concerning the effect of postmenopausal estrogen on breast cancer risk. Epidemiological studies have concluded that long-term (i.e., 10 yr or longer) use may result in as little as no increase to as much as a 40% increase in breast cancer risk. Within the month of this writing, two careful and well-conducted studies have shown variously that long-term estrogen use is associated with close to a 50% increase *(56)* or absolutely no change *(57)* in breast cancer risk. It seems likely that additional case-control or observational studies short of a randomized clinical trial will not materially change this conclusion. Review of this complex field is beyond the scope of this chapter. To my reading, it appears to be a fair summary to state that **if** there is an effect of estrogen on breast cancer risk, it is not particularly large. If one of nine women is destined to develop invasive breast cancer, a 40% increase in risk would change an individual's chance from 0.11 to 0.154%. Nonetheless, women with personal or family histories of breast cancer should be fully informed of the issues and be prepared to undergo continuing aggressive mammographic surveillance if they are to embark on estrogen replacement. There are many patients for whom **any** added breast cancer risk is unacceptable, regardless of other health issues. If such women need skeletal protection, it is certainly prudent to consider other antiresorptive agents.

7. CONCLUSIONS, CONCERNS, AND FUTURE DIRECTIONS

Despite persistent ambiguity surrounding aspects of this problem, I find the conclusion to be compelling that timely and sustained administration of estrogen to menopausal women offers substantial protection against bone loss and fragility fractures. In consideration of evidence that antifracture efficacy is lost for "past users," even if duration of use exceeded 10 yr *(30)*, estrogen replacement should ideally be considered a lifelong strategy for skeletal health. It is a fact of life, however, that women who are initially prescribed estrogen generally take it for only a few months. North American pharmaceutical industry surveys suggest that the "half-life" of estrogen therapy is not much more than 6 mo, a trend that has been stable for the past decade. To some degree, this may reflect the fact that many women are prescribed estrogen for short-term control of vasomotor instability rather than as a long-term health maintenance strategy, but it must also reflect the controversy and public uncertainty that surrounds the entire topic of hormone replacement.

There has never been a time that more than about 30% of the potential estrogen consumers in the US or other industrialized nations have taken estrogen, and consumption figures are far lower for Asian and Third World countries. Reasons for this are complex, and involve a dislike for taking medication, reluctance to continue vaginal bleeding, and, particularly, concerns about breast cancer. In recognition of these various issues, it is encouraging to note that compounds are under development whose actions mimic those of 17β-estradiol on bone and on lipoproteins, but seem not to lead to potentially adverse effects on the endometrium or the breast. Raloxifene is an example of such an agent. This compound acts either as an estrogen agonist or antagonist, depending on the specific tissue. Administered to oopholectomized rats, raloxifene mimics the skeletal protection actions of 17β-estradiol, but does not stimulate endometrial hyperplasia and antagonizes estrogen action on the breast *(58)*. Clinical trials of raloxifene in postmenopausal osteoporotic women are currently in progress. It is to be hoped that this or similar agents may prove acceptable and effective for many women who are unable or unwilling to take long-term estrogen.

REFERENCES

1. Heaney RP, Recker RR, Saville PD. Calcium balance and calcium requirements in middle-aged women. *Am J Clin Nutr* 1977; 30: 1603–1611.
2. Hui SL, Slemenda CW, Johnston CC Jr. Baseline measurement of bone mass predicts fracture in white women. *Ann Intern Med* 1989; 111: 355–361.
3. Cummings SR, Black DM, Nevitt MC, Browner WS, Cauley JA, Genant HK, Mascioli SR, Scott JC, Seeley DG, Steiger P, Vogt T, for the SOF Research Group. Appendicular bone density and age predict hip fracture in women. *JAMA* 1990; 263: 665–668.
4. Melton LJ III, Atkinson EJ, O'Fallon WM, Wahner HW, Riggs BL. Long-term fracture prediction by bone mineral assessed at different skeletal sites. *J Bone Miner Res* 1993; 8: 1227–1234
5. Heaney RP, Recker RR, Saville PD. Menopausal changes in bone remodeling. *J Lab Clin Med* 1978; 92: 964–970.
6. Gallagher JC, Riggs BL, DeLuca HF. Effect of estrogen on calcium absorption and serum vitamin D metabolites in postmenopausal osteoporosis. *J Clin Endocrinol Metab* 1980; 51: 1359–1364.
7. Cheema C, Grant BF, Malcus R. Effects of estrogen on circulating "free" and total 1,25-dihydroxyvitamin D and on the parathyroid-vitamin D axis in postmenopausal women. *J Clin Invest* 1989; 83: 537–542.
8. Recker RR, Davies KM, Hinders SM, Heaney RP, Stegman MR, Kimmel DB. Bone gain in young adult women. *JAMA* 1992; 268: 2403–2408.
9. Ravn P, Hetland ML, Ovelgaard K, Christiansen C. Premenopausal and postmenopausal changes in bone mineral density of the proximal femur measured by dual-energy x-ray absorptiometry. *J Bone Miner Res* 1994; 9: 1975–1980.
10. Christiansen C, Riis BJ, Rødbro P. Prediction of rapid bone loss in postemenopausal women. *Lancet* 1987; i: 1105–1107.
11. Blunt BA, Klauber MR, Barlett-Connor EL, Edelstein SL. Sex differences in bone mineral density in 1653 men and women in the sixth through tenth decades of life: the Rancho Bernardo Study. *J Bone Miner Res* 1994; 9: 1333–1338.
12. Greenspan S, Maitland LA, Myers ER, Krasnow MB, Tamiko HK. Femoral bone loss progresses with age: a longitudinal study in women over age 65. *J Bone Miner Res* 1994; 9: 1959–1965.

13. Harris S, Dallal GE, Dawsoll-Hughes B. Influence of body weight on rates of change in bone density of the spine, hip, and radius in postmenopausal women. *Calcif Tiss Int* 1992; 50: 19–23.
14. Lindsay R, Hart DM, Aitken JM, MacDonald EB, Anderson JB, Clarke AC. Long-term prevention of postmenopausal osteoporosis by oestrogen. Evidence for an increased bone mass after delayed onset of oestrogen treatment. *Lancet* 1976; i: 1038–1040.
15. Lindsay R, Hart DM, Forrest C, Baird C. Prevention of spinal osteoporosis in oophorectomised women. *Lancet* 1980; ii: 1151–1153.
16. Genant HK, Christopher CE, Ettinger B, Gordan GS. Quantitative computed tomography of vertebral spongiosa: a sensitive method for detecting early bone loss after oophorectomy. *Ann Int Med* 1982; 97: 699–705.
17. Recker RR, Saville PD, Heaney RP. Effect of estrogens and calcium carbonate on bone loss in postmenopausal women. *Am Int Med* 1977; 87: 649–655.
18. Horsman A, Gallagher JC, Simpson M, Nordin BEC. Prospective trial of oestrogen and calcium in postmenopausal women. *Brit Med J* 1977; 2: 789–792.
19. Christiansen C, Christensen MS, McNair P, Hagen C, Stocklund A, Transbøl I. Prevention of early postmenopausal bone loss: controlled 2-years study in 315 normal females. *Eur J Clin Invest* 1980; 10: 273–279.
20. Lindsay R, Tolame JF. Estrogen treatment of patients with established postmenopausal osteoporosis. *Obstet Gynecol* 1990; 76: 290–295.
21. Quigley MET, Martin PL, Burnier AM, Brooks P. Estrogen therapy arrests bone loss in elderly women. *Am J Obstet Gynecol* 1987; 156: 1516–1523.
22. Holland EPN, Leather AT, Studd JWW. Increases in bone mass of older postmenopausal women with low mineral bone density after one year of percutaneous oestradiol implants. *Brit J Obstet Gynecol* 1995; 102: 238–242.
23. The PEPI Investigators. The Postmenopausal Estrogen/Progestins Interventions Trial: rationale, design, and conduct. *Control Clin Trials* 1995; 16(Suppl.): S3–S19.
24. Marcus R. For the PEPI Trial Investigator s. Effects of hormone replacement therapies on bone mineral density results from the postmenopausal estrogen and progestin interventions trial. Program of the 17th Annual Mtg, American Society for Bone & Mineral Research. *J Bone Miner Res* 1995; Suppl I, Abstract P276, S197.
25. Nachtigall LE, Nachtigall RH, Nachtigall RD, Beckmann EM. Estrogen replacement therapy I: a 10-year prospective study in the relationship to osteoporosis. *Obstet Gynecol* 1979; 53: 277–281.
26. Hutchinson TA, Polansky SM, Feinstein AR. Post-menopausal oestrogens protect against fractures of hip and distal radius. A case-control study. *Lancet* ii: 705–709.
27. Weiss NS, Ure CL, Ballard JH, Williams AR, Darling JR. Decreased risk of fractures of the hip and lower forearm with postmenopausal use of estrogen. *N Eng J Med* 1980; 303: 1195–1198.
28. Kanis JA, Johnell O, Gullberg B, Allander E, Dilsen G, Gennari C. Evidence for efficacy of drugs affecting bone metabolism in preventing hip fracture. *Brit Med J* 1992; 305: 1124–1128.
29. Felson DT, Zhang Y, Hannon MT, Kiel DP, Wilson PW, Anderson JJ. The effect of postmenopausal estrogen therapy on bone density in elderly women. *N Engl J Med* 1993; 329: 1141–1146.
30. Cauley JA, Seeley DG, Enstrud K, Ettinger B, Black D, Cummings SR. For the Study of Osteoporotic Fractures Research Group. Estrogen replacement therapy and fractures in older women. *Ann Int Med* 1995; 122: 9–16.
31. Horsman A, Jones M, Francis R, Nordin BEC. The effect of estrogen dose on postmenopausal bone loss. *N Engl J Med* 309: 1405–1407.
32. Ettinger B, Genant HK, Steiger P., Madvig P. Low-dosage micronized 17β-estradiol prevents bone loss in postmenopausal women. *Am J Obstet Gynecol* 1992; 166: 479–488.
33. Ettinger B, Genant HK, Cann CE. Postmenopausal bone loss is prevented by treatment with low-dosage estrogen with calcium. *Ann Int Med* 1987; 106: 40–45.
34. Gallagher JC, Baylink D. Effect of estrone sulfate on bone mineral density of the femoral neck and spine. Program of the American Society for Bone & Mineral Research, 12th annual meeting. *J Bone Miner Res* 1990; Suppl 2, Abstract 802.
35. Studd J, Smith R. The dose–response of percutaneous oestradiol implants on the skeletons of postmenopausal women. *Br J Obstet Gynecol* 1994; 101: 787–791.
36. Stevenson JC, Cust MP, Gangar KF, Hillard TC, Lees B, Whitehead MT. Effects of transdermal versus oral hormone replacement therapy on bone density in spine and proximal femur in postmenopausal women. *Lancet* 1990; ii: 265–269.

37. Field CS, Ory SJ, Washner HW, Herrmann RR, Judd HL, Riggs BL. Preventive effects of transdermal 17β-estradiol on ostseoporotic changes after surgical menopause: a two-year placebo-controlled trial. *Am J Obstet Gynecol* 1993; 168: 114–121.

38. Riis BJ, Thomsen K, Strom V, Christiansen C. The effect of percutaneous estradiol and natural progesterone on postmenopausal bone loss. *Am J Obstet Gynecol* 1987; 156: 61–65.

39. Studd JW, Holland EF, Leather AT, Smith RN. The dose-response of percutaneous oestradiol implants on the skeletons of postmenopausal women. *Brit J Obstet Gynaecol* 1994; 101: 787–791.

40. Ho KHY, Weissberger AJ. Impact of short-term estrogen administration on growth hormone secretion and action: distinct route-dependent effects on connective and bone tissue metabolism. *J Bone Miner Res* 1992; 7: 821–827.

41. Barnard R, Ng KW, Martin TJ, Waters MJ. Growth hormone (GH) receptors in clonal osteoblast-like cells mediate a mitogenic response to GH. *Endocrinology* 1991; 128: 1459–1464.

42. Ernst M, Froesch ER. Growth hormone dependent stimulation of osteoblast-like cells in serum-free cultures via local synthesis of insulin-like growth factor 1. *Biochem Biophys Res Commun* 1988; 151 142–147.

43. Lindsay R, Hart DM, MacLean A, Clarke AC, Kraszewski A, Garwood J. Bone response to termination of estrogen treatment. *Lancet* 1978; i: 1325–1327.

44. Christiansen C, Christensen MS, Transbøl I. Bone mass in postmenopausal women after withdrawal of oestrogen/gestagen replacement therapy. *Lancet* 1981; i: 459–461.

45. Minkoff JR, Young G, Grant B, Marcus R. Interactions of medroxyprogesterone acetate with estrogen on the calcium-parathyroid axis in post-menopausal women. *Maturitas* 1985; 8: 35–45.

46. Christiansen C, Riis BJ. 17β-estradiol and continuous norethisterone: a unique treatment for established osteoporosis in elderly women. *J Clin Endocrinol Metab* 1990; 71: 836–841.

47. Prior JC, Vigna YM, Schechter MT, Burgess AE. Spinal bone loss and ovulatory disturbances. *N Engl J Med* 1990; 323: 1221–1227.

48. Prior JC, Vigna YM, Barr SI, Rexworthy C, Lentle BC. Cyclic medroxyprogesterone treatment increases bone density: as controlled trial in active women with menstrual cycle disturbances. *Am J Med* 1994; 96: 521–530.

49. Gallagher JC, Kable WT, Goldgar D.. Effect of progestin therapy on cortical and trabecular bone: comparison with estrogen. *Am J Med* 1991; 90:171–178.

50. Gotfredsen A, Christiansen C, Palshof T. The effect of tamoxifen on bone mineral content in premenopausal women with breast cancer. *Cancer* 1984; 53: 853–857.

51. Love R, Mazess R, Tormey D, Barden H, Newcomb P. Jordan V. Bone mineral density in women with breast cancer treated with adjuvant tamoxifen for at least two years *Breast Cancel Res Treat* 1988; 12: 297–301.

52. Turken S, Siris E, Seldin D, Flaster E, Hyman G, Lindsay R. Effects of tamoxifen on spinal bone density in women with breast cancer. *J Natl Cancer Inst* 1989; 81: 1086–1088.

53. Bush TL, Barrett-Connor E, Cowan LD, et al. Cardiovascular mortality and noncontraceptive use of estrogen in women: results from the Lipid Research Clinics Program Follow-Up Study. *Circulation* 1987; 75: 1102–1109.

54. Stampfer MJ, Colditz GA. Estrogen replacement and coronary heart disease: a quantitative assessment of the epidemiologic evidence. *Prev Med* 1991; 20: 47–63.

55. Grady D, Rubin SM, Petitti DB, Fox CS, Black D, Ettinger B, Ernster VL, Cummings SR. Hormone therapy to prevent disease and prolong life in postmenopausal women. *Ann Int Med* 1992; 117: 1016–1037.

56. Colditz GA, Hankinson SE, Hunter DJ, Willett WC, Manson JE, Stampfer MJ, Hennekens C, Rosner B, Speizer FE. The use of estrogens and progestins and the risk of breast cancer in postmenopausal women. *N Engl J Med* 1995; 332: 1589–1593.

57. Stanford JL, Weiss NS, Voigt LF, Daling JR, Habel LA, Rossing MA. Combined estrogen and progestin hormone replacement therapy in relation to risk of breast cancer in middle-aged women. *JAMA* 1995; 274: 137–142.

58. Black LJ, Sato M, Rowley ER. Raloxifene (LY139481HCL) prevents bone loss and reduces serum cholesterol without causing uterine hypertrophy in ovariectomized rats. *J Clin Invest* 1994; 93: 62–69.

15 Drug Therapy

John L. Stock, MD

1. INTRODUCTION

Previous chapters have reviewed the importance of lifestyle changes, adequacy of calcium and vitamin D stores, and the use of hormone replacement therapy for the prevention and treatment of osteoporosis. The recent burgeoning interest in osteoporosis stems not only from an increased awareness of women's health issues and the important effects of lifestyle on health, but also from the related explosion of knowledge about the pathophysiology of osteoporosis. This has been the result of advances in basic science, new noninvasive techniques for measuring bone turnover and bone density, and the development of many new promising drugs for the prevention and treatment of bone loss *(1–4)*.

The first aim of this chapter is to classify the available drugs and those under study. Drugs will be classified regarding their:

1. Ability to inhibit bone resorption vs enhance bone formation;
2. Efficacy in preventing the vertebral fractures of type I osteoporosis compared with the hip fractures of type II osteoporosis;
3. Role in preventing fractures in subjects with a low bone density vs treating patients with existing fractures; and
4. Current status of US Food and Drug Administration (FDA) approval and availability *(5)*.

Individual drugs will then be reviewed. This will include the historical background; review of controlled studies investigating efficacy on bone density, fracture rate, and quality of life; dosing, side effect profile, and cost; and current as well as anticipated future use patterns. Given the complexity of this rapidly changing field, the reader will be offered guidelines for the use of drug therapy. Finally, no discussion would be complete in this era of cost consciousness without an analysis of the costs and benefits of these drugs and their place in managed care plans. How should patients with osteoporosis on

From: *Osteoporosis: Diagnostic and Therapeutic Principles*
Edited by: C. J. Rosen Humana Press Inc., Totowa, NJ

drug therapy be followed? What is the role of the primary care physician, and when should consultants be involved in their care?

2. CLASSIFICATION OF DRUGS ACTIVE IN PATIENTS WITH OSTEOPOROSIS

2.1. Effects on Bone Resorption and Bone Formation

As described in Chapter 1, bone is constantly undergoing remodeling at bone remodeling units in which osteoclasts are resorbing bone or osteoblasts are forming new bone (6). Patients lose bone when resorption exceeds formation, and these changes may be magnified by the overall rate of bone turnover, which is determined by the number of active remodeling units. Estrogen deficiency in early postmenopausal women leads to increased osteoclast activity and increased bone resorption that is particularly noticeable in the vertebral trabecular bone. The more gradual decrease in osteoblastic activity that occurs with aging may result in weakness of cortical as well as trabecular bone.

The drugs to be discussed have been classified as to their ability to decrease bone resorption (antiresorptive) or increase bone formation. Most of the currently available drugs decrease bone resorption, but owing to the coupling of bone resorption and formation, those drugs may also decrease bone formation. The efficacy of antiresorptive therapy most likely depends on the more rapid effects on bone resorption compared to bone formation, allowing a period of decreased resorption prior to the onset of decreased formation, leading to small increases in bone mass.

Studies have suggested that baseline bone turnover might predict drug efficacy. For example, the vertebral bone density was found to increase in a subset of postmenopausal women with elevated bone turnover treated with parenteral salmon calcitonin (7). This finding led some clinicians to select patients for calcitonin therapy using measurements of bone turnover markers (8). However, although these markers are of great value in studying the mechanism of drug action and in following large groups of patients, the benefit of this approach has not been proven in the individual patient given the variability and cost of bone turnover markers (9). The recent advances in bone turnover marker technology may lead to new proposals for algorithms for selecting patients for drug treatment and following their responses to therapy.

2.2. Prevention of Vertebral and Hip Fractures

Drugs have also been classified by their ability to prevent the vertebral fractures seen most commonly as a result of estrogen deficiency in postmenopausal women (Type I osteoporosis), compared with the hip fractures associated with aging in both men and women (Type II osteoporosis). Because the trabecular bone found more plentifully in the vertebrae than femur is more responsive to pharmacologic agents and because vertebral fractures are more easily studied in a younger population, vertebral bone density and fracture rates have been the end points for most clinical studies. However, given the increasing incidence of costly hip fractures in our aging society, it is becoming increasingly important to demonstrate drug efficacy for Type II as well as Type I osteoporosis.

2.3. Prevention and Treatment

Another distinction that has been made among drugs is their use in preventing bone loss in patients at risk for fracture because of a low bone density, as compared to their efficacy in treating established osteoporosis in patients with existing fractures. This distinction has become somewhat less important given the recent acceptance of the World Health Organization definition of osteoporosis as a bone density more than 2.5 SD below young normal *(10)* and the proven relationship between bone density and fracture risk *(11)*. However, patients who have already had one vertebral fracture are more likely to have future fractures *(12)*, so that the presence of fracture may be a useful parameter in selecting drugs for patients at increased risk. In the future, other measures, such as bone strength measured by ultrasonography *(1)*, may be used along with bone density and fracture history as guidelines for choosing pharmacologic therapy.

2.4. FDA-Approved Drugs

The selection of drugs available for the treatment of osteoporosis is currently limited, but should be rapidly expanding given the large number of ongoing research studies. Although estrogen, calcitonin, and alendronate are currently the only FDA-approved therapies, additional drugs should be available in the near future. The FDA Endocrinologic and Metabolic Drugs Advisory Committee has recommended that the FDA approve slow-release sodium fluoride. Such drugs as the first-generation bisphosphonate etidronate and the calcium-sparing diuretic hydrochlorothiazide may also be appropriate for some treatment regimens. Other drugs, such as calcitriol, anabolic steroids, and growth hormone, are available, but should not be used other than in a research setting given concerns regarding efficacy and side effects.

3. REVIEW OF DRUGS ACTIVE
IN PATIENTS WITH OSTEOPOROSIS

3.1. Calcitonin

Calcitonin is a 32 amino acid polypeptide hormone made in the C-cells present in the thyroid. Although probably a vestigial hormone in humans, pharmacologic doses of this hormone have potent bone resorption-inhibiting properties. Salmon calcitonin is more potent than human calcitonin and has been approved by the FDA for parenteral administration, and more recently was approved as a nasal spray for the treatment of postmenopausal osteoporosis. The use of calcitonin has been reviewed *(13–16)*.

Controlled studies of parenterally administered calcitonin over 1–2 yr in postmenopausal women with osteoporosis have shown small increases in total body bone density *(17)* and vertebral bone density *(7,18)*, and variable effects on the density of the distal forearm *(17,19)* and femur *(17,18)*, which contain more cortical bone. Effective doses range from 50 IU every other day to 100 IU daily given by the sc or im route. Controlled studies using calcitonin administered nasally to healthy early postmenopausal women *(20–24)* or to women with established osteoporosis *(25,26)* at doses ranging from 50 to 400 IU daily over 1–3.5 yr show increases in vertebral bone density of approx 2%, but results have ranged from 0.2 to as much as 9.3%. Variable effects have been seen on bone density of the distal forearm *(20,21,25–27)*. Higher doses may be necessary to achieve significant effects, particularly in early postmenopausal women *(21)*. Other studies have failed to find significant effects even at higher doses in this population *(27)*. Nasal calcitonin has recently been approved at a dose of 200 IU daily for treatment of women at least 5 yr postmenopausal with a low bone density who are not candidates for hormone replacement therapy.

Preliminary evidence suggests fracture efficacy as well. Several controlled studies have demonstrated a decrease in the incidence of both vertebral and peripheral fractures in postmenopausal women with established osteoporosis treated with calcitonin administered over 2 yr by the parenteral *(28,29)* or nasal *(26)* routes. A retrospective study also suggested benefit of calcitonin in preventing hip fractures *(30)*.

One of the major advantages of calcitonin is the lack of serious side effects *(31)*. There is no long-term accumulation of calcitonin in bone, and calcitonin does not affect bone quality *(32)*. Bothersome side effects of the parenteral preparation, such as nausea or flushing, may limit its use, but often resolve after several days of treatment. Nasally administered calcitonin appears to have fewer side effects than the parenteral form *(33)*. The difficulty of parenteral administration has decreased the enthusiasm for the use of this drug in the past, but the recent availability of the easily administered nasal preparation may lead to increased acceptability. Another potential advantage of calcitonin therapy is its acute analgesic effect, unrelated to effects on bone metabolism. Several controlled studies have demonstrated that patients with acute vertebral fractures treated with parenteral *(34)* or nasal *(35)* calcitonin have less pain than appropriate control groups.

Controversies still remain with regard to the most effective use of nasal calcitonin. The most cost-effective dose of nasal calcitonin has not been established. The duration of effect of calcitonin also remains controversial. It has been suggested that calcitonin may be most effective in postmenopausal women with high bone turnover *(7)*, and some have used markers of bone turnover to select patients for calcitonin treatment. These findings do not appear consistent with some studies showing lack of efficacy in early postmenopausal women who usually have high bone turnover *(27)*.

The average wholesale price of a 1-mo supply of parenterally administered salmon calcitonin at a dose of 100 IU given 3 times/wk ranges from $264 to $424 *(36)*. The wholesale acquisition price of a 1-mo supply of nasal calcitonin at a dose of 200 IU daily is $45 (personal communication, Sandoz Pharmaceuticals Corp.).

3.2. Bisphosphonates

The use of bisphosphonates in the treatment of osteoporosis has been extensively reviewed *(37–41)*. Bisphosphonates are analogs of pyrophosphates, which naturally inhibit bone resorption. They contain a P-C-P instead of P-O-P moiety, and therefore undergo less degradation. Their affinity for hydroxyapatite leads to a long skeletal half-life. Osteoclast function is inhibited by ingestion of bone on resorptive surfaces containing the bisphosphonate.

Bisphosphonates have been useful in treating many skeletal disorders characterized by increased bone turnover, including Paget's disease, primary hyperparathyroidism, hypercalcemia of malignancy, and metastatic bone disease. Most of the bisphosphonates are poorly absorbed and should be administered on an empty stomach. Simultaneous calcium ingestion particularly interferes with absorption. The drugs are rapidly cleared by bone and kidney. The short circulating half-life leads to few systemic side effects other than gastrointestinal intolerance at high doses. However, since the bisphosphonates reside in bone for long periods of time, some have expressed concern about the potential for long-term side effects, although none have been documented. Occasional hypocalcemia has been described, but is mild and asymptomatic. At high doses or with continuous administration, etidronate may cause mild asymptomatic hyperphosphatemia, and may inhibit mineralization and cause osteomalacia. Fever and leukopenia have been described after administration of pamidronate.

Studies investigating the utility of bisphosphonates for the prevention and treatment of osteoporosis began with etidronate. The use of this drug has been limited by its potential for inhibiting mineralization. The newer bisphosphonates do not inhibit mineralization at the doses used, and appear to increase bone density and bone strength and decrease fracture incidence. The potency, side effect profiles, effects on bone formation, and duration of action of individual agents are under investigation.

Two placebo-controlled studies have documented the efficacy of cyclic low-dose etidronate in postmenopausal patients with vertebral osteoporosis. Both studies utilized a regimen of 400 mg given daily for 2 wk every 3 mo, but the details of calcium, phosphorus, and vitamin D supplementation differed. In a group of patients with severe osteoporosis, a 5.3% increase in vertebral bone density compared with a 2.7% loss in the placebo group over 3 yr was demonstrated *(42)*. A decrease in the vertebral fracture rate was shown in the second and third year, and no adverse effects were seen on bone biopsies *(43)*. In an open 2-yr extension of crossover design, patients previously treated with etidronate maintained their bone density. Using a similar regimen, others demonstrated a 3–4% increase in vertebral bone density over 2 yr *(44)*. There were also fewer vertebral fractures, a small increase in hip bone density, and no adverse effects on bone histology *(45)*. Further studies up to 4-yr of treatment showed maintenance of bone density changes, but fracture protection persisted only in high-risk patients *(46)*. No significant side effects were noted with this regimen in either study. In summary, etidronate appears to be safe and effective over 2–3 yr in increasing vertebral bone density and in preventing vertebral fractures. The long-term efficacy has not been proven, so, although the drug is available, it has not received FDA approval for this indication. The average wholesale price of 1 cycle (3 mo) of etidronate is $49 *(36)*.

Several other bisphosphonates are currently under investigation for the treatment of osteoporosis. These compounds are more potent than etidronate and are not associated with mineralization abnormalities. Alendronate was recently approved by the FDA for treatment of postmenopausal osteoporosis *(47)*. In a 2-yr double-blind, placebo-controlled trial of alendronate in 188 postmenopausal women with low spinal bone density, but no fracture, a 10 mg dose of alendronate was associated with a rapid decrease in markers of bone turnover, a 7.2% increase in lumbar spine, and 5.3% increase in total hip bone density after 2 yr *(48)*. In a subset of patients treated for 1 yr and then observed for a followup year on placebo, increases in bone density were sustained. Although gastrointestinal side effects were noted at higher doses, the 10-mg dose was well tolerated. In a similar international study of 516 postmenopausal women with osteoporosis, the 10 mg dose of alendronate given for 2 yr was well tolerated, and led to a 6.0% increase in lumbar spine and 3.5% increase in femoral neck bone density *(49)*. Preliminary results of an international multicenter study of 994 postmenopausal women with low bone density show that those women treated with calcium supplementation and with varying doses of alendronate for 3 yr had 48% fewer new vertebral fractures, less progression of vertebral deformity, and less loss in height than those women treated with calcium supplementation alone *(50)*. Animal studies show that alendronate treatment leads to an increase in bone strength without any adverse histomorphologic changes *(51)*. The wholesale price of a 1-mo supply of alendronate is $42 (personal communication, Merck & Co., Inc.). Studies are in progress with other bisphosphonates, including tiludronate *(52)*, pamidronate *(53)*, clodronate, and risedronate.

3.3. Sodium Fluoride

Sodium fluoride potently stimulates bone formation and increases trabecular bone mass, but there have been concerns regarding the structural quality of the new bone formed. The initial positive results led to its widespread use despite lack of FDA approval. Concerns about antifracture efficacy and side effects led to a 4-yr NIH-sponsored prospective, placebo-controlled trial of sodium fluoride (75 mg) daily in postmenopausal women with vertebral fracture *(54)*. All patients received 1500 mg calcium supplementation daily. As expected, the bone density of trabecular sites, such as the vertebrae, increased by as much as 35%, but cortical bone density appeared to decrease. There was no difference in the incidence of new vertebral fractures, but nonvertebral fractures were more common in the treatment group as were side effects including gastrointestinal symptoms and lower extremity pain. Similar results were found in a smaller randomized trial *(55)*. These studies ended the widespread use of sodium fluoride in the US outside of clinical trials and confirmed concerns that bone density data alone is an insufficient end point for efficacy of osteoporosis drugs.

The possibility that lower doses of sodium fluoride *(56)* or other preparations, such as slow-release sodium fluoride, might be more effective in the treatment of osteoporosis is currently under study. In a 4-yr placebo-controlled randomized trial using intermittent slow-release sodium fluoride, 25 mg bid, a 4.8%/yr increase in lumbar spine bone mass and a 2.4%/yr increase in femoral neck hip bone density were noted, and there was a decrease in the vertebral fracture rate *(57)*. Both treatment and control groups received calcium citrate supplements, and there are currently no data published using less expensive calcium carbonate. However, this regimen appeared to be ineffective in patients with severe bone loss. There was also no effect on the rate of recurrent fracture in already fractured vertebrae, and there was no improvement in the rate of appendicular fracture. The FDA Endocrinologic and Metabolic Drugs Advisory Committee has recommended that the FDA approve slow-release sodium fluoride for the treatment of postmenopausal osteoporosis, and full approval is expected in the near future. The specific indications for use and price information are not yet available.

3.4. Other Drug Therapy

In women who decline or who are not candidates for hormone replacement therapy, salmon calcitonin or the bisphosphonates are the first choices for antiresorptive therapy and slow-release sodium fluoride may soon be available. Women with a history of breast cancer are generally not candidates for estrogen and may be treated with tamoxifen. This drug acts as an estrogen antagonist on the breast, but may have estrogen agonist effects on bone, with studies demonstrating increased vertebral *(58,59)* and proximal femoral bone density *(59)*. There are currently no fracture data, and this drug should not be used in women who do not have a history of breast cancer, given the potential increased risk for endometrial carcinoma.

Calcium balance may be improved by treatment with thiazide diuretics in patients with hypertension or hypercalciuria, and physiologic replacement of nonactivated vitamin D preparations in elderly patients at risk for vitamin D deficiency. The remainder of the pharmacologic options should be considered experimental. Despite the potential anabolic effects and general availability of activated vitamin D analogs, anabolic steroids, and growth hormone, issues regarding efficacy and side effects preclude their current general use. Other experimental agents, including skeletal growth factors and parathyroid hormone show potential for causing increased bone formation. Newer estrogen analogs may selectively decrease bone resorption without effects on other estrogen-sensitive tissues.

3.4.1. THIAZIDE DIURETICS

Thiazide diuretics are a cost-effective treatment for hypertension and have the additional benefit of decreasing urinary calcium excretion and improving calcium balance. Although no placebo-controlled, prospective studies have been performed, some observational studies have demonstrated positive effects on bone density and fracture rates. For example, thiazide use is associated with an increase in bone density of the os calcis (heel) in men *(60)* and distal radius in older women *(61)*. In a prospective study of men and women over age 65, treatment with thiazide caused a reduction of approx 1/3 in the risk of hip fracture *(62)*, but a case-controlled study of elderly patients hospitalized with hip fracture failed to find any protection *(63)*. A recent meta-analysis showed that current thiazide use or previous thiazide use of long duration were associated with a 20% reduction in hip fracture risk *(64)*. It is unlikely that the very large prospective randomized trial necessary to confirm these findings will be performed. Thiazides should certainly be considered as a first-line antihypertensive treatment in appropriate patients with or at risk for osteoporosis, and should also be considered in the treatment of patients with hypercalciuria and osteoporosis.

3.4.2. VITAMIN D METABOLITES

As previously discussed, alterations in vitamin D metabolism are common in aging populations. Most commonly this includes vitamin D deficiencies owing to inadequate intake, malabsorption, and decreased sun exposure. This leads to secondary hyperparathyroidism and increased bone resorption, and should be corrected by repletion of vitamin D stores and assurance of adequate calcium intake as previously discussed. For example, in elderly ambulatory women living in nursing homes or in the community, treatment with 800 IU vitamin D_3 and 1.2 g elemental calcium daily for 18 mo decreased the incidence of hip fracture by 43% compared with control subjects *(65)*.

There is also evidence that irrespective of vitamin D stores, renal production of $1,25(OH)_2D_3$ and the number of vitamin D receptors in the intestinal mucosa decline with aging. This would also contribute to a decline in calcium absorption, along with potential secondary hyperparathyroidism and increased bone resorption. Thus, treatment with $1,25(OH)_2D_3$ itself might be effective in delaying bone loss. This active metabolite also has potent effects in vitro in promoting cell differentiation, collagen synthesis, and alkaline phosphatase production, and theoretically might be useful as a stimulation of bone formation. Several controlled studies have demonstrated the efficacy of $1,25(OH)_2D_3$ in increasing calcium absorption and decreasing bone resorption *(66,67)*. Studies have shown positive effects on trabecular bone volume *(52)* and bone density *(68,69)*, but others have failed to show any changes *(70)*. One prospective study of 622 postmenopausal women with vertebral fractures showed that treatment with $1,25(OH)_2D_3$ (0.25 µg bid) and supplemental calcium was effective in reducing the rate of new vertebral and nonvertebral fractures during the second and third year of study compared with patients given calcium alone *(71)*. A smaller study of 80 postmenopausal Japanese women with osteoporosis showed similar results after 1 yr of treatment with 1α-hydroxyvitamin D_3 (1 µg daily) *(72)*. However, other studies of similar design have failed to show any fracture protection *(70,73)*. One of the major concerns regarding $1,25(OH)_2D_3$ or its related metabolites is the potential for hypercalcemia and hypercalciuria noted in some studies *(68,70,73)*, but not others *(71)*. This effect might be minimized by using lower doses, avoiding excessive calcium supplementation, or perhaps by using newer vitamin D analogs that have similar effects on bone but cause less hypercalcemia *(72,74)*. Until dependable dose–response relationships are established with existing analogs or until newer and more selective effective analogs are developed, treatment with activated vitamin D metabolites should be considered experimental. However, given the safety, cost-effectiveness, and efficacy of low-dose vitamin D replacement for maintenance of normal stores, it is reasonable for all patients with osteoporosis and all elderly subjects at risk to receive 400–800 IU supplemental vitamin D_3 daily.

3.4.3. ANABOLIC STEROIDS

Anabolic steroids are derivatives of testosterone with anabolic activity, but fewer virilizing side effects *(75)*. These drugs increase bone cell proliferation and differentiation in vitro, and also inhibit bone resorption. Although previously approved for use in the US, the approval was withdrawn by the FDA because of adverse effects, including virilization, hepatic dysfunction, and decrease in HDL cholesterol. A number of double-blind, placebo-controlled studies have shown the efficacy of these drugs in increasing bone density in patients with osteoporotic fractures, but there are few data with fracture as the end point. The total body calcium increased by 2% in postmenopausal women with vertebral fractures given methandrostenolone for 26 mo, compared with a 3% loss in the placebo group *(76)*. Similar results were found in 23 postmenopausal women treated with stanozolol for 29 mo, but 76% of the treated subjects developed an increase in SGOT levels and 30% an increase in facial hair growth *(77)*. The bone mineral content (BMC) of the radius increased by 3.3% in 34 men and women completing a 2-yr study of imnandrolone given every 3 wk, and there was also biochemical evidence for decreased bone turnover *(78)*. Vertebral bone density increased by 2.9% in 32 postmenopausal women with osteoporosis treated with parenteral nandrolone for 18 mo compared with a 2.3 loss in the placebo group, but increased facial hirsutism was noted in 16% of patients and a significant reduction in HDL cholesterol was seen *(79)*. The small effects on bone density, lack of fracture data, and side effect profile preclude the general use of these agents at this time. The current use of testosterone continues to be as replacement therapy for men with hypogonadism.

3.4.4. GROWTH HORMONE

Another currently available drug that may have anabolic effects on bone is growth hormone. This hormone has anabolic effects on multiple organs, including bone, but acts mainly by increasing synthesis of insulin-like growth factor I (IGF-I) by the liver *(80)*. IGF-I has been shown to have potent mitogenic effects on osteoblasts. Patients with growth hormone deficiency may have decreased bone density, which may be increased by growth hormone treatment *(81)*. Elderly patients may also demonstrate a physiological decline in pituitary growth hormone secretion and in circulating concentrations of IGF-I that might contribute to bone loss and a decrease in lean body mass. Growth hormone supplementation for 6 mo in a group of elderly healthy men was found to cause a 1.6% increase in lumbar vertebral bone density, but no change at cortical sites compared with controls, and was associated with an increase in lean body mass and skin thickness and a decrease in adipose tissue mass *(82)*. A similar 6-mo study of growth hormone in healthy elderly females failed to show changes in lean body mass, but showed increased markers of bone turnover. Bone density of the hip and spine was unchanged compared with a small decline in the placebo group. The use of growth hormone in these subjects was associated with bothersome side effects, including fluid retention and carpal tunnel syndrome *(83)*. The lack of substantial effects on bone mass and the side effects associated with the systemic effects of growth hormone treatment make it unlikely that this treatment alone will be an effective therapy for osteoporosis, although it might be useful in association with other pharmacologic agents.

3.4.5. OTHER DRUGS UNDER INVESTIGATION

Many other pharmacologic agents not generally available are currently under preliminary investigation for the treatment of osteoporosis. Skeletal growth factors, such as the IGFs, transforming growth factor β, fibroblast growth factors, platelet-derived growth factors, bone morphogenetic proteins, and cytokines of the hematological and immune systems are secreted in multiple tissues, including bone cells *(80,84)*. They have complex local effects on bone formation and resorption, and may be further regulated by systemic hormones, such as estrogen. Clinical studies of these agents are limited. IGF-I was given to postmenopausal women in a short-term study and increased markers of bone turnover and was associated with orthostatic hypotension, edema, and other side effects at higher doses *(85)*. As with growth hormone, the multiple effects of IGF-I on different tissues will probably limit its systemic administration as a viable treatment for osteoporosis, although it is possible that a certain low dose may be found with specific effects on bone.

Another experimental approach is to stimulate synthesis of the skeletal growth factors locally and specifically in bone. This approach would theoretically limit systemic side effects. The actions of estrogen and anabolic steroids may be at least partially mediated by such effects. Another example of this approach is the intermittent parenteral administration of parathyroid hormone (PTH). Although grossly and tonically elevated levels of PTH are associated with increased bone resorption and hypercalcemia in primary hyperparathyroidism, the intermittent administration of low-dose PTH stimulates increased bone formation that may be mediated by local increased production of skeletal growth factors *(80)*. Most of the experience with this agent has been using the 1–34 fragment of human PTH (PTH[1–34]) in small, uncontrolled trials *(71)*. These studies generally show an increase in normal quality cancellous bone, but concerns about loss of cortical bone during treatment and a waning of the positive effect on cancellous bone over time may limit the use of PTH(1–34) monotherapy *(71)*. Preliminary results from a placebo-controlled trial of PTH(1–34) in postmenopausal osteoporotic women treated with estrogen did reveal a 10.1% increase in lumbar spine bone density after 18 mo of treatment, compared with no change in the placebo group or in the bone density of cortical sites *(86)*. In another controlled study, 20 women with hypogonadism as a result of gonadotropin-releasing hormone treatment for endometriosis were treated with PTH(1–34) for 6 mo and maintained lumbar spine bone density compared with a control group who lost bone mass *(87)*. Thus, PTH(1–34) may be useful for prevention of cancellous bone loss in both estrogen-replete and deficient patients. Concerns still remain regarding the potential effects on cortical bone and need for parenteral administration, and there are no data regarding fracture incidence. Larger, placebo-controlled trials are required for full evaluation of this promising therapy, as well as the related hormone PTHrP.

A large number of other pharmacologic agents are in even earlier stages of testing in the prevention and treatment of osteoporosis. These include $KHCO_3$, which may affect bone turnover by its action on Ca and P balance *(88)*, the flavenoids, such as ipriflavone *(89,90)*, strontium *(71)*, the bioactive peptide echistatin *(91)*, the nonsteroidal anti-inflammatory drug diclofenac sodium *(92)*, silicon-containing compounds, such as the zeolites *(71)*, cytokine antagonists *(84)*, and more bone-specific estrogen agonists, such as raloxifene *(93)*. There are few clinical data on these compounds in well-controlled studies, but their use either as single agents or in combination with other drugs active on bone metabolism appears promising.

4. GUIDELINES FOR USE OF DRUG THERAPY

Given the efficacy of estrogen in increasing vertebral and hip bone density and decreasing fractures at these sites, as well as the additional cardiovascular and quality of life benefits, hormone replacement therapy should be considered in all postmenopausal women with established osteoporosis, osteoporosis, or osteopenia *(1,2,6)*. For each patient, the decision regarding whether to use hormone replacement therapy should be an individual one, considering risks and benefits. The average wholesale price of a 3-mo supply of conjugated estrogen (as Premarin 0.625 mg daily) and medroxyprogesterone (2.5 mg daily) is \$62 *(36)*. In patients declining or not considered candidates for hormone replacement therapy, decisions concerning treatment with other drugs will depend on the severity of bone loss and presence of fracture *(8)*. Guidelines are currently being formulated. All patients with any degree of bone loss, particularly the elderly and those in northern climates, should receive at least 400 U of vitamin D daily. Thiazide diuretics should be considered in patients with hypertension or hypercalciuria. In those patients presenting with acute vertebral fracture and pain, nasal salmon calcitonin may be used for 1–3 mo prior to or in addition to other pharmacologic therapy for its analgesic effects, as well as positive effects on vertebral bone density. The additional cost may be offset by savings from decreased length of hospitalization and rehabilitation, and earlier return to normal function.

Patients with established osteoporosis should receive pharmacologic therapy. The nonhormonal treatments most effective in increasing vertebral and hip bone density are alendronate and slow-release sodium fluoride. The future use of these drugs will depend on well-controlled studies demonstrating comparative efficacy in preventing vertebral and hip fractures, as well as cost. The efficacy of combination treatment using alendronate and hormone replacement therapy is currently under investigation and studies investigating combination treatment with slow-release sodium fluoride would be of interest. Concerns about the bisphosphonates include the potential for side effects given the long half-life in bone and the inconvenience of administration on an empty stomach. Concerns about the use of slow-release sodium fluoride in patients with established osteoporosis relate to its lack of efficacy in preventing recurrent vertebral fractures *(57)*, and its use in patients with severe osteoporosis with multiple compression fractures should probably be limited until more data are available. If a bisphosphonate or slow-release sodium fluoride is not indicated or tolerated, such as in patients with active gastrointestinal disease or renal insufficiency, nasal salmon calcitonin should be considered, given its efficacy in increasing vertebral bone density in women more than 5 yr postmenopausal, its potential fracture efficacy, and its long safety record. Concerns about nasal calcitonin include the long-term effectiveness of this drug and its lack of benefit in some studies. The only direct comparison of a bisphosphonate vs nasal salmon calcitonin revealed that 10 mg of alendronate given daily increased lumbar spine bone density 4.7% and femoral neck bone density 3.1% compared with no effect of 100 IU nasal calcitonin given daily, relative to placebo *(94)*. However, this dose of nasal calcitonin may have been suboptimal *(24)*.

Treatment of patients with osteoporosis, but without fracture is not as clear. Given the lack of long-term data and cost–benefit analyses, guidelines are not currently available. There are also few data on the effect of these drugs on quality of life, which may be an important determinant in drug selection *(95)*. Nonpharmacologic intervention, including nutrition and exercise counseling, psychosocial support, and fall prevention, should be considered in every patient. There are 12–17 million postmenopausal women in the US with osteopenia and 6–7 million with osteoporosis by World Health Organization definitions *(96)*. Major issues in developing cost-effective guidelines for treatment are: At what bone density should preventive, nonhormonal therapy be instituted at the menopause *(97)*? What is the value of screening elderly women? Since hip fractures have the greatest cost, given the increasing evidence that pharmacologic treatment decreases hip fracture risk, it has been suggested that the elderly be aggressively screened and treated *(98)*.

There are also numerous issues related to following patients on drug treatment, including compliance, drug efficacy, and duration of treatment. The use of bone markers and followup bone density studies has been suggested in order to make these decisions. Bone markers are not yet a cost-effective, specific approach for decision making in individual patients *(9)*. Followup bone density determinations at 1–2 yr intervals are reasonable for following effects of drug treatment given the multiple choices for therapy now available and the possible variabilities of response to specific agents in any individual patient. Specific guidelines concerning frequency and sites to measure are not yet available.

Primary care physicians are well positioned to diagnose osteoporosis and osteopenia, institute nonpharmacologic prevention and treatment, and discuss the risks and benefits of hormone replacement therapy and other drugs. However, currently few primary care physicians even treat with hormone replacement therapy for osteoporosis *(99)*, so that further physician education will be important. For complex patients, diagnostic issues, patients intolerant of drugs, or those patients requiring extra time, subspecialty consultations should be considered.

This is an exciting time for patients with osteoporosis and for those physicians with an interest in the prevention and treatment of osteoporosis, since we now have accurate tools to measure bone loss and many new available and investigational treatment modalities.

REFERENCES

1. Recker RR. Current therapy for osteoporosis. *J Clin Endocrinol Metab* 1993; 76: 14–16.
2. Consensus Development Conference: diagnosis, prophylaxis, and treatment of osteoporosis. *Am J Med* 1993; 94: 646–650.
3. Rodan GA. Emerging therapies in osteoporosis. *Ann Rep Med Chem* 1994; 29: 275–285.
4. Reginster JY. Treatment of bone in elderly subjects: calcium, vitamin D, fluor, bisphosphonates, calcitonin. *Horm Res* 1995; 43: 83–88.
5. Cooper C, Kanis JA, Compston J. How to assess drug efficacy in osteoporosis. *Lancet* 1995; 345: 743–744.
6. Riggs BL, Melton LJ III. The prevention and treatment of osteoporosis. *N Engl J Med* 1992; 327: 620–627.
7. Civitelli R, Gonnelli S, Zacchei F, et al. Bone turnover or postmenopausal osteoporosis. Effect of calcitonin treatment. *J Clin Invest* 1988; 82: 1268–1274.
8. Kleerekoper M. Extensive personal experience: the clinical evaluation and management of osteoporosis. *J Clin Endocrinol Metab* 1995; 80: 757–763.

9. Eriksen EF, Brixen K, Charles P. New markers of bone metabolism: clinical use in metabolic bone disease. *Eur J Endocrinol* 1995; 132: 251–263.

10. World Health Organization. Assessment of fracture risk and its application to screening for postmeno-pausal osteoporosis. Technical Report Series WHO, Geneva 1994.

11. Melton LJ III, Atkinson EJ, O'Fallon WM, et al. Long-term fracture prediction by bone mineral assessed at different skeletal sites. *J Bone Miner Res* 1993; 8: 1227–1233.

12. Silman AJ. The patient with fracture: the risk of subsequent fracture. *Am J Med* 1995; 98 (suppl 2A): 12S–16S.

13. McDermott MT, Kidd GS. The role of calcitonin in the development and treatment of osteoporosis. *Endocr Rev* 1987; 8: 377–390.

14. Carstens JH Jr, Feinblatt JD. Future horizons for calcitonin: a U.S. perspective. *Calcif Tissue Int* 1991; 49 (suppl 2): S2–S6.

15. Reginster JY. Effect of calcitonin on bone mass and fracture rates. *Am J Med* 1991; 91 (suppl 5B): 19S–22S.

16. Avioli LV. Calcitonin in the prevention and therapy of osteoporotic syndromes. *Endocr Pract* 1995; 1: 33–38.

17. Gruber HE, Ivey JL, Baylink DJ, et al. Long-term calcitonin therapy in postmenopausal women. *Metabolism* 1984; 33: 295–303.

18. Gennari C, Chierichetti SM, Bigazzi S, et al. Comparative effects on bone mineral content of calcium and calcium plus salmon calcitonin given in two different regimens in postmenopausal osteoporosis. *Curr Ther Res* 1985; 38: 455–464.

19. Mazzuoli GF, Passeri M, Gennari C, et al. Effects of salmon calcitonin in postmenopausal osteoporosis: a controlled double-blind clinical study. *Calcif Tissue Int* 1986; 38: 3–8.

20. Overgaard K, Riis BJ, Christiansen C, et al. Effects of salcatonin given intranasally on early postmeno-pausal bone loss. *BMJ* 1989; 299: 477–479.

21. Overgaard K. Effect of intranasal salmon calcitonin therapy on bone mass and bone turnover in early postmenopausal women: a dose-response study. *Calcif Tissue Int* 1994; 56: 82–86.

22. Reginster JY, Meurmans L, Deroisy R, et al. A 5-year controlled randomized study of prevention of postmenopausal trabecular bone loss with nasal salmon calcitonin and calcium. *Eur J Clin Invest* 1994; 24: 565–569.

23. Lyritis GP, Magiasis B, Tsakalakos N. Prevention of bone loss; in early nonsurgical and nonosteoporotic high turnover patients with salmon calcitonin: the role of biochemical bone markers in monitoring high turnover patients under calcitonin treatment. *Calcif Tissue Int* 1995; 56: 38–41.

24. Reginster JY, Deroisy R, Lecart MP, et al. A double-blind, placebo-controlled, dose-finding trial of intermittent nasal calcitonin for prevention of postmenopausal lumbar spine bone loss. *Am J Med* 1995; 98: 452–458.

25. Overgaard K, Riis BJ, Christiansen C, et al. Nasal calcitonin for treatment of established osteoporosis. *Clin Endocrinol* 1989; 30: 435–442.

26. Overgaard K, Hansen MA, Jensen SB, et al. Effect of salcatonin given intranasally on bone mass and fracture rates in established osteoporosis: a dose-response study. *BMJ* 1992; 305: 556–561.

27. Campodarve I, Drinkwater BL, Insogna KL, et al. Intranasal salmon calcitonin (INSC) 50–200 IU does not prevent bone loss in early postmenopausal women. 1994; *J Bone Miner Res* 9 (suppl 1): S391 (abstract).

28. Rico H, Hernandez ER, Revilla M, et al. Salmon calcitonin reduces vertebral fracture rate in postmeno-pausal crush fracture syndrome. *Bone Miner* 1992; 16: 131–138.

29. Rico H, Revilla M, Hernandez ER, et al. Total and regional bone mineral content and fracture rate in postmenopausal osteoporosis treated with salmon calcitonin: a prospective study. *Calcif Tissue Int* 1995; 56: 181–185.

30. Kanis JA, Johnell O, Gullberg B, et al. Evidence for efficacy of drugs affecting bone metabolism in preventing hip fracture. *BMJ* 1992; 305: 1124–1128.

31. Wimalawansa SJ. Long- and short-term side effects and safety of calcitonin in man: a prospective study. *Calcif Tissue Int* 1993; 52: 90–93.

32. Wallach S, Farley JR, Baylink DJ, et al. Effects of calcitonin on bone quality and osteoblastic function. *Calcif Tissue Int* 1993; 52: 335–339.

33. Reginster JY, Albert A, Lecart MP, et al. 1-year controlled randomized trial of prevention of early postmenopausal bone loss by intranasal calcitonin. *Lancet* 1987; ii: 1481–1483.

34. Lyritis GP, Tsakalakos N, Magiasis B, et al. Analgesic effect of salmon calcitonin in osteoporotic vertebral fractures: a double-blind placebo-controlled clinical study. *Calcif Tissue Int* 1991; 49: 369–372.

35. Pun KK, Chan LWL. Analgesic effect of intranasal salmon calcitonin in the treatment of osteoporotic vertebral fractures. *Clin Ther* 1989; 11 : 205–209.

36. Drug Topics Red Book 1995; Medical Economics, Montvale, NJ.

37. Lombardi A, Santora AC. Clinical trials with bisphosphonates. *Bone Miner* 1993; 22 (suppl): S59–S70.

38. Ott S. Clinical effects of bisphosphonates in involutional osteoporosis. *J Bone Miner Res* 1993; 8 (suppl 2): S597–S606.

39. Fleisch H. New bisphosphonates in osteoporosis. *Osteoporosis Int* 1993; 2 (suppl): S15-S22.

40. Compston JE. The therapeutic use of bisphosphonates. *BMJ* 1994; 309: 711–715.

41. Bijvoet OLM, Valkema R, Lowik CWGM, et al. Bisphosphonates in osteoporosis? *Osteoporosis Int* 1993; 1 (suppl): S230–S236.

42. Storm T, Thamsborg G, Steiniche T, et al. Effect of intermittent cyclinical etidronate therapy on bone mass and fracture rate in women with postmenopausal osteoporosis. *N Engl J Med* 1990; 322: 1265–1271.

43. Storm T, Steiniche T, Thamsborg G, et al. Changes in bone histomorphometry after long-term treatment with intermittent, cyclic etidronate for postmenopausal osteoporosis. *J Bone Miner Res* 1993; 8: 199–208.

44. Watts NB, Harris ST, Genant HK, et al. Intermittent cyclical etidronate treatment of postmenopausal osteoporosis. *N Engl J Med* 1990; 327: 73–79.

45. Ott SM, Woodson GC, Huffer WE, et al. Bone histomorphometric change after cyclic therapy with phosphate and etidronate disodium in women with postmenopausal osteoporosis. *J Clin Endocrinol Metab* 1994; 78: 968–972.

46. Harris ST, Watts NB, Jackson RD, et al. Four-year study of intermittent cyclic etidronate treatment of postmenopausal osteoporosis. Three years of blinded therapy followed by one year of open therapy. *Am J Med* 1993; 95: 557–567.

47. Kanis JA, Gertz BJ, Singer F, et al. Rationale for the use of alendronate in osteoporosis. *Osteoporosis Int* 1995; 5: 1–13.

48. Chesnut CH III, McClung MR, Ensrud KE, et al. Alendronate treatment of the postmenopausal osteoporotic woman: effect of multiple dosages on bone mass and bone remodeling. *Am J Med* 1995; 99: 144–152.

49. Seeman E, Nagant de Deuxchaisnes C, Meunier P, et al. Treatment of postmenopausal osteoporosis with oral alendronate. *Bone* 1995; 16 (suppl 1): 120S (abstract).

50. Liberman UA, Weiss SR, Broll J, et al. Effect of alendronate on bone mineral density and the incidence of fractures in postmenopausal osteoporosis. *N Engl J Med* 1995; 1437–1443.

51. Balena R, Toolan BC, Shea M, et al. The effects of 2-year treatment with the aminobisphosphonate alendronate on bone metabolism, bone histomorphometry, and bone strength in ovariectomized non-human primates. *J Clin Invest* 1993; 92: 2577–2586.

52. Reginster JY, Deroisy R, Denis D, et al. Prevention of postmenopausal bone loss by tiludronate. *Lancet* 1989; ii: 1469–1471.

53. Reid IR, Wattie DJ, Evans MC, et al. Continuous therapy with pamidronate, a potent bisphosphonate, in postmenopausal osteoporosis. *J Clin Endocrinol Metab* 1994; 79: 1595–1599.

54. Riggs BL, Hodgson SF, O'Fallon WM, et al. Effect of fluoride treatment on the fracture rate in post-menopausal women with osteoporosis. *N Engl J Med* 1990; 322: 822–809.

55. Kleerekoper M, Peterson EL, Nelson DA, et al. A randomized trial of sodium fluoride as a treatment for postmenopausal osteoporosis. *Osteoporosis Int* 1991; 1: 155–161.

56. Riggs BL, O'Fallon WM, Lane A, et al. Clinical trial of fluoride therapy in postmenopausal osteoporotic women: extended observations and additional analysis. *J Bone Miner Res* 1994; 9: 265–275.

57. Pak CYC, Sakhaee K, Adams-Huet B, et al. Treatment of postmenopausal osteoporosis with slow-release sodium fluoride. *Ann Int Med* 1995; 123: 401–408.

58. Love RR, Mazess RB, Barden HS, et al. Effects of tamoxifen on bone mineral density in postmenopausal women with breast cancer. *N Engl J Med* 1992; 326: 852–856.

59. Ward RL, Morgan G, Dalley D, et al. Tamoxifen reduces bone turnover and prevents lumbar spine and proximal femoral bone loss in early postmenopausal women. *Bone Miner* 1993; 22: 87–94.

60. Wasnich RD, Benfante RJ, Yano K, et al. Thiazide effect on the mineral content of bone. *N Engl J Med* 1983; 309: 344–347.

61. Cauley JA, Cummings SR, Seeley DG, et al. Effects of thiazide diuretic therapy on bone mass, fractures, and falls. *Ann Int Med* 1993; 118: 666–673.

62. LaCroix AZ, Weinpahl J, White LR, et al. Thiazide diuretic agents and the incidence of hip fracture. *N Engl J Med* 1990; 322: 286–290.

63. Heidrich FE, Stergachis A, Gross KM. Diuretic drug use and the risk for hip fracture. *Ann Int Med* 1991; 115: 1–6.

64. Jones G, Nguyen T, Sambrook ON, et al. Thiazide diuretics and fractures: can meta analysis help? *J Bone Miner Res* 1995; 10: 106–111.

65. Chapuy MC, Arlot ME, Duboeuf F, et al. Vitamin D_3 and calcium to prevent hip fractures in elderly women. *N Engl J Med* 1992; 327: 1637–1642.

66. Gallagher JC, Jerpbak CM, Jee WSS, et al. 1,25-dihydroxyvitamin D_3: short- and long-term effects on bone and calcium metabolism in patients with postmenopausal osteoporosis. *Proc Natl Acad Sci USA* 1982; 79: 3325–3329.

67. Riggs BL, Nelson KI. Effect of long term treatment with calcitriol on calcium absorption and mineral metabolism in postmenopausal osteoporosis. *J Clin Endocrinol Metab* 1985; 61: 457–461.

68. Aloia JF, Vaswani A, Yeh JK, et al. Calcitriol in the treatment of postmenopausal osteoporosis. *Am J Med* 1988; 84: 401–408.

69. Gallagher JC, Goldgar D. Treatment of postmenopausal osteoporosis with high doses of synthetic calcitriol. *Ann Int Med* 1990; 113: 649–655.

70. Ott SM, Chesnut CH III. Calcitriol treatment is not effective in postmenopausal osteoporosis. *Ann Int Med* 1989; 110: 267–274.

71. Tilyard MW, Spears GFS, Thornson J, et al. Treatment of postmenopausal osteoporosis with calcitriol or calcium. *N Engl J Med* 1992; 326: 357–362.

72. Orimo H, Shiraki M, Hayashi Y, et al. Effects of 1α-hydroxyvitamin D_3 on lumbar bone mineral density and vertebral fractures in patients with postmenopausal osteoporosis. *Calcif Tissue Int* 1994; 54: 370–376.

73. Falch JA, Odegaard OR, Finnanger AM, et al. Postmenopausal osteoporosis: no effect of three years treatment with 1,25-dihydroxycholecalciferol. *Acta Med Scand* 1987; 221: 199–204.

74. Gallagher JC. Prevention of bone loss in postmenopausal and senile osteoporosis with vitamin D analogues. *Osteoporosis Int* 1993; 1 (suppl): S172–S175.

75. Riggs BL. Formation-stimulating regimens other than sodium flouride. *Am J Med* 1993; 95 (suppl 5A): 62S–68S.

76. Chesnut CH III , Nelp WB, Baylink DJ, et al. Effect of methandrostenolone on postmenopausal bone wasting as assessed by changes in total bone mineral mass. *Metabolism* 1977; 26: 267–277.

77. Chesnut CH III, Ivey JL, Gruber HE, et al. Stanozolol in postmenopausal osteoporosis: therapeutic efficacy and possible mechanisms of action. *Metabolism* 1983; 32: 571–580.

78. Geusens P, Dequeker J. Long-term effect of nandrolone decanoate, 1 hydroxyvitamin D_3 or intermittent calcium infusion therapy on bone mineral content, bone remodeling and fracture rate in symptomatic osteoprosis: a double-blind controlled study. *Bone Miner* 1986; 1: 347–357.

79. Passeri M, Pedrazzoni M, Pioli G, et al. Effects of nandralone decanoate on bone mass in established osteoporosis. *Maturitas* 1993; 17: 211–219.

80. Canalis E. Growth hormone, skeletal growth factors and osteoporosis. *Endocr Pract* 1995; 1: 39–43.

81. O'Halloran DJ, Tsatsoulis A, Whithouse RW, et al. Increased bone density after recombinant human growth hormone (GH) therapy in adults with isolated GH deficiency. *J Clin Endocrinol Metab* 1993; 76: 1344–1348.

82. Rudman D, Feller AG, Nagraj HS, et al. Effects of growth hormone in men over 60 years old. *N Engl J Med* 1990; 323: 1–6.

83. Holloway L, Butterfield G, Hintz FL, Gesundheit N, Marcus R. Effects of recombinant human growth hormone on metabolic indices, body composition, and bone turnover in healthy elderly women. *J Clin Endocrinol Metab* 1994; 79: 470–479.

84. Manolagas SC, Jilka RL. Bone marrow, cytokines, and bone remodeling. *N Engl J Med* 1995; 332: 305–311.

85. Ebeling PR, Jones JD, O'Fallon WM, et al. Short-term effects of recombinant human insulin-like growth factor I on bone turnover in normal women. *J Clin Endocrinol Metab* 1993; 77: 1384–1387.

86. Lindsay R, Cosman F, Nieves J, et al. A controlled clinical trial of the effects of 1–34 h PTH in estrogen treated osteoporotic women. *J Bone Miner Res* 1993; 8 (suppl 1): S130.

87. Finkelstein JS, Klibanski A, Schaefer EH, et al. Parathyroid hormone for the prevention of bone loss induced by estrogen deficiency. *N Engl J Med* 1994; 331: 1618–1623.

88. Sebastian A, Harris ST, Ottaway JH, et al. Improved mineral balance and skeletal metabolism in post-menopausal women treated with potassium bicarbonates *N Engl J Med* 1994; 330: 1776–1781.

89. Brandi ML. New treatment strategies: ipriflavone, strontium, vitamin D metabolites and analogs. *Am J Med* 1995 (suppl 5A): 69–74.

90. Maugeri D, Panebianco P, Russo MS, et al. Ipriflavone-treatment of senile osteoporosis: results of a multicenter, double-blind clinical trial of 2 years. *Arch Gerontol Geriatr* 1994; 19: 253–263.

91. Oursler MJ. Echistatin, a potential new drug for osteoporosis. *Endocrinology* 1993; 132: 939–940 (editorial).

92. Bell NH, Hollis BW, Shary JR, et al. Diclofenac sodium inhibits bone resorption in postmenopausal women. *Am J Med* 1994; 96: 349–353.

93. Black LJ, Sato M, Rowley ER, et al. Raloxifene (LY 139481 HC1) prevents bone loss and reduces serum cholesterol without causing uterine hypertrophy in ovariectomized rats. *J Cin Invest* 1994; 93: 63–69.

94. Adami S, Baroni MC, Broggini M, et al. Treatment of postmenopausal osteoporosis with continuous daily oral alendronate in comparison with either placebo or intranasal salmon calcitonin. *Osteoporosis Int* 1993; 3 (suppl): 21–27.

95. McClung MR, Love B, Rosen CT, et al. Evaluation of a new osteoporosis quality of life questionnaire (OQLQ) for women with osteoporosis and back pain. *J Bone Miner Res* 1995; 10 (suppl 1): S255.

96. Looker AC, Johnston Jr CC, Wahner HW, et al. Prevalence of low femoral bone density in older US women from NHANES III. *J Bone Miner Res* 1995; 10: 796–802.

97. Christiansen C. What should be done at the time of menopause? *Am J Med* 1995; 98 (suppl 2A): 56S–59S.

98. Kanis JA. Treatment of osteoporosis in elderly women. *Am J Med* 1995; 98 (suppl 2A): 60S–66S.

99. Grisso JA, Baum CR, Turner BJ. What do physicians in practice do to prevent osteoporosis? *J Bone Miner Res* 1990; 5: 213–219.

16 Nonpharmacologic Therapy for Osteoporosis

Michael R. McClung, MD, FACE and Kristi Spencer, PT

1. INTRODUCTION

Osteoporosis is a disorder of skeletal fragility. Fractures are the complications of osteoporosis that result in the patient's symptoms, and their physical, functional, and psychosocial problems. The primary objectives in the management of patients with established osteoporosis are the following:

1. Prevent new fractures
   a. Preserve or increase bone mass
   b. Prevent falls and injuries;
2. Minimize acute and chronic symptoms; and
3. Improve physical and psychologic function.

We have an expanding set of effective pharmacologic options to prevent bone loss and to reduce the incidence of fractures. However, with the possible exception of the use of calcitonin in the treatment of patients with acute fractures, there is no basis on which to expect pharmacologic therapy to accomplish the other therapeutic objectives. In a comprehensive management program, the prevention of injuries and falls, the control of symptoms, and the attempt to improve the patient's function are best accomplished by a structured program of exercise and education. Collaboration between a physician and a physical therapist experienced in treating patients with osteoporosis is a model with

From: *Osteoporosis: Diagnostic and Therapeutic Principles*
Edited by: C. J. Rosen Humana Press Inc., Totowa, NJ

which we have had several years' experience. This chapter will discuss our physical therapy intervention program for patients with osteoporosis, including the role of weight-bearing exercises, education in posture, body mechanics and fall prevention, the rehabilitation of patients following fractures of the spine and hip, and the management of chronic back pain in patients who have experienced vertebral fractures.

EXERCISE

That exercise is an important determinant of skeletal health is widely believed by clinicians and the general public. Weight-bearing exercise is always included as one of the most important steps to be taken by postmenopausal women for the prevention of bone loss. However, the data on which this recommendation is made is relatively weak. The original notion that weight-bearing is a determinant of skeletal health came from observing the rapid and marked bone loss in immobilized individuals or in the weightless environment of space. Subsequent studies comparing athletes and sedentary adults have demonstrated that bone mass is almost always higher in athletes, sometimes as much as 20–30% (1). This difference is certainly of clinical significance. The results comparing athletes to sedentary controls may be owing either to sampling bias (perhaps persons with stronger bones are better athletes) or to the fact that most athletes begin their physical training during their growth years when bone mass can be substantially influenced by exercise. Certainly, physical activity during childhood and adolescence can be a factor in maximizing the growth potential of bone during those years. It is also true that physical activity is one of the important correlates if not determinants of bone mass in the proximal femur in young adults (2). In both young adults and postmenopausal women, statistical correlation between muscle mass or muscle strength and bone density has been observed.

Despite these observations, the association of physical activity with bone health in older adults or in patients with osteoporosis is less clear and less convincing. Walking is frequently recommended as the safest and most practical weight-bearing activity for older adults. While aerobic exercise such as walking will increase endurance, most studies have shown no or only weak correlations between measures of cardiovascular fitness and bone density in older adults (3). In a prospective study, a program of brisk walking did not slow bone loss in postmenopausal women (4). Other studies have confirmed that exercise is not capable of preventing bone loss in early menopause, which is a result of estrogen deficiency (5). In a study by Sinaki in osteoporotic women, strengthening of extensor back musculature was not accompanied by increased spinal bone density (6). Weight lifting and resistance exercises result in greater loading of the spine than does walking. In an intense program of weight-bearing exercise combining walking, jogging, and resistance exercises to strengthen the back, lumbar spine density increased by 6.1% after about two years (7). After returning to their pre-exercise program activity for 13 mo, the average spinal bone density value was only 1.1% higher than baseline. Thus, a combination of weight-bearing activities may be able to increase bone mass modestly or perhaps to slow the process of age-related bone loss, but the exercises must be both intense and sustained for those objectives to be accomplished. Such a program is probably not acceptable or practical for most adults and may be fraught with risk in the frail elderly.

That the skeletal effects of low-to-moderate levels of exercise in adults is at best modest does not detract from the importance of exercise in the therapeutic plan for patients with or at risk for osteoporosis. Both the strength and level of physical activity are important risk factors for fractures, independent of bone density. Even modest exercise is associated with improvements in many of the parameters that characteristically decline with aging (8). These benefits include increased muscle strength of the back, buttocks, and legs, better balance, greater endurance, improved functional ability, decreased injury potential, and increased sense of well being.

Regarding the role of exercise in the prevention and treatment of osteoporosis, these conclusions can be drawn:

1. Physical activity during growth years helps maximize peak bone mass potential.
2. Exercise is not a substitute for estrogen or other antiresorptive therapy in preventing bone loss in postmenopausal women.
3. While exercise may slow age-related bone loss in older individuals, the major target of an exercise program should not be the skeleton. Rather, the objectives of this program for patients with osteoporosis are to increase strength, decrease the risk of falling, retard the infirmity and frailty (which characterizes advancing age), minimize symptoms, and enhance both function and quality of life.
4. An exercise program for older adults must be practical and individualized. Each patient must be adequately educated regarding the value and intent of the exercise program, and the program must address functional targets that the patients themselves help identify. Physicians are often poorly equipped to either prescribe an appropriate exercise program or to instruct patients in its use. This is an area where other health professionals such as physical therapists, nurses, and health educators can be of special value to our practice.

3. INJURY PREVENTION

While low bone mass, usually assessed by low bone density, is the major determinant of fracture risk, extraskeletal factors also play important roles. Indeed, there is a very large overlap in the bone density values of persons who have fractures compared to those of similar age who have not fractured. This suggests that factors such as injuries, the frequency and severity of falls, the manner of falling, and patients' ability to protect themselves from the impact of falls are important determinants of whether a fracture occurs. By age 75, most women and many men have experienced age-related bone loss to the extent they are at risk for fractures with only minor injury. Current pharmacologic and nutritional therapy may prevent the progression of bone loss and decrease the incidence of hip fractures in patients with osteoporosis, but we are not yet capable of correcting the quantitative and qualitative deficits in osteoporotic bone. Consequently, patients with osteoporosis will remain at increased risk for fracture even if pharmacologic therapy is initiated. Appropriate management of patients with osteoporosis needs to include attempts to reduce the important injury component to fracture risk since one of our major therapeutic goals is to decrease the incidence of new fractures.

Because hip fractures are almost always acute events requiring hospitalization, factors that predispose an individual to fracture are better understood with respect to hip fracture than with other fractures. In the Study of Osteoporotic Fractures, the most important risk fractures for hip fracture were low BMD and factors known to enhance the frequency of falls (including weakness, physical inactivity, and therapy with sedative drugs) (9). In addition, other factors, such as a history of previous hip fracture or a maternal history of hip fracture, were found to be important determinants of fracture risk. This information confirmed the important relationship between falls and fractures. Indeed, more than 90%

of hip fractures are associated with falls, as are virtually all Colles' fractures. The role of injury as a proximate cause of spinal fractures is less clear; vertebral fractures are usually described as being nontraumatic. However, Cooper described 335 men and women who experienced vertebral fractures that led to medical attention (10). He noted that 47 (14%) were related to severe trauma, and 276 (82%) were associated with mild-to-moderate injury. The remainder were classified as pathologic fractures. It is our experience, too, that most patients who present with an acute vertebral fracture will associate it with some traumatic episode, most commonly a fall or a lifting injury. Strategies to minimize injury are important considerations in the management of patients with osteoporosis.

Several studies have identified the factors associated with the risk of falling (11–15). The most important of these include impairments of strength, gait, balance, mobility, or vision. Recognizing these risk factors provides strategies for intervention. These fall into three major categories:

1. Exercises to promote strength, improve balance and gait;
2. Correction of age or disease-related problems affecting balance such as orthostatic hypotension, sedative drugs including alcohol; and
3. The provision of ambulatory supports such as hand rails (on stairs, in the bathroom), walkers, or canes.

While exercise programs do result in improved strength, flexibility, and functional performances, the effects of these changes on the frequency or response to fractures has not yet been carefully evaluated. It is our opinion that such exercise programs are indicated for the frail elderly who are at the greatest risk of falling as well as for healthy individuals in whom we attempt to prevent the functional deficits that accompany aging.

Environmental hazards are frequently identified as important factors affecting fracture risk. Most falls, though, are not related to such hazards, and aggressive attempts to remove such hazards from the home environment have not significantly reduced the risk of falls (16).

Since only 2% of falls results in fractures in older people, it is clear that factors other than low bone density and fall frequency are determinants of fracture risk. Cummings and Nevitt described four factors that must be present for a fall to result in a hip fracture:

1. Fall must result in landing on or near the hip;
2. Patient's protective measures must be inadequate to lessen the impact of the fall;
3. Local shock absorbers (clothing, adipose tissue, surface onto which the fall occurs) must inadequately absorb enough energy to prevent injury; and
4. Bone strength in the proximal femur must be insufficient to resist the damage from the residual energy (17).

There is recent research regarding the nature of and mechanics of falls that are most apt to result in fracture, and we may soon be able to use this information for fracture prevention (18).

From a practical standpoint, we acknowledge that bone mass deficit in osteoporotic patients cannot be corrected and that all falls will not be prevented. An additional line of defense for hip fracture is to minimize the impact of the fall through the use of cushioning of the landing surface or of the trochanteric region of the patient. Having padded landing surfaces for all falls is impractical; however, there is increased interest in the use of hip pads. In an early study, nursing home residents assigned to wear hip pads had a marked reduction in the frequency of hip fractures (19). In fact, the only hip fractures that occurred in the group assigned to wear hip pads, occurred when they were not wearing them. The design of a comfortable, effective, energy-absorbing protective garment and its use in the frail elderly is a strategy that deserves careful evaluation.

The types of falls most often associated with vertebral fractures are those in which the patient lands on the buttocks. While not carefully assessed, it is probable that factors affecting strength, balance, and gait are also important in the frequency of these type falls. Of special importance for the prevention of vertebral fractures is the avoidance of excessive weight loading of the spine under conditions of flexion or torsion. Lifting a grandchild, a heavy or awkward object, a sack of groceries from the trunk of a car or a garage door are activities that patients who have fractures frequently describe as being associated with acute onset of back pain. These lifting injuries most often cause anterior compression fractures of the thoracic spine, while falls in the seated position most frequently result in central body or crush fractures of the lumbar spine. There have been no studies evaluating the usefulness of therapeutic programs to reduce the frequency of these injuries. However, avoidance of flexion exercises and activities, education about proper body mechanics, and exercises to strengthen the extensor muscles of the back are reasonable strategies to pursue.

4. REHABILITATION AFTER ACUTE FRACTURES

4.1. Vertebral Fracture

Fractures of the vertebral bodies define, in the minds of most patients, the clinical picture of osteoporosis. They are the most common fractures associated with postmenopausal osteoporosis, and they also occur with increased frequency in men with age-related bone loss (20). Most of these fractures are associated with some traumatic event, albeit minor. Some patients with vertebral deformities and fractures never, however, have an episode of acute back pain, and their fractures are discovered only when height loss or radiographic evidence of vertebral deformity is noted.

The symptoms associated with acute vertebral fractures may be mild or quite severe (21). For patients with mild symptoms, often interpreted as only muscle strain, analgesic therapy and nonsteroidal anti-inflammatory drugs coupled with transient limitation of physical activity is often sufficient. More often, patients with acute vertebral fractures experience moderate to severe back pain, which significantly limits their activities. These patients often benefit from a program of pain control measures and education, activity education, and exercises for stretching and gentle strengthening of their back musculature. The patient can be referred to the physical therapist immediately, using home health therapists, if necessary. The therapist can provide education and be a resource in the use of heat, ice, positioning for support, and activity modification for pain control. Recommendations often cover such items as the avoidance of prolonged unsupported sitting or standing, optimal sleeping positions, the use of lumbar supports while sitting, proper body mechanics, and spinal stabilization during daily activities such as getting into and out of bed or a chair and lifting. Although resolution of bone-related pain will not be enhanced by a physical therapy program, early intervention will speed the improvement of paraspinal muscle spasms and the related pain from new strain on segmental soft tissues. Early intervention can also prevent the establishment of chronic soft-tissue dysfunction.

Bedrest for 1–7 d may be necessary for patients with more severe back pain following a fracture, especially if complicated by muscle spasm. Appropriate administration of analgesics is important and should be accompanied by adequate fluid intake and high fiber diet to minimize the occurrence of constipation, which complicates the analgesic therapy. Muscle spasms frequently complicate acute spinal fracture and are often the most difficult part of the acute management. Muscle relaxants are not usually effective in this situation. Local heat or ice packs are often helpful, while electrical stimulation, ultrasound, and massage are salutary for some patients. The purpose of these modalities is to decrease spasms and increase comfort, allowing the patient to perform the necessary exercises. Our experience is that ice and electrical stimulation are often most effective in decreasing the acute spasm cycle, but the other modalities seem to be more helpful in individual cases. The splinting and protective guarding by the muscle spasms, in addition to creating pain, result in decreased trunk motion, particularly rotation, during ambulation and bed mobility. This contributes to decreased tolerance of activity and decreased balance recovery ability when challenged. Exercises such as bringing the knee to the chest can be taught as pain relieving "tools." These are often momentarily but highly effective. Assisted transfer from the bed to a comfortable chair and subsequent support of ambulation should be accomplished as early as possible to avoid the deconditioning that occurs quickly with bedrest. The use of a lumbar support or thoracolumbar corset is often helpful at this stage. The use of a rigid brace may sometimes afford symptomatic relief, but its use should be limited in duration to a maximum of only a few weeks to avoid the loss of muscle strength in the back, for the ultimate goal of management will be to increase muscle strength through an appropriate exercise program. The role of subcutaneous calcitonin for pain relief in this setting of acute vertebral fractures is primarily supported by anecdotal descriptions. Controlled clinical trials do suggest that calcitonin has analgesic properties in some patients *(22,23)*. The intensity of the fracture pain may resolve more quickly with calcitonin therapy, but the ultimate outcome does not seem to be affected.

Flexion activities, especially with thoracic fracture, are to be avoided. Instructions and education regarding appropriate transfer techniques and proper body mechanics should be instituted as the acute symptoms begin to subside and may actually hasten improvement. Ultimately, exercises to stretch and strengthen the spinal extensor muscles are appropriate to bring about the long-term improvement in symptoms and should be started early in the course of therapy. Gentle sustained stretches and slow motions to decrease tightness and muscle spasm reduce the pain level, improve spinal mobility, prevent residual muscle dysfunction, and speed the recovery process. Strengthening the support muscles around the site of the vertebral fracture may begin early, even before the back is pain free. The rhythmical contract–relax cycles of strengthening exercises are also effective in decreasing the frequency and intensity of muscle spasms. The treating physical therapist needs to be savvy in timing the introduction and progression of strengthening exercises, for an exacerbation of symptoms can be easily provoked by a regimen that is too vigorous. As improving symptoms allow, the patient will progress through some or all of the strengthening exercises used in the management of chronic back pain in these patients.

The acute pain for most vertebral fractures related to osteoporosis usually improves within a few days and abates by 6–12 wk. Worsening or persistent pain should increase concern about osteomalacia or pathologic fractures related to malignancy or other medical problems. The management of patients with chronic back pain subsequent to vertebral fractures is discussed later.

4.2. Hip Fractures

While less common than vertebral fracture or Colles' fractures, hip fractures represent the most serious and debilitating consequence of osteoporosis in both men and women. The average age of patients with hip fractures is greater than 75 yr. As a group, these patients are weak, frail, have other age-related illnesses, and may have cognitive defects. The in-hospital mortality following hip fracture is about 6%, and the total excess mortality adjusted for age is 12–20% after 12 mo *(24)*. The incidence of complications following hip fracture is influenced by the patient's age, nature of coexisting medical problems, the level of physical fitness before the fracture, and their psychosocial function and support. Only 12–23% of patients regain their prefracture ambulatory status or functional ability. The occurrence of a hip fracture, then, places intense strain on not only the patient, but his/her family and the entire health system.

The details of a hip fracture rehabilitation program are beyond the scope of this chapter, but have been reviewed by a number of authors *(25)*. In general, the program includes instruction in proper transfer techniques, early ambulation with appropriate supportive devices, exercise to strengthen the muscles about the hip, quadriceps and lower leg, and training and guidance with daily activities such as dressing and bathing. In the current health-care environment with emphasis on short hospital stay, patients are frequently transferred to a nursing home facility to complete their recuperation. It is very important that the rehabilitation program be maintained throughout the recovery phase. The ability to return home and ultimately assume independent living may be related to the completeness and intensity of this postoperative rehabilitative program.

The great majority of patients over the age of 65 who have hip fractures have osteoporosis. Most of those patients have not received pharmacologic therapy for osteoporosis prior to their fracture. The occurrence of any fracture after age 50 is an independent risk factor for a second hip fracture *(9)*. Consequently, patients who have experienced a hip fracture are at quite high risk for having another fracture. A program of rehabilitation following hip fracture is not complete without instituting measures to prevent the progression of bone loss and to minimize the risk of falls, injuries, and future fractures.

5. MANAGEMENT OF CHRONIC SYMPTOMS

After an acute vertebral fracture, many patients experience complete resolution of their back symptoms. Other patients, however, continue to have chronic symptoms, primarily pain associated with activity and maintaining unsupported erect or upright postures *(26–28)*. The cause of this chronic back pain is not well understood and is probably related to multiple factors. Chronic bone tenderness or pain is quite unusual in patients with uncomplicated osteoporosis. Fortunately, nerve compressive syndromes are quite rare in patients with vertebral fractures. Vertebral deformity may result in facet joint arthropathy. Concomitant but unrelated degenerative disk disease may be a major contributor to symptoms in some patients. In our experience, the most common cause of back discomfort is muscle or soft tissue dysfunction related to the vertebral deformities. Most patients experience little or no pain when at rest, either lying in bed or sitting in a supportive chair. When standing or sitting unsupported, pain is experienced over a wide area across the back and is not localized to a discrete area like the pain of an acute fracture. Symptoms are precipitated by activities such as standing in one position for any length of time, particularly if coupled with sustained forward or downward oriented activities such as bending over the stove, sink, or bed to perform regular household chores. These symptoms are usually described as an ache and feeling of tightness across the upper or lower back and/or a burning, painful sensation between the shoulder blades. Unless the activity is curtailed, the intensity of the symptoms continues to increase owing to soft-tissue overload and fatigue. Ultimately, muscle spasm and severe pain occur. The symptoms gradually subside over a few minutes after sitting or lying down. Activities can then be resumed for another, shorter interval of time before symptoms recur.

Tightness and tenderness is frequently observed in the paravertebral muscles of the lower back and in the intrascapular region of these patients. Muscle weakness in older individuals is a common phenomenon. Studies by Sinakai and others have demonstrated that women with osteoporosis have decreased extensor muscle strength in their back compared to age-matched controls *(29)*. Whether this weakness is a characteristic of the patients with osteoporosis or the result of deconditioning of back muscles in patients who have decreased their activity following a vertebral fracture is not clear. This muscle weakness contributes significantly to the back pain experienced by older osteoporotic patients. Decreased strength causes muscle fatigue and aching with only modest activity. These symptoms are often interpreted as being harmful or destructive. Patients then curtail their activity to alleviate the backache. This decreased activity results in progressive muscle weakness and increases susceptibility to muscle fatigue and pain with even less exertion. It is this vicious cycle of weakness causing pain, which contributes to weakness, which must be addressed in the symptomatic management of this group of patients. Prominent kyphosis increases the work of extensor back muscles and decreases the capacity to perform functions requiring forward bending. Individuals who have had vertebral deformity seem to be particularly susceptible to the muscle dysfunction associated with regular daily activities.

The area most affected by chronic pain is typically at or immediately below the apex of the kyphosis because of the increased compensatory forces required. Once chronic, symptoms in the thoracic and lumbar areas are often interrelated. In patients such as these, both regions of the spine need to be addressed, regardless of where the fracture occurred. Goals in the chronic stage are as follows:

1. To decrease or relieve soft tissue pain and postural muscle fatigue;
2. To increase tolerance for daily activities; and
3. To promote or restore an active lifestyle to maintain strength, balance, function, and quality of life.

These goals are accomplished through exercise and education, with the help of an experienced physical therapist.

Patients with symptomatic osteoporosis are usually very motivated and eager to improve and be physically active but are often reluctant to engage in a program of exercise for fear of worsening their symptoms or experiencing a new fracture. Physicians often contribute to that anxiety by prescribing restricted activity. Explanation by the physician about the nature of the symptoms and the rationale of an exercise program are important for the patient's acceptance of the program.

Exercises can be approached more aggressively when the symptoms are chronic. Relief of symptoms results from improved extensor stabilizer strength and endurance and stretching of tightened tissues and joints. We employ exercises aimed at the extensor muscles of the upper, middle, and lower back, similar to a program described by Dr. Sinakai and her colleagues *(30)*. (Examples of these exercises are available in *Boning Up,* a booklet about osteoporosis available from the National Osteoporosis Foundation.) All flexion exercises, particularly those involving flexion of the midthoracic spine, should be avoided *(31)*. Such exercises increase the mechanical strain on the anterior portion of the vertebral body and may increase the occurrence of fractures in patients with severe skeletal fragility. Nonflexion or isometric abdominal strengthening can be used for increased spinal support. Exercise programs may take many forms and may include the use of resistance bands, free weights, Nautilus equipment, and so on. Despite being challenged, patients experiences noticeable improvement from the exercises, which easily motivates them to continue with the program. Designing the exercises to be performed at home or at a fitness center is important. We have also used organized biweekly group exercise classes for these patients, primarily as a means of training them to perform their exercises at home on a regular basis. These group sessions add variety and interest to the exercise regimen and often serve as an important time for socialization. The education and sharing that occur in this setting contribute to the psychosocial support of the patients as discussed in this volume by Love and Overdorf.

Exercises in symptomatic patients need to be done daily and can progress as rapidly as the patient's tolerance allows. Improvement usually begins within a few weeks, sometimes within days. Depending on the level of initial weakness and the presence of complicating factors such as scoliosis or arthritis, 6–12 wk or more of graduated exercises may be needed to accomplish our goals. Ideally, some combination of the exercises will be continued long term to maintain the results.

Education at this stage mainly focuses on the need for continued participation in the exercise activities, on functional body mechanics training, and injury prevention. Other family members may also need information and counseling so that they understand the rationale, objectives, and even the details of the program so as to assist rather than resist the patient's efforts to become more active and to work through her symptoms.

The effects of muscle strengthening programs and rehabilitative programs in patients with osteoporosis have only just begun to be evaluated, but the results described by others are also encouraging *(32,33)*. Additionally, experience with rehabilitation of other groups of elderly individuals lends credence to such an approach. The ability of exercise to improve muscle strength seems to be as good in older women as it is in younger women *(34)*. Furthermore, the intensity of the exercise program does not need to be marked. It is encouraging to note that the gains in muscle strength and endurance achieved with an exercise program can be maintained by short sessions of exercise 2–3 times each week *(35)*.

6. SUMMARY

Osteoporosis is a heterogeneous, multifactorial disease in which fractures occur that impair both function and quality of life in many patients, especially in older individuals. For some patients, the effects of osteoporosis are the most significant factors contributing to physical and psychological decline. With the availability of new diagnostic and therapeutic tools, we are now in a position to prevent osteoporosis and its complications. However, many patients have already experienced bone loss and fractures. For them, strategies of management to minimize the discomfort, to enhance their level of activity and function, and to decrease the risk of further skeletal injury and fracture need to be employed. With the combined efforts of a health-care team, including nurses, physical therapists, and counselors as well as physicians, the quality of life and activity of these patients can be enhanced.

REFERENCES

1. Pirnay F, Bodeux M, Crielaard JM. Bone mineral content and physical activity. *Int J Sports Med* 1987; 8: 331–335.
2. Pocock NA, Eisman JA, Yeates MG, Sambrook PN, Eberl S. Physical fitness is a major determinant of femoral neck and lumbar spine bone mineral density. *J Clin Invest* 1986; 78: 618–621.
3. Dalsky G, Stocke KS, Ehsani AA. Weight-bearing exercise training and lumbar bone mineral content in postmenopausal women. *Ann Int Med* 1988; 108: 824–828.
4. Nelson ME, Fisher EC, Dilmanian FA, Dallal GE, Evans WJ. A 1-year walking program and increased calcium in postmenopausal women: effects on bone. *J Bone Miner Res* 1991; 53: 1304–1311.
5. Prince RL, Smith M, Dick IM, Price RI, Webb PG, Henderson NK, Harris MM. Prevention of postmenopausal osteoporosis: a comparative study of exercise, calcium supplementation, and hormone-replacement therapy. *NEJM* 1991; 325: 1189–1195.
6. Sinaki M, Wahner HW, Offord KP, Hodgson SF. Efficacy of nonloading exercises in prevention of vertebral bone loss in postmenopausal women: a controlled trial. *Mayo Clin Proc* 1989; 6: 762–769.
7. Dalsky GP, Stocke KS, Ersani AA, et al. Weight bearing exercise training and lumbar bone mineral content in postmenopausal women. *Ann Intern Med* 1988; 108: 824–828.
8. Edward K, Larson EB. Benefits of exercise in older adults. *Clin Geriat Med* 1992; 8: 35–113.
9. Cummings SR, Nevitt MC, Browner WS, Stone K, Fox KM, Ensrud KE, Cauley J, Black D, Vogt TM. Risk factors for hip fracture in white women. *NEJM* 1995; 332: 767–773.
10. Cooper C, Atkinson EJ, O'Fallon WM, Melton LJ. Incidence of clinically significant vertebral fractures: a population-based study in Rochester, Minnesota, 1885–1989. *J Bone Miner Res* 1992; 7: 221–227.
11. Tinetti ME, Speechley M, Ginter F. Risk factors for falls among elderly persons living in the community. *N Engl J Med* 1988; 319: 1701–1707.
12. Campbell AJ, Borrie MG, Spears GF. Risk factors for falls in a community-based prospective study of people 70 years old and older. *J Gerontol* 1989; 44: 112–117.
13. Speechley M, Tinetti M. Falls and injuries in frail and vigorous community elderly persons. *J Am Geriat Soc* 1991; 39: 46–52.
14. Grisso JA, Kelsey JL, Strom BL, Chiu GY, Maislin G, O'Brien LA, Hoffman S, Kaplan F. Risk factors for falls as a cause of hip fractures in women. *N Engl J Med* 1991; 324: 1326–1331.
15. Lipsitz LA, Jonsson PV, Kelly MM, Koestner JS. Causes and correlates of recurrent falls in ambulatory frail elderly. *J Gerontol* 1991; 46: M114–M122.
16. Hornbrook MC, Stevens VJ, Wingfield DJ, Hollis JF, Greenlick MR, Ory MG. Preventing falls among community-dwelling older persons: results of a randomized trial. *Gerontologist* 1994; 34: 16–23.
17. Cummings SR, Nevitt MC. A hypothesis: the cause of hip fractures. *J Gerontol* 1989; 44: M107–M111.
18. Hayes WC, Myers ER, Morris JN, Gerhart TN, Yett HS, Lipsitz LA. Impact near the hip dominates fracture risk in elderly nursing home residents who fall. *Calcif Tissue Int* 1993; 52: 192–198.
19. Lauritzen JB, Petersen MM, Lund B. Effect of external hip protectors on hip fractures. *Lancet* 1993; 341: 11–13.
20. Cooper C, Atkinson EJ, Jacobsen SJ, O'Fallon M, Melon L. Population-based study of survival after osteoporotic fractures. *Am J Epidemiol* 1993; 137: 1001–1005.
21. Patel U, Skingle S, Campbell GA, Crisp AJ, Boyle IT. Clinical profile of acute vertebral compression fractures in osteoporosis. *Br J Rheum* 1991; 30: 418–421.
22. Paul KK, Chan LWL. Analgesic effect of intranasal salmon calcitonin in the treatment of osteoporotic vertebral fractures. *Clin Ther* 1989; 11: 205–209.
23. Lyritis GP, Tsakalakos N, Magiasis B, Karachalio T, Viazides A, Tsekoara M. Analgesic effect of salmon calcitonin in osteoporotic vertebral fractures: a double-blind placebo-controlled clinical study. *Calcif Tissue Int* 1991; 49: 369–372.
24. White BL, Fisher WD, Laurin CA. Rate of mortality for elderly patients after fracture of the hip in the 1980. *J Bone Joint Surg* 1987; 69A: 1335–1339.
25. Mehta AJ, Nastasi AE. Rehabilitation of fractures in the elderly. *Clin Geriat Med* 1993; 9: 717–730.
26. Ross PD, Ettinger B, Davis JW, Melon L, Wasnich RD. Evaluation of adverse health outcomes associated with vertebral fractures. *Osteopor Int* 1991; 1: 134–140.

27. Silverman SL. The clinical consequences of vertebral compression fracture. Bone 1992; 13: S27–S31.

28. Lyles KW, Gold DT, Shipp KM, Pieper CF, Martinez S, Mulhausen PL. Association of osteoporotic vertebral compression fractures with impaired functional status. *Am J Med* 1993; 94: 595–601.

29. Sinaki M, Khosla S, Limbur PJ, Rogers JW, Murtaugh PA. Muscle strength in osteoporotic versus normal women. *Osteoporosis Int* 1993; 3: 8–12.

30. Sinaki M. Postmenopausal spinal osteoporosis; physical therapy and rehabilitation principles. *Mayo Clin Proc* 1982; 57: 699–703.

31. Sinaki M, Mikkelsen BA. Postmenopausal spinal osteoporosis: flexion versus extension exercises. *Arch Phys Med Rehabil* 1984; 65: 593–596.

32. Gold DT, Stegmaier BS, Bales CW, Lyles KW, Westlund RE, Drezner MK. Psychosocial functioning and osteoporosis in late life: results of a multidisciplinary intervention. *J Women's Health* 1993; 2: 149–155.

33. Harrison JE, Chow R, Dornan J, Goodwin S, Strauss A, the Bone and Mineral Group of the University of Toronto. Evaluation of a program for rehabilitation of osteoporotic patients (PRO): 4-year follow-up. *Osteoporosis Int* 1993; 3: 13–17.

34. Fiaterone M, Marks E, Ryan, ND, High-intensity strength training in nonagenarians: effects on skeletal muscle. *JAMA* 1990; 263: 3029–3034.

35. Tucci JT, Carpenter DM, Pollock ML, Graves JE, Leggett SH. Effect of reduced frequency of training and detraining on lumbar extension strength. *Spine* 1992; 17: 1497–1501.

V Case Presentations

17

Prevention of Osteoporosis

Robert M. Levin, MD

CASE STUDY

A 53-yr-old Caucasian woman presents to her primary care physician for advice regarding her concerns about developing osteoporosis. The reason she is anxious is that her mother has osteoporosis, a great deal of back pain, and a prominent thoracic spine deformity (dowager's hump). The patient's menopause occurred 12 mo ago, and has been associated with minimal vasomotor symptoms. She is generally in good health. Her only medications are L-thyroxine (0.15 mg daily) for hypothyroidism and 25 mg daily of hydrochlorozide for mild hypertension. The patient has a good appetite, but she cannot tolerate dairy products owing to lactose intolerance. A dietary history reveals that her daily calcium intake is about 700 mg.

Her family history is noteworthy in that one brother died at age 49 of a myocardial infarction; her dad died at age 50 of lung cancer; and her mother is 80 and, apart from her osteoporosis, is well.

Physical exam reveals a BP of 150/85, pulse 90 and regular but with a bounding quality, weight 140 lbs, height 62 in. There are no clinical stigmata of Cushing's syndrome or acromegaly. She has a slight dorsal kyphosis. Her deep tendon reflexes are slightly hyperactive. There is no tremor of the outstretched hands. Examination of her heart, lungs, and abdomen is within normal limits. There is no thyroid enlargement.

Laboratory tests: Serum creatinine 1.0 mg/dL, fasting blood sugar 100 mg/dL, serum calcium 8.8 mg/dL, alkaline phosphatase 100 IU/L (normal 40–120), serum albumin 4.0 g/dL, hematocrit 38, serum T4 11.4 µg/dL (normal 4–12), urinalysis within normal limits.

From: *Osteoporosis: Diagnostic and Therapeutic Principles*
Edited by: C. J. Rosen Humana Press Inc., Totowa, NJ

Table 1
Dietary Dairy Sources of Calcium[a]

Milk	1 cup	300 mg
Yogurt	1 cup	
Plain		415 mg
Fruited		345 mg
Cheeses, hard	1 oz.	
American		175 mg
Cheddar		200 mg
Monterey		200 mg
Swiss		270 mg

[a]Dairy products comprise 75% of the calcium intake of the average American diet.

Questions to be addressed:

1. What instructions would you give to the patient regarding supplemental calcium?
2. What exercise program would you recommend?
3. Should estrogen replacement therapy be started? If so, why and how? The patient heard that estrogens may increase her chance of getting breast cancer. How would you respond to her?
4. Do you need any further tests or information before finalizing your management plan for this patient?

1. REPLY TO QUESTION NO. 1

A careful history of the patient's dietary calcium intake is essential. For most individuals, you do not need a nutrition consultation. Since 75% of the average American's calcium intake is ingested in dairy products, a reasonable estimate can be made of an individual's calcium intake by asking how much milk, yogurt, and hard cheese are consumed daily. Table 1 lists the best dietary dairy sources of calcium.

Osteoporosis is characterized by a disturbed balance between bone resorption and bone formation. This results in a progressive loss of skeletal calcium and bone mass. Part of the loss is owing to a decrease in the intestinal absorption of calcium. Vitamin D deficiency impairs the gastrointestinal absorption of calcium. Therefore, your dietary history should include questions about the availability of vitamin D. Does the patient drink milk regularly? Each quart of milk contains about 400 U of vitamin D. A serum 25-hydroxyvitamin D level is indicated to exclude a deficiency of vitamin D.

Vitamin D deficiency should be considered in all elderly individuals. The production of vitamin D by the skin is an important source of this vitamin. Does your patient spend sufficient time exposed to the sun? An exposure of as little of 10–15 min daily, two to three times weekly, is ample (1). The amount of vitamin D made by the skin varies considerably depending on the season of the year. For example, if you live in the Northeast, no vitamin D is made during the months of November through March. In our patient, because she had a number of risk factors for osteoporosis, I would obtain a serum 25-hydroxyvitamin D level, and, even if the value returned over 20 ng/mL, I would recommend two multivitamin tablets daily to ensure a daily intake of 800 U of vitamin D.

Can a negative calcium balance be corrected by increasing the intake of calcium? Over the past few years, there have been a number of clinical trials that have focused on the

Table 2
Recommended Daily Calcium Intake for Women

Age group, yr	Calcium intake, mg/d
6–10	800–1200
11–24	1200–1500
25–50	1000
Postmenopausal <65	
On estrogen	1000
No estrogen	1500
Postmenopausal >65	1500
Pregnant	
Specific age group	400 additional

effectiveness of different drugs in women with well-established osteoporosis, such as bisphosphonates, vitamin D, and fluoride. Calcium supplements were used as the placebo arm in these studies. An often overlooked, but significant observation of these studies is that the "placebo" (calcium)-treated women maintained their bone mass during the 2–4-yr periods of the studies (2–4). A true placebo arm, not calcium, may well have shown a steady decline in bone mass.

Robert Heaney and his colleagues, 17 yr ago, reported that premenopausal women needed to ingest 1000 mg of calcium daily, and postmenopausal women 1500 mg daily in order to remain in calcium balance (5). During the past year, a Consensus Conference was convened by the National Institutes of Health, and a group of experts in mineral metabolism met to establish optimal calcium intake levels for various age groups (6). Their recommendations were not very different from those made earlier by Heaney et al. The levels for women are summarized in Table 2.

Do calcium supplements, or an increase in dietary calcium, benefit bone in elderly women with well-established osteoporosis? Dawson-Hughes reported that elderly women (six or more years postmenopausal), whose baseline calcium intake was <400 mg daily, can slow their rate of bone loss by increasing their calcium intake to 800 mg daily (7). This beneficial effect of calcium supplements could not be demonstrated in women who were <6 yr postmenopausal. Matkovic et al. reported a 60%–75% reduction in hip fractures in Yugoslavian women who lived in an area with a high calcium-water content, compared to Yugoslavian women who lived in an area with a low calcium-water content (8). Reid and associates also demonstrated a reduction in bone loss in women taking calcium supplements (9).

Based on the above observations, what recommendations regarding calcium intake are reasonable? Young individuals during their rapid growth phase (ages 11–24) need 1200–1500 mg of calcium daily. This is a period during which there is a large deposition of calcium into the skeleton, and an increased calcium intake may result in a higher peak bone mass (see Fig. 1). In other words, the greater the reservoir of skeletal calcium achieved in youth, the longer it will take to deplete bone of enough calcium to levels that may result in fractures in the elderly. Postmenopausal estrogen-deprived women need to ingest 1500 mg of calcium daily in order to avoid being in negative calcium balance. However, if a woman is taking estrogen, her recommended calcium intake is only 1000

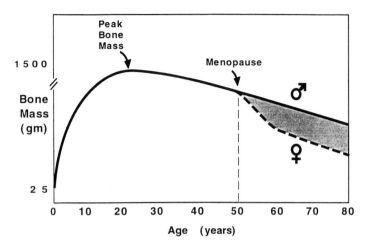

Fig. 1. Rise and decline of bone mass with age.

mg daily. A dietary history is necessary to determine an individual's daily calcium intake. For example, our patient, who is 53-yr old and currently ingests only 700 mg of calcium daily, is 800 mg shy of the amount needed to be in calcium balance. Food sources of calcium are preferred, if possible. However, our patient may be unable to tolerate dairy products in sufficient quantities. Therefore, 500 mg calcium carbonate tablets, each containing 200 mg of elemental calcium, may be taken with meals. Our patient should ingest a total of four tablets of calcium carbonate daily.

2. REPLY TO QUESTION NO. 2

I inquire from the patient about her daily activities and, particularly, if she does any regular exercising, whether it be jogging, bicycling, aerobic classes, or walking. In my effort to "sell" an exercise program, I explain that bone is a living tissue, metabolically active, and needs exercise to keep it healthy. I try to motivate my patients to exercise by explaining to them that one of the major health problems of the astronauts in our space program is bone loss induced by weightlessness. It is difficult to exercise adequately in a weightless environment.

Most bone experts agree that exercise is an important determinant of bone mass, but there is little agreement about how much and what type of exercise is required to result in benefit to bone. Numerous studies, prospective and retrospective, intended to define the role of exercise in preserving bone mass have been published. Some demonstrate a benefit of exercise on bone health, and others fail to show any benefit *(10–12)*. There are many possible explanations for these differing conclusions, such as different age groups studied, different exercise protocols used, and differences in the tools used to measure outcomes.

A recent paper by Kannus and colleagues demonstrated that not only does exercise increase bone mass, but the earlier it is begun, the better *(13)*. They studied national-level women tennis and squash players, who began their athletic careers before the menarche, and demonstrated that these women had a greater bone mass than those who began their careers after their menarche. In addition, these athletes had a greater bone mass in the dominant, compared to nondominant, arm. Similar observations have been made by

Table 3
Prescription for Exercise

Walk 15 min daily × 1 wk
Walk 20 min daily × 1 wk
Walk 25 min daily × 1 wk
Continue to increase walking by 5 min weekly until
    1 h is reached; then one hour at least 5 d weekly.

Jones and colleagues, who demonstrated significant hypertrophy of the humeri of professional tennis players in response to exercise *(14)*.

Growing bone is more responsive to exercise than is the bone of elderly individuals, yet most of the literature on this topic is concerned with the treatment of well-established osteoporosis in the elderly *(15)*. More effort should be made to increase an individual's peak bone mass early in adolescence. What is the role then of exercise in adults? Many of the published studies of exercise and the measurement of bone mass in adults conclude that the role of exercise is to preserve bone mass rather than to add new bone. Even a modest commitment to a regular exercise program might stimulate bone formation. Unfortunately, we do not know the best type of exercise or exactly how much activity is optimal for bone health, but regular walking seems a reasonable start. I write a prescription of how much to walk daily (Table 3). I believe patients take your advice more seriously if you write it on one of your prescription pads. I also recommend to the patient to purchase high-quality jogging or walking shoes. I even recommend the names of the top shoes and which stores are nearby where experienced salespersons will help choose the best fitting shoe for that person. Even if the patient does not walk a sufficient distance to benefit her skeleton, it may be that the most valuable aspect of an exercise program is to increase muscle tone, strength, and agility, and thereby reduce the frequency of falls. Falls are an important cause of fractures *(16)*. Approximately one-third of elderly fall each year, and 10%–15% of these falls result in a serious injury. Hip fractures occur in up to 1% of these individuals. More than 250,000 hip fractures occur each year in the US, and the perioperative mortality rate is as high as 20%. Among those who survive the fracture, up to 50% end up invalids, unable to live independently, and many are moved to nursing homes. Presenting these facts to our patients may motivate them to practice preventive medicine. At the same time, I recommend other practical measures to prevent falls (Table 4). Some of these suggestions are more appropriate for our more fragile elderly patients.

3. REPLY TO QUESTION NO. 3

"Should I start estrogen replacement therapy?" This is the most frequently asked question of the primary care physician, and the most difficult to answer. Some physicians feel a great passion about the importance of estrogen replacement therapy (ERT), and others feel it is such a controversial issue that they choose not to become involved in the debate with their patients. I will present the pros and cons of ERT, and conclude with a discussion of implementation.

The list of risk factors for the development of osteoporosis is quite lengthy, but far and away, the most important risk factor is estrogen deficiency. As depicted in Fig. 1, between the ages of 20 and 50, men and women lose bone at about the same rate, approx 0.3%/yr.

Table 4
Helpful Hints to Prevent Falls

Advise against wearing unsafe shoes, i.e., high heels, straps, backless
Use night-lights as a precaution to avoid accidently falling
Avoid use of scatter or loose rugs, unless they have a rubber back or secure
    padding underneath
Install handrails in bathtub/shower
Avoid drugs that cause postural hypotension, confusion, or sedation
Educate the patient how to bend and lift
Do exercises to improve flexibility and agility

The rate of bone loss increases by 10-fold in women at the time of the menopause. During the first 6–8 yr following the menopause, bone loss increases dramatically. By the age of 70, the slope of the curve of bone loss between men and women is similar. Therefore, if ERT is to be instituted, it should be started at the time of the menopause.

There are contraindications, some more important than others, to the use of ERT. These include a history of unexplained deep venous thrombosis and/or pulmonary embolic disease, liver disease, history of breast or endometrial cancer, unexplained vaginal bleeding, migraine headaches, and symptomatic uterine fibroids. These are not all hard and fast contraindications. For example, there is considerable controversy about when ERT should be restarted in a woman following a hysterectomy and oophorectomy for endometrial cancer. Migraine headaches are a relative contraindication depending on the frequency and severity. Deep vein phlebitis is a relative contraindication, depending on whether or not there was a well-recognized precipitating event. If there was none, then future use of ERT is contraindicated.

The major benefits of ERT are as follows:

- Contributes to the treatment of hot flashes, urogenital atrophy and dyspareunia, cystitis, urinary incontinence, and various nonspecific complaints, such as mood swings, depression, and insomnia.
- Slows the rate of bone loss and decreases the incidence of fractures (17,18). ERT is, in fact, the gold standard to which new treatments are compared when studying the effectiveness of new agents. Although ERT is most effective if started promptly at the time of the menopause, there is evidence that ERT is effective, although somewhat less so, even in women in their 70s (19).
- Slows the progression of cardiovascular disease. A number of epidemiologic studies have demonstrated a 40–50% reduction in the incidence of major cardiovascular events in estrogen users, compared to nonusers (20–22). The explanations for the cardioprotective effect of estrogen include:
  a. Estrogen reduces LDL cholesterol levels by 10–15%;
  b. Increases HDL cholesterol levels;
  c. Increases blood flow in major organs, including coronary vasodilatation; and
  d. Increases prostacyline levels and decreases thromboxane levels.

The major disadvantages of ERT are as follows:

- Menstrual bleeding is the major reason why most women refuse to consider ERT. Menstrual periods usually cease at about age 50, and many women do not want to have any further periods. Approximately one-third of the women who agree to continuous hormonal therapy, which eliminates cyclical bleeding, quit because of unpredictable spotting that may occur during the first 6–8 mo.

• The fear of developing breast cancer. There is no more controversial topic in this field than the following question asked by your patient: "What is my risk of developing breast cancer, if I take estrogen?" Unfortunately, the answer is not clear. There have been a few meta-analyses, which have summarized most of the important papers published on the association of ERT and breast cancer *(23–25)*. Of the more than 30 studies reported, most failed to show a significant increase in the risk of breast cancer in women on ERT. There are a number of conclusions which can be drawn from these studies:

   a. The increase in risk of breast cancer is small for past users of ERT, particularly if use was <5 yr;

   b. The risk may be increased by 15–30% in individuals who had taken ERT for >10 yr; and

   c. The addition of a progestin does not increase or decrease the incidence of breast cancer.

A very recent paper by Colditz and associates reported their followup of the Nurses' Health Study Cohort, covering 725,550 patient-years of followup in women on ERT *(26)*. They observed that the risk of breast cancer in women who formerly used ERT was no different than women who had never used ERT. On the other hand, women currently on ERT for more than 5 yr had an increased risk of breast cancer. The incidence of breast cancer was particularly increased among older women taking estrogen, e.g., relative risk (RR) of 1.46 for those aged 50–54, and an RR of 1.69 for those aged 65–69. It is important to point out that despite the impressive size of the cohort of women followed by the Nurses' Health Study Cohort, it was not designed to be a randomized, double-blinded, placebo-controlled study. It is unclear why the women in this study who chose to take ERT did so or why the women who elected not to take ERT made that decision. The final answer to this debate may have to await completion of the prospective, ongoing Women's Health Initiative studies by the National Institutes of Health.

What do we tell our 53-yr-old patient, who is eager to practice preventive medicine, but is fearful of the risk of breast cancer? To advise this particular patient, consider the advantages and disadvantages of ERT for her. For example, our patient has a strong family history of coronary artery disease, and she has hypertension. In addition, her mother has osteoporosis (an important risk factor for our patient). Let us assume for the moment that a baseline bone mineral density (BMD) study in our patient showed significant bone loss compared to a healthy young adult, and there is no history of breast cancer in the family. I would advise this woman to take ERT because her risk for coronary artery disease and osteoporosis appears greater than her risk of developing breast cancer. The advice may be to avoid ERT in another patient who has no cardiovascular risk factors, but who has two sisters with breast cancer.

My recommendation to our patient would be to take ERT. I prescribe 0.625 mg of a conjugated equine estrogen (CEE) daily for the first 25 d of each month, and 5–10 mg of a progestational agent, e.g., medroxy progesterone acetate (MPA), from days 12 through 25. This regimen will result in monthly withdrawal bleeding. If the bleeding begins prior to the 11th day of the progestational agent, the dose of MPA should be increased from 5 to 10 mg. There is also a transdermal patch available that must be applied twice weekly. If the patient chooses the patch, and 50 mcg is a reasonable starting dose, a progestin must still be prescribed. If our patient requests a regimen that is not associated with withdrawal

Table 5
Risk Factors for Osteoporosis

Genetic	White, thin, female, family history of osteoporosis
Nutrition	Low calcium diet, excess alcohol
Drugs	Loop diuretics, glucocorticoids, thyroxine
Life-style	Physical inactivity, cigaret smoking
Endocrinopathies	Hypogonadism Hyperprolactinemia, Hyperparathyroidism, Thyrotoxicosis, Cushing's syndrome

bleeding, 0.625 mg of CEE and 2.5 mg of MPA are taken uninterrupted, daily. Unpredictable spotting occurs in up to one-third of the women who choose this regimen, but such spotting is unusual after 6–8 mo.

4. REPLY TO QUESTION NO. 4

The most important information you need to know when evaluating a person for osteoporosis can be learned from a careful history. What are the risk factors for osteoporosis (Table 5)? Our patient has five that are readily apparent. She is Caucasian, postmenopausal, has a positive family history for osteoporosis, has been on a low calcium diet most of her life, and has been on a relatively large dose of thyroxine. Is this reason enough to obtain a BMD study? Table 6 lists the indications for bone densitometry, but the one that is most relevant here refers to the patient's decision regarding whether to start on estrogen. If she is undecided, measurements revealing a low BMD may help her decide to start estrogen therapy, since this is our most sensitive risk factor for osteoporosis (27). On the other hand, with her positive family history of coronary artery disease, she may feel strongly about taking estrogen regardless of the results of a BMD study. In that case, I would not order a BMD study. In short, there are two important points to be made: first, order a BMD only when the results of the study will help direct your therapy, and second, a significant reduction in BMD is the most sensitive risk factor for osteoporosis.

Is our patient on too much thyroid hormone and, if so, is that harmful to her bones (28)? If the thyroid-stimulating hormone (TSH) level is maintained within normal limits by administering a proper replacement dose of levothyroxine, bone mass is unaffected. However, doses of levothyroxine that are large enough to suppress the TSH level have been reported to increase bone turnover and lead to bone loss. For example, women with a past history of thyroid cancer, who have been operated on and require suppressive doses of levothyroxine, are at risk for increased bone loss. They should be monitored annually with BMD. Estrogen replacement therapy for such patients may prevent excessive bone loss. If ERT is not an option, consider the use of other antiresorptive agents (see Chapter

Table 6
Indications for Bone Mineral Densitometry

For the undecided estrogen-deficient woman, BMD may help her decide to take estrogens
For patients about to start on prolonged gluco-corticoid therapy, BMD measurements may help
    in considering additional therapy to prevent bone loss
It is used to determine effectiveness of therapy
In patients with asymptomatic hyperparathyroidism, BMD measurement may help determine who
    should have surgical intervention

15). However, still unanswered is whether patients on suppressive thyroid hormone are at increased risk of fracture compared to otherwise normal individuals.

In our patient, a serum TSH is clearly indicated, particularly in view of those clinical features suggesting hyperthyroidism, such as resting tachycardia, bounding pulse, and hyperactive reflexes. If her TSH is suppressed, the dose of thyroid hormone should be lowered and rechecked in 2 mo. The issue of her thyroid disease is another reason why a BMD study might be helpful in the management of our patient.

Our patient has lactose intolerance, and it has been hypothesized that such patients have avoided dairy products (calcium sources) and, therefore, may have a reduced bone mass. An excellent study by Slemenda and his colleagues of a cohort of adult female twins, discordant for lactase activity, demonstrated no significant difference in bone mass between the twin pairs *(29)*.

REFERENCES

1. Holick MF. Vitamin D requirements for the elderly. *Clin Nutr* 1986; 5: 121–129.
2. Watts NB, Harris ST, Genant HK, et al. Intermittent cyclical etidronate treatment of postmenopausal osteoporosis. *N Engl J Med* 1990; 323: 73–79.
3. Ott SM, Chestnut CH III. Calcitriol treatment is not effective in postmenopausal osteoporosis. *Ann Int Med* 1989; 110: 267–274.
4. Riggs BL, Hodgson SF, O'Fallon WM, et al. Effect of fluoride treatment on the fracture rate in post-menopausal women with osteoporosis. *N Engl J Med* 1990; 322: 802–809.
5. Heaney RP, Recker RR, Saville PD. Menopausal changes in calcium balance performance. *J Lab Clin Med* 1978; 92: 953–963.
6. NIH Consensus Conference. Optimal calcium intake. *JAMA* 1994; 272: 1942–1948.
7. Dawson-Hughes B, Dallal GE, Kroll EA, et al. A controlled trial of the effect of calcium supplementation on bone density in postmenopausal women. *N Engl J Med* 1990; 323: 878–883.
8. Matkovic V, Kostal K, Simonvic I, et al. Bone status and fracture rates in two regions of Yugoslavia. *Am J Clin Nutr* 1979; 32: 540–549.
9. Reid IR, Ames RW, Evans MC, et al. Effective calcium supplementation on bone loss in postmenopausal women. *N Engl J Med* 1993; 328: 460–464.
10. Dalsky GP, Stocke KS, Ehsani AA, et al. Weight-bearing exercise training and lumbar bone mineral content in postmenopausal women. *Ann Intern Med* 1988; 108: 824–828.
11. Cavanaugh DJ, Cann CE. Brisk walking does not stop bone loss in postmenopausal women. *Bone* 1988; 9: 201–204.
12. Aloia JF, Cohn SH, Ostuni JA, et al. Prevention of involutional bone loss by exercise. *Ann Intern Med* 1978; 84: 356–358.
13. Kannus P, Haapasalo H, Sankelo M, et al. Effect of starting age of physical activity on bone mass in the dominant arm of tennis and squash players. *Ann Intern Med* 1995; 123: 27–31.
14. Jones HH, Priest JD, Hayes WC, et al. Humeral hypertrophy in response to exercise. *J Bone Jt Surg* 1977; 59–A: 204–208.
15. Forwood MR, Burr DB. Physical activity and bone mass: exercises in futility? *Bone Miner* 1993; 21: 89–112.

16. Sattin RW. Falls among older persons: a public health perspective. *Ann Public Health* 1992; 13: 489–508.
17. Kiel DP, Felson DT, Anderson JJ, et al. Hip fracture and the use of estrogens in postmenopausal women: the Framingham study. *N Engl J Med* 1987; 317: 1169–1174..
18. Lindsay R, Hart DM, Aitken JM, et al. Long-term prevention of postmenopausal osteoporosis by oestrogen. *Lancet* 1976: 1038–1040.
19. Lindsay R, Tohme JF. Estrogen treatment of patients with established postmenopausal osteoporosis. *Obstet Gynecol* 1990; 76: 290–295.
20. Bush TL, Barrett-Conor E, Cowan LD, et al. Cardiovascular mortality in noncontraceptive use of estrogen in women: results from the Lipid Research Clinics Program Follow-up Study. *Circulation* 1987; 75: 1102–1109.
21. Stampfer MJ, Colditz GA, Willett WC, et al. Postmenopausal estrogen therapy and cardiovascular disease. Ten year follow-up from the Nurses' Health Study. *N Engl J Med* 1991; 325: 756–762.
22. Sullivan JM, Vander Zwaag R, Lemp GF, et al. Postmenopausal estrogen use and coronary atherosclerosis. *Ann Int Med* 1988; 108: 358–363.
23. Brinton LA, Schairer C. Estrogen replacement therapy and breast cancer risk. *Epidemiol Rev* 1993; 15: 66–79.
24. Dupont WD, Page DL. Menopausal estrogen replacement therapy and breast cancer. *Arch Intern Med* 1991; 151: 67–72.
25. Steinberg KK, Thacker SB, Smith JS, et al. A meta-analysis of the effect of estrogen replacement therapy on the risk of breast cancer. *JAMA* 1991; 265: 1985–1990.
26. Colditz GA, Hankinson SE, Hunter DJ, et al. The use of estrogens and progestins and the risk of breast cancer in postmenopausal women. *N Engl J Med* 1995; 332: 1589–1593.
27. Hui SL, Slemenda CW, Johnston CC. Baseline measurements of bone mass predicts fracture in white women. *Ann Intern Med* 1989; 111: 355–361.
28. Wartofsky L. Levothyroxine therapy and osteoporosis. *Arch Int Med* 1995; 155: 1130–1131.
29. Slemenda CW, Christian JC, Hui S, et al. No evidence for an effect of lactase deficiency on bone mass in pre- or postmenopausal women. *J Bone Miner Res* 1991; 6: 1367–1371.

18

The Diagnosis and Treatment of Postmenopausal Osteoporosis

Clifford J. Rosen, MD

CONTENTS

INTRODUCTION
ESTABLISHING THE DIAGNOSIS OF POSTMENOPAUSAL OSTEOPOROSIS
THERAPY FOR ESTABLISHED POSTMENOPAUSAL OSTEOPOROSIS
NONPHARMACOLOGIC INTERVENTION WITH PARTICULAR EMPHASIS
    ON EXERCISE
SUMMARY
REFERENCES

CASE STUDY

TW is a 68-yr-old retired white female who presents to your office with a 4-wk history of upper thoracic back pain. The pain began in the morning as intense-knife-like discomfort between her shoulder blades. This followed a strenuous day of moving and rearranging furniture. There was a pleuritic component to this pain, and over the course of 3 wk, it remained relatively intense. In the past 1 wk, her pain has subsided somewhat. The patient underwent spontaneous menopause at age 41 and has never been on hormone replacement therapy. She has been well all her adult life, although she suffered a wrist fracture at age 58 after falling onto ice during a storm. Currently, she states she weighs 105 lbs and is 5 ft 4 in. in height. This is her first episode of back pain, and it has interfered with her lifestyle, which includes thrice weekly walking and once weekly tennis. The patient has never smoked, does not drink, and maintains a healthy lifestyle, including regular milk consumption daily. She had three children and two grandchildren. Her mother suffered a hip fracture at age 89 and died 1 wk later of pulmonary embolism last year. Her husband teaches history at a nearby university.

Initial physical exam revealed mild paraspinal muscle spasm in the upper back, but no other abnormalities. Her height was 5 ft 2 in. and weight was 106 pounds. Heart and lung exam were normal, and the thyroid gland measured only 15 g. PA chest X-ray was normal, but on lateral there was a compression fracture of T8 with mild osteopenia noted in the other vertebrae. Bone density of the spine (L2-L4) was reported as a t-score of –2.5 (0.860 g/cm^2).

From: *Osteoporosis: Diagnostic and Therapeutic Principles*
Edited by: C. J. Rosen Humana Press Inc., Totowa, NJ

1. INTRODUCTION

The case of TW illustrates what could be considered a "classic" presentation of post-menopausal osteoporosis. Even though this diagnosis appears relatively straightforward, the subtleties of this disorder, its differential diagnosis, and subsequent management can be complex. These issues will be explored in this chapter.

2. ESTABLISHING THE DIAGNOSIS
OF POSTMENOPAUSAL OSTEOPOROSIS

This 68-yr-old woman has several risk factors that would predispose her to primary (involutional or Type I) postmenopausal osteoporosis. First, she went through menopause at any early age. Ovarian failure before the age of 45 is considered early menopause. Although not well understood, premature estrogen withdrawal accelerates age-related bone loss (1). The relatively strong inverse relationship between age of menopause and rate of bone loss suggests that TW suffered rather significant bone loss during and after her spontaneous menopause.

Do all women lose bone after premature estrogen deprivation? In general, the answer is probably yes, although there are few prospective studies that have examined this question in detail. Estrogen deprivation during the reproductive years is associated with low bone mass (1–3). Moreover, in older women who went through menopause early (and were not replaced with estrogens), mean spine bone densities are consistently lower than age-matched controls who entered menopause between the ages of 48 and 55 (1–3). Also, young women who suffer from primary or secondary amenorrhea in their teens exhibit very low t-scores especially in the spine (4). However, whether this is a function of rapid bone loss or impaired bone acquisition is uncertain. Certainly, when 17 β-estradiol levels fall consistently below 60 pg/mL in perimenopausal women, bone loss begins.

We can conclude TW suffered from bone loss during and immediately after her menopause. In addition to premature estrogen deprivation, TW is a slender woman. Even though low body weight represents a strong independent risk factor for osteoporotic fractures, the reasons for the close association between body weight and bone mineral density (BMD) are probably multifactorial (5–7). First, low body mass leads to a reduced total surface area to protect the skeleton. Since trauma produces fractures, the less fat and connective tissue surrounding bone, the more likely fractures are to occur following injury. Second, low body fat in thin women produces profound metabolic changes in testosterone metabolism. Endogenous estrogens are generated from androgens in bone marrow by aromatase enzymes found in fat cells. Reduced total body fat is associated with a reduction in aromatase activity and, therefore, less estrogenic activity adjacent to the remodeling unit. Since gonadal steroids inhibit osteoclastogenesis within the bone marrow (see Chapter 1), reduced " skeletal" estrogens in thin women could lead to enhanced bone resorption (6). Third, the relatively small size of TW's skeleton (e.g., the diameter of the bone or the frame size) may, in itself, be a predictor of future fracture (7).

Irrespective of the pathogenetic factors surrounding early menopause and thinness, we could conclude that TW is at high risk for osteoporosis even without knowing her BMD. Still, the sum of all risk factors for osteoporotic fractures does not come close to approximating the power of bone density to predict osteoporosis (8,9). Bone density measurements in TW also provide three additional pieces of important information:

1. The severity of disease: A spine BMD that is 2.5 standard deviations below peak bone mass (t-score) represents moderate to severe osteoporosis by WHO criteria *(9,10)*.
2. The scope of the disease: A low BMD confirms that osteoporosis is a diffuse disorder not purely confined to the area where her fracture has occurred.
3. The predictive nature of BMD: One bone mass measurement allows a prediction of future fractures with relative confidence, as well as solidifying the decision to treat TW.

From several studies, it is clear that BMD predicts fractures better than cholesterol predicts heart disease or blood pressure predicts stroke *(9,10)*. A measurement by densitometry at any bone site that is more than 1 SD below peak bone mass means that the relative risk of a future spine fracture is approximately two *(8–10)*. Since TW's BMD is more than −2.0 SD from mean young normal, her relative risk for another fracture is >3. More importantly, the presence of a new compression fracture independently doubles her relative risk of fracture and, combined with low bone mass, places her at approximately an eightfold higher risk for future spine fractures *(11)*. These are compelling numbers for TW, especially if therapy is delayed or not instituted (*see* Chapter 7).

Is the case of TW unusual? In other words, how often is premature menopause the principle cause of low bone mass and subsequent fractures? That answer varies from geographic area to area probably because of different practice patterns. However, in a recent study of nearly 1000 women in our metabolic bone clinic who presented with osteopenia, premature menopause was the principal etiologic factor for osteopenia in nearly 1/3 of the patients (steroid-induced osteoporosis was second at 25%) *(12)*. Therefore, this piece of historical information alone may alert the physician to the strong possibility that TW is suffering from postmenopausal osteoporosis.

Osteoporotic fractures result from trauma and low bone mass. Absent treatment, the natural course for TW almost certainly will be recurrent vertebral and nonspine fractures, often with minimal trauma. Indeed, as has been pointed out repeatedly in this book, previous fractures of the spine (or other sites) predispose individuals to future fractures independent of bone mass *(11)*. The combination of one spine fracture and very low bone density places TW at extremely high risk for recurrent osteoporotic fractures *(9,11)*.

TW suffered bone loss owing to premature estrogen deprivation, but she also may have been at risk for osteoporosis because of genetic determinants. Her strong family history of hip fracture (i.e., her mother) may suggest there is a heritable component to her disease. Although age, body mass index, and menopausal status are very strong predictors of bone mass, emerging studies of twins have established that as much as 60% of adult bone mass is determined by genetic factors *(13,14)*. The heritable determinants of bone mass primarily exert their control during the bone acquisition phase of a person's life *(15)*. In the case of TW, her potential to acquire optimal bone mass (45–50 yr prior to her fracture) may have been impaired by genetic factors contributed by her mother. Over her life, the combination of reduced peak bone mass and accelerated bone loss could have produced her osteopenic state. Although this is little consolation to TW, understanding the genetic components of this disorder is important for family counseling and for prevention. Indeed, one could make the case that early intervention (at age 41) to minimize bone loss (e.g., estrogens) would at least have allowed TW to maintain her bone mass at a level that could have prevented her subsequent fractures. Therefore, identification of all possible risk factors are important in the total management of patients with postmenopausal osteoporosis.

TW has significant midthoracic back pain, which was her presenting complaint. Although the initial diagnosis of osteoporosis is made by a radiographic interpretation of osteopenia or a bone density, the first fracture, especially in the spine, is a common manifestation of underlying osteoporosis. Bone pain from such a compression fracture is often severe, especially during the first month. Depending on its site of origin, pain can manifest itself in different ways. However, the lack of a history for a particular traumatic event is usual. In up to 50% of postmenopausal women with osteoporotic fractures, the patient cannot remember the cause, or for that matter, even the time of onset of back pain. Often "asymptomatic" spine fractures are reported by the radiologist. Careful questioning, however, may uncover episodes of pain that the patient cannot relate to a specific cause. On the other, an acute thoracic vertebral fracture can be associated with severe bone and muscle pain often localized to the midline area between the scapulae. A pleuritic component is sometimes reported as is pain radiating to the anterior chest. After the first fracture, 3–4 wk of severe pain followed by dull aching for 6–8 wk is very common.

This is the first compression fracture for TW but it is not her first osteoporotic fracture. Her remote history of a wrist fracture points away from a new pathologic process and toward a more generalized metabolic state which has been smoldering for years. In general, a previous osteoporotic fracture at any site increases that individual's risk for future fractures (11). Still, it is essential that after the first compression fracture, secondary causes of osteoporosis be considered. For TW the workup should include a general chemistry screening study (Chem-20, SMAC-20, or the equivalent) to exclude other obvious causes for osteoporotic fractures. In particular, an elevated serum calcium would suggest primary hyperparathyroidism or metastatic neoplasm. On the other hand, a low serum calcium might suggest coexistent osteomalacia owing to malabsorption (e.g., coeliac sprue). Alkaline phosphatase levels may also provide useful information (normal concentrations are consistent with osteoporosis, whereas high levels are seen in vitamin D deficiency, hyperthyroidism, osteomalacia, and healing osteoporotic fractures). An elevated total protein level would be suggestive of multiple myeloma. Although many clinicians routinely obtain a serum immunoelectrophoresis to exclude myeloma, this might be optional in the workup of TW, especially in view of her other risk factors. Since there are no published guidelines as to the relative value of a screening serum immuno-electrophoresis for osteoporosis, obtaining these studies in TW would depend on the provider. In general, a one-time evaluation to exclude myeloma would likely be considered cost-effective if this patient was followed on a continuous basis by the same person.

A complete blood count is a necessity, since anemia can also be an indicator of a hematologic malignancy associated with pathologic fractures. A serum TSH level will exclude hyperthyroidism, a disorder associated with bone loss especially during the postmenopausal period (16). Finally, an FSH level would tell us about the state of her pituitary. By history the patient underwent spontaneous menopause at an early age. Yet there was no history of hot flushes and the patient was never placed on HRT. Her FSH concentration, even at age 68, should be in the menopausal range (>20 mIU/L). A low FSH, on the other hand, would suggest a primary pituitary/hypothalamic etiology for her early menopause, and would prompt consideration of a CT or MRI scan to exclude a slow-growing space-occupying tumor (such as a pituitary adenoma).

This would be the minimal workup to exclude secondary causes of osteoporosis in TW. Examination of her X-rays is mandatory in order to be sure that the compression fracture is not associated with vertebral destruction or disk-space disease (suggestive of osteomyelitis, infiltrative processes, Paget's disease, or neoplasm) and to exclude possible lesions in the lung. On the other hand, a Tc^{99} bone scan would add little to the workup (except cost!). In the multicenter trials of anti-osteoporosis drugs, Tc^{99} bone scans are never used to confirm the diagnosis of an osteoporotic fracture. Although commonly employed in clinical practice, scant data support its use as a principal tool for diagnosing osteoporosis. Bone scans can, however, help establish the presence of metastatic bone disease if the clinical suspicion is high. In most cases, these scans become positive 1–2 wk after an osteoporotic fracture and remain positive for up to 6 mo. A negative scan would suggest another etiology or a misinterpretation of the plain films.

An equally important question is whether further studies of bone turnover are necessary in TW. At a minimum, TW should have a 25-hydroxyvitamin D$_3$ (25-OH-D) level. As noted in earlier chapters, vitamin D deficiency is common among older postmenopausal women. In part, this is a function of reduced sunlight exposure, especially in the winter months. Among healthy elders living in New England during the winter months, serum 25-OH-D concentrations average 19 ng/mL (10–55 ng/mL) *(17)*. This value is 24% lower than during summer and represents concentrations that can trigger parathyroid hormone release. Most investigators believe that serum levels of 25-OH-D should range between 30 and 50 ng/mL in order to prevent secondary hyperparathyroidism and potential hypovitaminosis D. Strong epidemiologic evidence (from randomized placebo-controlled studies) now have demonstrated that correction of low serum 25-OH-D levels in older postmenopausal women (by vitamin D supplementation) can prevent bone loss, especially during the winter months *(18–20)*.

The issue of whether measurements of other biochemical markers would be useful in this case is not mundane considering our cost-conscious environment. If secondary causes of bone loss have been excluded, this patient has postmenopausal osteoporosis and needs some form of antiresorptive therapy. Measurement of collagen crosslinks, or osteocalcin in TW might demonstrate increased bone turnover, or these studies might be entirely normal. Such tests would cost the patient approx $100 each and would be unlikely, based on her history and risk factors, to change your basic management strategy. On the other hand, if this patient did not have access to another bone mass measurement, or TW was to be placed on HRT, then a baseline N-telopeptide level followed by another one in 3 mo might predict spinal bone mineral density at yr one or two (*see* Chapter 11). By contrast, if the patient is to be placed on alendronate, the chance of skeletal nonresponsiveness appears to be slim. Therefore, serial markers would not be particularly useful (unless the provider was measuring compliance).

In summary, the role of biochemical markers in the case of TW remains up in the air. A single test for a biochemical marker could identify patients with very high bone turnover, although in this case (TW), it would not change your management. Serial measurements may help the provider predict, with some confidence, bone density changes following therapy. Whether certain indices of bone resorption will prove to be independent risk markers for future hip fractures will require further longitudinal studies.

Finally, use of a tetracycline-labeled bone biopsy as a diagnostic tool should be considered. This procedure (*see* Chapter 1) provides useful information about skeletal dynamics (such as the mineralization time, the number of osteoclasts, and the degree of bone turnover). However, little information could be gained from a bone biopsy in TW that could not be obtained by close and careful followup. Furthermore, the test is invasive (although needle biopsies in the hands of qualified personnel are relatively benign) and the cost ranges from $300 to $800 depending on whether the provider has access to a physician who can perform percutaneous needle biopsy under local anesthesia. On the other hand, bone biopsies can provide extremely useful information when considering the diagnosis of osteomalacia, osteolgenesis imperfecta, Paget's disease, neoplastic infiltration, or other metabolic bone disorders.

3. THERAPY
FOR ESTABLISHED POSTMENOPAUSAL OSTEOPOROSIS

The diagnosis of postmenopausal osteoporosis in TW has been established by:

1. Excluding secondary causes;
2. Demonstrating diffuse osteopenia by bone density;
3. Confirming that a compression fracture has occurred; and
4. Assessing her risk factors to confirm the presence of a systemic metabolic disorder.

Almost everyone would agree that the next step in this process would be to treat TW. These are the following options currently available to the practitioner:

1. Calcium + vitamin D;
2. HRT;
3. A bisphosphonate;
4. Calcitonin.

The efficacy of calcium and vitamin D in age-related osteoporosis has already been noted in several chapters of this book. Suffice it to say that calcium and vitamin D are essential components of TW's therapeutic plan; 1500 mg of calcium carbonate (or calcium citrate maleate) plus at least 400 IU of vitamin D/d are minimal therapy for this patient. These numbers are based on several randomized double-blinded placebo-controlled studies, which confirm that older women (>5 yr after menopause) who consume <500 mg of calcium per day benefit from calcium supplementation and vitamin D *(18– 20)*. During winter, when bone loss appears to be the greatest (and vitamin D is the lowest), some investigators would recommend 700 IU of vitamin D/d for 6–8 mo *(18)*. However, by itself, calcium and vitamin D probably are not enough. If the serum 25-OH-D level is <15 ng/mL at baseline, then a 6-mo trial of 50,000 U of cholecalciferol (vitamin D_3)/wk or 800–1200 IU/d of cholecalciferol could be considered prior to antiresorptive treatment. A followup serum 25-OH-D should be employed for two reasons: (1) to detect hypervitaminosis D, or (2) to determine if there is vitamin D malabsorption, which would point towards coeliac sprue or other malabsorptive states.

Most clinicians would support the use of calcium and vitamin as supplementary measures in TW, to be used along side at least one drug that has antiresorptive properties. Three types of antiresorptive drugs could be considered for TW: estrogens, calcitonin, or bisphosphonates. The choice depends on the background of the physician, and his/her previous experience with a specific medication or treatment regimen.

3.1. Estrogens

An extensive review of HRT is noted in Chapter 14. This section will deal only with the use of estrogens ± progesterone in the case of TW. In general, institution of HRT (or estrogen replacement therapy [ERT]) remains a decision for both the provider and the patient. The pros and cons of this form of therapy must be shared with the patient. In the case of TW, several trials have convincingly demonstrated the efficacy of estrogens in preserving bone mass. In particular, two studies of older postmenopausal women with established osteoporosis have shown that bone density can increase by as much as 8% after the first year of treatment *(21,22)*. Moreover, from large cohort studies, continuous HRT can effectively reduce the number of spine and hip fractures *(23–25)*. Therefore, if the skeleton is considered alone, HRT might be a wise choice for TW.

However, several factors might mitigate against this choice of treatment for TW. First, noncompliance with HRT is common. Some studies suggest that up to 20% of patients will not even fill their prescription for HRT after leaving a physician's office *(26)*. Moreover, up to 40% of women will stop HRT within 1 yr of treatment *(26)*. Various reasons have been given for premature discontinuation of HRT. The most common are mastalgia, weight gain, and resumption of menses *(27)*. In patients receiving continuous estrogen + low dose progesterone (2.5 mg/d) some women will have significant and unpredictable breakthrough bleeding *(28)*. Furthermore either cyclic or continuous progesterone can be associated with other side effects, including changes in mood and behavior. These alone may be enough to discourage patients from continuing HRT. For TW with an intact uterus, HRT therapy would mean both estrogen and progesterone.

The second factor that might prevent a provider from prescribing HRT is a patient's fear of breast cancer. Even assuming the mammograms on TW are normal, her concerns about the long-term use of estrogen and breast cancer may be well founded, and certainly represent one of the most important reasons why women do not want to start hormone replacement. Although estrogens significantly reduce the relative risk of heart disease in postmenopausal women, recent data suggest that long-term use of HRT (>5 yr) **may be** associated with a modest increase in the relative risk for breast cancer, especially in women over age 60 (i.e., TW's chance of developing breast cancer if she remained on HRT for 5 yr or more would increase from 1:292 women to 1:209) *(29,30)*. Despite the lack of family history for breast cancer, it is certain that TW will be concerned about her relative risk for breast neoplasm if she takes HRT. Hence, these issues would need to be thoroughly discussed with the patient so that TW could make an informed decision.

The third consideration that might mitigate against the choice of HRT for TW is the long-term commitment to followup required for the provider and the patient. HRT is only effective on the skeleton when it is taken on a regular basis and probably for at least 7 yr *(25)*. Thus, regular provider visits during the course of therapy are indicated. At these followups, yearly mammograms, pap smears, and possibly endometrial sampling would be required. Also, the patient should have at least one more bone density to establish skeletal responsiveness to HRT, since as many as 10% of postmenopausal women are "nonresponders' to HRT (i.e., they exhibit slight or continued loss of BMD on estrogen therapy) *(31)*. Hence, sequential indicators of bone turnover (such as N-telopeptide) or bone density would be necessary to establish both compliance and efficacy These tests may turn out to be a greater burden to TW than originally projected by the provider.

In conclusion, HRT therapy would be beneficial to TW because it would reduce her fracture risk (assuming she is one of the 90+% responders, she remains compliant and she does not have serious menstrual irregularities). In addition, HRT would decrease her likelihood of heart disease (*see* Chapter 14). However, side effects and compliance issues might limit the usefulness of HRT. Again, the final decision would lie with both the provider and the patient.

3.2. Bisphosphonates

Alendronate and etidronate are two possible therapeutic options for this woman with established osteoporosis. Both are bisphosphonates with good safety profiles and few compliance issues. Etidronate is prescribed as a 400-mg tablet once/d on an empty stomach for 2 wk every 3 mo. In between these 90 d cycles, calcium and vitamin D (1500 mg of calcium + 400 IU vitamin D) are recommended. Two relatively small multicenter trials confirmed that etidronate increases spine and hip BMD after 3 yr of therapy *(32,33)*. Moreover, there are few side effects from the bisphosphonates in general and etidronate in particular. Most complaints center around gastrointestinal effects of these drugs (e.g., nausea and heartburn). Although cyclic regimens require careful attention by the patient to time of treatment, compliance in practice has been quite high. Yet despite its widespread use in North America and Europe, this drug has not been approved by the US Food and Drug Administration.

Alendronate (Fosomax) is a third-generation bisphosphonate recently approved by the FDA for the treatment of osteoporosis (*see* Chapter 15). Although the precise mechanism of action for any of the bisphosphonates is not clearly defined, the second- and third-generation agents (such as alendronate) strongly inhibit osteoclastic activity at the remodeling surface. Ten milligrams of alendronate effectively suppress bone resorption (i.e., a 40–50% reduction in N-telopeptide excretion) and leads to a significant increase in bone density at the spine, hip and radius *(34)*. More importantly, there is a statistically significant reduction in both spine and nonvertebral fractures in postmenopausal women followed for 5 yr on alendronate *(34)*. Moreover, bone biopsies up to 4 yr in these women have not demonstrated any evidence of osteomalacia as a result of continuous' therapy. Finally, gastrointestinal side effects are relatively minor. Hence, for TW, alendronate may be a perfect therapeutic choice.

The provider must inform the patient, however, that alendronate is to be taken every day in the morning in an upright position with a glass of water 1/2 to 1 h prior to breakfast (owing to the poor bioavailability of all the bisphosphonates, it is recommended that these drugs be consumed on an empty stomach). In addition, this is an agent that must be taken every day, since discontinuation of alendronate leads to increased bone turnover within 30–90 d. Finally, there are no long-term safety data on alendronate beyond 5 yr. Since the bisphosphonates can stay in bone for a long time, caution must be used when prescribing this drug to young individuals. Still, in sum, alendronate probably represents the best therapeutic option for TW. If there is compliance with this regimen (and adequate calcium and vitamin D), she would be expected to have an increase in spine BMD after 2 yr of treatment, which would range between 5 and 8%. This change alone would likely reduce her fracture risk by 50%.

3.3. Calcitonin

Salmon calcitonin (sCT) is approved by the US Food and Drug administration for the treatment and prevention of osteoporosis Prior to late 1995, only parenteral calcitonin was available. That form can be administered either sc or im in doses from 25–200 IU/d. Although it has been shown that parenteral calcitonin may prevent bone loss in many individuals, the cost ($40–45/bottle [400 IU/bottle]), the inconvenience, and the possibility that cortical bone sites are not affected by sCT raise questions regarding whether TW would be a candidate for this treatment *(35,36)*. Furthermore, fracture efficacy with CT has not been well established either with continuous or intermittent therapy.

On the other hand, TW's chief complaint was back pain. Anecdotal reports suggest that sCT reduces back pain from osteoporotic crush fractures *(37)*. The mechanism of this action is not known, although sCT increases β-endorphin secretion and may have effects on local neurotransmitters *(37)*. Therefore, a trial of sCT may prove useful for TW, especially in increasing mobilization and reducing pain without the use of heavy narcotics or nonsteroidals. Unfortunately, many patients cannot tolerate more than 100 IU/d of parenteral sCT without significant nausea, headaches, flushes, or other gastrointestinal side effects.

Nasal salmon calcitonin (Miacalcin®) has recently been approved by the US FDA for the treatment of osteoporosis. Its cost (for 200 IU/d) is approximately the same as alendronate ($1.75/dose). Still, the overall role for this drug in the late 1990s needs to be defined. Probably most clear is the fact that patients can use larger doses of sCT by nasal administration without suffering significant side effects. Therefore, it may be an important adjunct for TW and might be used for 3–6 mo prior to initiation of either estrogens or bis-phosphonates.

4. NONPHARMACOLOGIC INTERVENTION WITH PARTICULAR EMPHASIS ON EXERCISE

Although drug therapy is the cornerstone of TW's management, supportive measures are also important. Pain management was discussed in light of calcitonin's possible effect on neurotransmitters. Narcotics and nonsteroidals are also helpful to relieve pain, although in this age group, the NSAIDs can cause significant gastrointestinal and renal difficulties. Physical therapy may be helpful in some patients. Generally, back braces are not recommended, and early mobilization is the key to successful rehabilitation. In a broader sense, an active exercise program may be one goal for a preventive therapy program.

Studies on the effects of exercise on bone mass have been fraught with many confounding variables. Although physical activity can stimulate osteoblastic activity (probably through a "mechanostat" located in the osteon), in vivo effects are much more difficult to quantify. Cross-sectional studies that have demonstrated that active exercisers have higher bone mass suffer from ascertainment bias (i.e., people who exercise over many years are fundamentally different in many ways from sedentary people; these differences include body mass, health habits, genetic predispositions, as well as a greater likelihood of being involved in longitudinal exercise studies). Also, in many cross-sectional studies, age is an important confounder (i.e., young exercisers tend to have a greater skeletal response to exercise than elders) *(38)*. Therefore, critical analysis of the data require an examination of long-term randomized controlled trials with exercise of which there are few. In general, the best studies show only a modest (0–2%) increase in bone mass among elders or postmenopausal women during prolonged aerobic or anaerobic exercise programs *(39)*. Still, these changes multiplied over a long period of time may be enough to prevent osteoporotic fractures. Certainly, the preservation of bone mass during states of accelerated bone loss, may be highly desirable. Yet there are unresolved issues about exercise, including the following:

1. Does exercise enhance bone mass only in estrogen-replete subjects?
2. Are there skeletal benefits to weight-lifting exercises, which exceed those noted with running or simple weight-bearing activities?
3. Is there a critical threshold for exercise-induced changes in bone mass?

These answers will have to await further studies. In this case, however, it is strongly recommended that TW at least become involved in a modest activity program to supplement her pharmacologic therapy and to enhance her sense of general well-being.

5. SUMMARY

TW has established postmenopausal osteoporosis, almost certainly as a result of early menopause, and possibly aggravated by physical stature and family history. Aggressive therapy is warranted in order to prevent subsequent hip and spine fractures. Choices (in addition to supplemental calcium and vitamin D) include the bis-phosphonates, estrogens, or the calcitonins. That decision can be made by a primary care provider as long as the patient's options are clear and the patient participates in the decision-making process. Overall, even more than medication, the physician–patient relationship will define the eventual outcome for TW. Osteoporosis is a chronic disease that will require continued care and surveillance for as long as TW remains a patient. Close attention to the medical as well as the psychosocial aspects of her disease (*see* Chapter 6) will guarantee a successful outcome for both the provider and the patient.

REFERENCES

1. Cann CE, Genant HK, Ettinger B, Gordon GS. Spinal mineral loss in oophorectomized women. Determination by quantitative computed tomography. *JAMA* 1980; 244: 2056–2059.
2. Ohta H, Masuzawa T, Ikeda T, Suda Y, Makita K, Nozawa S. Which is more osteoporosis-inducing menopause or oophorectomy? *Bone Miner* 1992; 19: 273–285.
3. Louis O, Devroey P, Kalender W, Osteaux M. Bone loss in young hypoestrogenimic women due to primary ovarian failure. *Fertil Steril* 1989; 52: 227–231.
4. Cann CE, Martin MC, Genant HK, Jaffe RB. Decreased spinal mineral content in amenorrheic women. *JAMA* 1984; 151: 626–629.
5. Bachrch LK, Katzman DK, Litt IF, Guido D, Marcus R. Recovery from osteopenia in adolescent girls with anorexia nervosa. *J Clin Endocrinol Metab* 1991; 72: 602–606.
6. Manolagas SC, Jilka RL, Cytokines, hematopoiesis, osteoclastogenesis and estrogens. *Calcif Tissue Int* 1992; 50,199–202.
7. Katzman DK, Bachrach LK, Carter DR, Marcus R. Clinical and anthropometric correlates of bone mineral acquisition in healthy adolescent girls. *J Clin Endocrinol Metab* 1991; 73: 1332–1339.
8. Cummings SR, Black DM, Rubin SM. Lifetime risks of hip, Colles' or vertebral fracture and coronary heart disease among, white postmenopausal women. *Arch Intern Med* 1989; 149: 2445–2448.
9. WHO Study Group. Assessment of Fracture Risk and its Application to screening for postmenopausal osteoporosis. Geneva: World Health Organization. 1994, pp. 50.
10. Miller PD, Rosen CJ, Bonnick IS. Guidelines for the Clinical Utilization of Bone Mass Measurements in the Adult Population. *Calcif Tissue Int* 1995; 57: 251–252.
11. Ross PD, David JW, Epstein RS, Wasnich RD. Preexisting fractures and bone mass predict vertebral fracture incidence in women. *Ann Int Med* 1991; 114: 191–193.
12. Rosen CJ, Holick MF, Millard PS. Premature graying of hair is a risk marker for osteopenia. *J Clin Endocrinol Metab* 1994; 79: 854–857.
13. Slemenda CW, Christian JC, Williams CJ, Norton JA, Johnston CC. Genetic determinants of bone mass in adult women: a reevaluation of the twin model and the potential importance of gene interaction on heritability estimates *J Bone Miner Res* 1991 ; 6: 561–567.
14. Slemenda CW, Christian JC, Reed T, Reister TK, Williams CJ, Johnston CC. Long term bone loss in men: effects of genetic and environmental factors. *Ann Int Med* 1992; 117: 286–291.
15. Kelly PJ, Hopper JUL, Macaskill GGT, Pocock NA, Sambrook PH, Eisman JA. Genetic factors in bone turnover. *J Clin Endocrinol Metab* 1991; 72: 808–814.
16. Wartofsky L. Osteoporosis and therapy with thyroid hormone. *The Endocrinologist* 1991: 1 : 57–61.
17. Rosen CJ, Morrison AM, Zhou H, Storm D, Hunter SJ, Musgrave KO, Chen T, Wen Wei T, Holick MF. Elderly women in northern New England exhibit seasonal changes in bone mass and calciotropic hormones. *Bone Miner* 1994; 25: 83–92.

18. Dawson-Hughes B, Harris S, Frall E. Rates of bone loss in postmenopausal women randomly assigned to one of two dosages of vitamin D. *Am J Clin Nutr* 1995; 61: 1140–1145.
19. Meunier PJ, Chapuy MC, Arlot ME, Delmas PD, Duboeuf F. Can we stop bone loss and prevent hip fractures in the elderly. *Osteoporosis Int* 1994; S1 76–78.
20. Chapuy MC, Arlot ME, Duboeuf F, Brun J, Crouzet B, Arnaud S, Delmas PD, Meunier PJ. Vitamin D and calcium to prevent hip fractures in elderly women. *N Engl J Med* 1992; 327: 1637–1642.
21. Lindsay R, Tohme JF. Estrogen treatment of patients with postmenopausal osteoporosis. *Obst Gynecol* 1991; 76: 290–295.
22. Lufkin EJ, Washner HW, O'Fallon WM. Treatment of postmenopausal osteoporosis with transdermal estrogen. *Ann Int Med* 1992; 117: 1–9.
23. Hutchinson TA, Polansky SM, Feinstein AR. Postmenopausal estrogens protect against fractures of hip and distal radius. A case-control study. *Lancet* 1979; ii: 705–709.
24. Weiss NS, Ure CL, Ballard JH, Williams AR, Daling JR. Decreased risk of fractures of the hip and lower forearm with postmenopausal use of estrogen. *N Engl J Med*; 1980; 303: 1195–1198.
25. Kiel DP, Felson DT, Anderson JJ. Hip fracture and the use of estrogens in postmenopausal women: the Framingham study. *N Engl J Med* 1987; 317: 1169–1174.
26. Jones MM, Francis RM, Nordin BEC. Five year follow-up of estrogen therapy in 94 women. *Maturitas* 1982; 4: 123–130.
27. Bush TL, Miller VT. Menopause: *Physiology and Pharmacology*. Chicago IL: Year Book Medical Publisher, 1987, pp. 191.
28. Writing group for the PEPI trial. Effects of estrogen or estrogen/progestin regimens on heard disease risk factors in postmenopausal women: the postmenopausal estrogen/progestin intervention trial. *JAMA* 1995; 273: 199–208.
29. Colditz GA, Hankinson SE, Hunter DJ, Willett WC, Manson JE, Stampfer MT, Hennekens C, et al. The use of estrogens and progestins and the risk of breast cancer in postmeneopausal women. *N Engl J Med* 1996; 332: 1589–1593.
30. Bush TL, Barrett-Connor E, Cowan LD. Cardiovascular mortality and noncontraceptive use of estrogen in women: results from the Lipid Research Clinics, Program follow-up study. *Circulation* 1987; 75: 1102–1109.
31. McClung MR, Fuleihan EH, LeBoff MS, Luciano AA, Gibbons WE, Slurry K, Ogrinc FG, Schoenfeld MJ. Comparison of sequential vs continuous estrogen/progesterone therapy on bone density. *J Bone Miner Res* 1991; 6: 784.
32. Storm T, Thamsborg G, Steiniche T, Genant HK, Sorensen OH. Effect of intermittent cyclical etidronate therapy on bone repass and fracture rate in women with postmenopausal osteoporosis. *N Engl J Med* 1990; 322: 265–271.
33. Harris ST, Watts NB, Jackson R. Four year study of intermittent cyclic etidronate treatment of postmenopausal osteoporosis: three years of blinded therapy followed by one year of open therapy. *Am J Med* 1993; 95: 557–567.
34. Recker RR, Karp DB, Quan H, et al. Three year treatment of osteoporosis with alendronate effect on vertebral fracture incidence. Endocrine Society 77th Annual Meeting, 1995, Endocrine Society, Bethesda, MD, p. 49.
35. Mazzuoli GF, Passeri M, Gennari C. Effects of salmon calcitonin in postmenopausal osteoporosis: a controlled double-blind clinical study. *Calcif Tissue Int* 1986: 38: 3–8.
36. Rico H, Hernandez ER, Revilla M, Gomex-Castresana F. Salmon calcitonin reduces vertebral fracture rate in the postmenopausal crush fracture syndrome. *Bone Miner* 1992; 16: 131–138.
37. Lyritis GP, Tsakalabos S, Magiasis B, Karachalios T, Yiatzides A, Tsekoura M. Analgesic effect of salmon calcitonin on osteoporotic vertebral fractures. Double blind, placebo-controlled study. *Calcif Tissue Int* 1991; 49: 369–372.
38. Smith EL. The role of exercise in the prevention and treatment of osteoporosis. *Top Geriatr Rehabil* 1995; 10: (4): 55–63.
39. Taafe DR, Marcus R. Longitudinal changes in bone mineral density in collegiate female gymnasts. *J Bone Miner Res* 1994; 9: S319.

19 The Approach to Osteoporosis in the Elderly Patient

Douglas P. Kiel, MD, MPH

CONTENTS

CASE STUDY

Mrs F. is a thin 85-yr-old widow living alone in a small apartment. She is independent in her activities of daily living, but receives some assistance with heavy housework. She manages all of her own affairs, has been in relatively good health, but her family has noted increasing forgetfulness. She has osteoarthritis in the right knee, hypertension treated with a calcium channel blocker, and insomnia treated with temazepam. Mrs F. underwent a hysterectomy at age 45 for fibroids and never received hormone therapy. She eats three meals a day, but has never tolerated milk or dairy products because of gastrointestinal distress, and she hesitates to go out into the direct sunlight because she is fair-skinned. She has never had a fracture. For several days, she had been experiencing urinary frequency. One morning, she awoke with an urgency to void and stood up quickly to proceed to the toilet. Because of the pain from her arthritic knee, she had trouble getting up and the rug next to her bed slid out from under her. She fell to the side, landing on the left hip, but was unable to get up to call for assistance because of pain. Her home health aid came to the house later that day and found her on the floor. She was taken to the hospital where an X-ray of the left hip revealed a femoral neck fracture. She was hospitalized for 4 d, and was discharged to a rehabilitation facility. By the end of her 30-d stay, she was able to ambulate with a walker, and was discharged to her own apartment with a visiting nurse

From: *Osteoporosis: Diagnostic and Therapeutic Principles*
Edited by: C. J. Rosen Humana Press Inc., Totowa, NJ

and health aid. However, she was no longer able to perform housework, go grocery shopping, or prepare meals without assistance. During the subsequent 6 mo, she fell repeatedly at home, sustaining minor injuries on several occasions. Her daughter felt that it was unsafe for her to remain at home. She was, therefore, placed in a nursing home after long discussions among the family. In the nursing home, she was despondent, ate poorly, and lost weight. Depression was diagnosed by her nursing home physician, and she was begun on an antidepressant medication. Her functional status continued to decline, and one day while ambulating to the toilet, she fell and fractured the right hip. During her hospitalization for the fracture, she developed a grade II pressure ulcer on the buttocks, and an episode of urosepsis from the indwelling foley catheter. By the time of discharge back to the nursing home, she was totally dependent on the staff for her ADLs, and was incontinent of urine. She currently resides at the nursing home.

1. DEMOGRAPHICS OF OSTEOPOROSIS AND RELATED FRACTURES IN THE ELDERLY POPULATION

Using the new World Health Organization definition of osteopenia and osteoporosis, overall, approx 16.8 million (54%) postmenopausal white women in the US have osteopenia and another 9.4 million (30%) have osteoporosis. Among women age 80 and older, 27% have osteopenia and 70% have osteoporosis. Given these figures, it is not surprising that the incidence of osteoporotic fractures rises so dramatically with age. Over 280,000 hip fractures occur each year in the US, and this number continues to grow as the average age of the population increases. In fact, the fastest growing segment of the US population is the group older than age 85.

The morbidity and mortality of hip fracture are greater in older persons for many of the same reasons that any acute insult results in less favorable outcomes in this population, namely frailty or the state of reduced physiologic reserve associated with increased susceptibility to disability. This reduced physiologic capacity results from biologic aging, chronic conditions, and disuse or abuse. These effects are often modified further by psychosocial and environmental factors, self-care, and medical/rehabilitative care available to elderly persons (1). It is important to remember, however, that age alone is not associated with poor outcomes of fracture when other age-related comorbidities are accounted for. Thus, in a large cohort study of 2812 individuals followed for 6 yr, both 6-mo mortality and institutionalization were more common in older individuals, but after accounting for the number of comorbid diagnoses, type of hip fracture, premorbid mental status, and perioperative complications, age was no longer a significant factor (2). This same concept of comorbidities probably explains the observation that the 5-yr survival following vertebral fracture is 15% less than expected (3).

The clinical case above highlights the coexistence of multiple comorbid diagnoses that may have contributed to Mrs. F's poor outcome. She suffered from mobility limitations secondary to her osteoarthritis, had early cognitive decline, was taking hypotensive drugs and sedative hypnotics, and became depressed, withdrawn, and nutritionally deficient after placement in the nursing home following her first hip fracture.

The concept of frailty is a unique aspect of osteoporosis in the elderly population. It contributes substantially to the prediction of rehabilitation outcomes following a hip fracture. Multiple studies have confirmed that older subjects with hip fracture have better rehabilitation outcomes if they have better prefracture health, mobility, cognitive func-

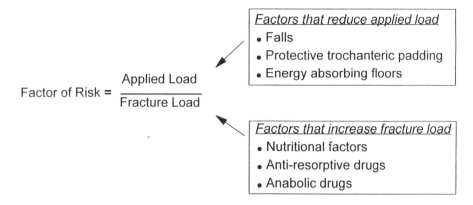

Fig. 1. The concept of "factor of risk" for fracture takes into account both the forces that impact the bone and the underlying forces required to fracture the bone. The forces that impact the bone derive from the fall energy that is actually delivered to the area of the body overlying a bone. The force required to fracture the bone is directly proportional to the strength of the bone. This figure is from ref. *34a*.

tion, and are living with someone. Poorer outcomes result from inadequate nutritional status and postoperative depression *(4–10)*. The recognition that such factors contribute to hip fracture outcomes has prompted some to attempt special geriatric-focused rehabilitative care after fractures of the proximal femur *(11,12)*. The use of a multidisciplinary team may result in shorter hospital stays, better short- and long-term (1-yr) functional recoveries, and better overall survival. Had Mrs. F's early rehabilitation process included a better understanding of her fall risk factors, she may have avoided institutionalization with its cascade of subsequent declines.

2. FACTORS CONTRIBUTING TO THE RISK OF FRACTURE IN ELDERLY PERSONS

2.1. The "Factor of Risk"

Another important concept for the understanding of osteoporosis and related fractures in elderly individuals is that decreased underlying bone strength as reflected by bone mineral density (BMD) measurement is probably not the most important contributor to fracture risk. Factors that contribute to the occurrence of hip fracture include propensity to fall, inability to correct a postural imbalance, the orientation of the fall, adequacy of local tissue shock absorbers, and underlying skeletal strength. For its part, the resistance of a skeletal structure to failure (i.e., fracture) depends on the geometry of the bone, the mechanical properties of the calcified tissue, and the location and direction of the loads to which the bone is subjected (i.e., during a fall). Estimations of the forces generated within the bone in response to a given load can be estimated using basic engineering principles. The forces can then be compared with the strengths of the tissue. The ratio of the force expected during normal activities, or during a fall, to the force required to cause the bone to fail may be thought of as the structure's "factor of risk" (*see* Fig. 1). When the factor of risk is high (close to or more than 1), the structure is at great risk of fracture.

In the elderly, simple stance and normal ambulation involve a factor of risk at the femoral neck of about 0.3. For stair climbing, it is about 0.6. In falls, the factor of risk probably ranges from 1 to >7. The calculations are complicated by considerable uncertainty about the loads to which hips are actually subjected during falls. For one thing, skeletal structures at high risk for age-related fracture, such as the hip, change their geometry with aging and bone remodeling. These changes snake it difficult to ascertain the force of failure in vivo.

Despite the difficulties of determining the force of failure in vivo, in vitro testing of femurs can provide data on the work required to fracture a bone. Recent studies have estimated the potential energies liberated by a fall from standing height to be close to 600 J. By the time the hip strikes the floor, 70% of the potential energy has been dissipated during the descent phase, leaving about 170 J of energy just before impact. This amount of energy is two orders of magnitude greater than the energy required to fracture elderly femurs during in vitro studies. These findings confirm that a simple fall is easily capable of fracturing the proximal femur. In the case of Mrs. F. her fall was to the side from a standing height. Her small body habitus contributed to her risk partly because of the absence of protective adipose tissue overlying her hip. She was predisposed to having reduced BMD from early surgical menopause without hormone replacement, causing perhaps 5 yr of premature estrogen deficiency, inadequate dietary calcium intake, and rare sunlight exposure, resulting in inadequate vitamin D levels. Thus, her factor of risk probably exceeded 1.

2.2. Falls

Over the past 5 yr, a number of prospective studies have confirmed many of the factors that had been implicated as risks for falling in older persons. Such factors include gait and mobility problems, leg and foot dysfunction (including balance problems), and medication use *(13–15)*. These findings set the stage for a series of intervention studies called the Frailty and Injuries: Cooperative Studies of Intervention Techniques (FICSIT studies). The FICSIT studies were comprised of a collection of eight independent clinical trials that assessed the efficacy and feasibility of a variety of intervention strategies, including exercise, balance training, and geriatric multidisciplinary interventions in reducing falls and/or frailty in the elderly. An overview of these studies revealed that elderly subjects who were assigned to some form of exercise reduced the risk of falls by about 10% *(16)*. It was not possible to identify which element of being in an exercise group conferred this protective effect or the specific types of exercise that were most effective. Similarly, studies that included balance training also reduced the risk of falls. One of the most notable results was that a multidisciplinary intervention that included behavioral changes, medication changes, education, as well as resistance, balance, and flexibility exercise for a period of 3 mo significantly reduced falls. These findings support the notion that fall-related risk factors for fracture can be modified. In the case of Mrs. F, attention to the osteoarthritis, choice of antihypertensive agent, elimination of benzodiazepines for the treatment of insomnia, and attention to the moving bedside throw rug could have prevented a hip fracture.

Obviously not all falls result in serious injury or fracture. Identifying those at risk for falls that are likely to result in fracture requires an understanding of the kinds of falls and their sequelae. An understanding of what constitutes a fall with a high risk of hip fracture and how factors related to fall severity compare to those related to bone fragility is now beginning to emerge. Falls on the hip, side of the leg, or falls straight down increase the risk of hip fracture up to 30-fold *(17,18)*. By contrast, the risk of hip fracture doubles for every standard deviation reduction in BMD or body mass index. Thus, in elderly persons who fall, most of whom have hip bone mineral well below "fracture threshold," fall severity (as reflected in falling to the side and impacting the hip) and body habitus are important risk factors for hip fracture, and touch on a domain of risk entirely missed by knowledge of BMD. In the most comprehensive evaluation of risk factors for hip fracture yet available, many of the risk factors associated with hip fracture, including reduced lower extremity strength and gait speed, were independent of bone mass and were the same factors known to be associated with a risk of falling. Several characteristics of Mrs. F (thin elderly woman with reduced lower extremity function who fell to the side) clearly contributed to the injurious nature of her fall.

Falls themselves are not simple events. In particular, the total energy of a fall is not entirely delivered to the trochanter. Potentially important factors that can influence the amount of force imposed include the presence of energy-absorbing soft tissues over the greater trochanter and the state of leg muscle contraction at the time of the fall. Threefold increases in the thickness of soft tissue overlying skeletal structures reduce the predicted peak impact force of a fall by 20% and may explain the observation that heavier persons have a reduced risk of hip fracture. Falling in a muscle-relaxed state reduces the peak force by more than 50%. It has been proposed that padding the trochanter may be an option for preventing hip fracture *(19)*. In fact, a few clinical trials are under way, as will be described.

2.3. Bone Density

Notwithstanding the less important role of bone density in the prediction of fracture risk when compared to fall severity, it contributes valuable information to the understanding of fracture risk. At least three longitudinal studies have confirmed that a single BMD measurement is associated with the risk of later fracture *(20–22)*. For each standard deviation decrease in BMD (regardless of the skeletal site measured), the risk of hip fracture increases 1.5- to 2.9-fold. This same predictive value was recently found to hold true for community-dwelling women 80 yr of age and older *(14)*, but was not as strong for residents of a retirement home who are older *(20)*. There have been no studies in nursing home residents.

Until recently, a commonly held belief about age-related bone loss was that as individuals age into their 70s, 80s, and beyond, the rate of bone loss either slows or plateaus. In fact, one study projected a small increase in radial BMD with advanced age *(23)*. These beliefs fueled the attitude that by the time one reached old age, "the horse was out of the barn." Many patients were told by their physicians that not much could be done at this point in life. This attitude still pervades some primary care environments. Recently new information has shed light on this long-held belief. It appears that the rate of bone loss in old age continues at the same rate *(24–26)* or may even increase *(27–29)* relative to bone loss rates seen in younger individuals.

3. FRACTURE PREVENTION IN ELDERLY PERSONS

The kind of information provided from the above-mentioned longitudinal studies of bone loss in the elderly population has important ramifications for therapy of osteoporosis among this age group. Obviously, fracture prevention is the goal of any therapeutic strategy. Older persons have lower bone density to begin with, are continuing to lose bone, and are in the age group most likely to fracture. Thus, interventions would be expected to be most cost-effective when initiated in older aged individuals. These interventions can be divided into two groups: (1) those interventions that reduce the factor of risk by reducing the applied load (fall prevention, passive protective systems) and (2) those interventions that reduce the factor of risk by increasing the force required to fracture the bone (therapies that preserve or increase bone density). This is shown in Fig. 1.

3.1. Interventions that Reduce the Factor of Risk by Reducing the Applied Load

3.1.1. FALL PREVENTION

A good primary care physician caring for older individuals should evaluate such patients for their risk of falling and should attempt to reduce the number of predisposing factors for falls. This need not be an elaborate process. All patients should be queried regarding the past history of falls, because a history of falls is the single most important risk factor for a subsequent fall. If there is a history of a fall, additional information should be obtained surrounding the events of the fall, including the activity of the faller at the time of the incident, prodromal symptoms (lightheadedness, imbalance, dizziness), and where and when the fall occurred. This previous fall information may identify important factors for targeting risk factor modification strategies. The medical history should ascertain whether there are any visual, vestibular, hearing, or peripheral neuropathic diseases, such as diabetes. Central nervous system diseases of interest include dementia and Parkinson's, disease, both of which affect the central processing of sensory information. Musculoskeletal diseases account for deficiencies in the effector system. Conditions, such as arthritis, cause pain and deformity, which result in joint instability and falls, especially when the knees are involved. Rheumatoid arthritis also can cause significant foot deformities that make it difficult to stand. Disorders of the feet should be included in the review of systems, because such deformities as calluses, bunions, toe deformities, such as hammertoes, and large, thick, deformed toenails can compromise gait and interfere with proprioception. Treatment of any of the above conditions may help to reduce this risk of a fall. This follows from the principle of geriatric care that small improvements in several chronic conditions can often result in improved functional status in older persons.

In the physical assessment of fall risk, vital sign measurement should include a careful assessment of orthostatic blood pressure changes and heart rate immediately after standing, and after a few minutes. The head and neck examination includes a careful assessment of visual acuity using best corrected vision with existing eyeglasses. Hearing can be assessed using the "whisper test" or a handheld audiometer. Eighth cranial nerve deficits may be associated with vestibular dysfunction, another risk factor for falls. Cardiac exam may identify arrhythmias or slow heart rate. Examination of the extremities may uncover deformities of the feet that may contribute to the risk of falling, such as those mentioned above. Footwear may be in poor repair, with unsafe soles, or may not fit properly.

The remainder of the physical examination assesses the three components of postural stability: sensory input, central integrative function, and effecter responses. A neurologic examination allows one to examine each of the three components separately, such as a test for lower extremity proprioceptive function, Mini-Mental Status Examination of cognitive function, or an examination of lower extremity muscle strength.

The postural stability system as a whole can be tested using any of several recently developed assessment tools. One of the more well known of these, the "Get Up and Go" test, consists of a subject rising from a standard arm chair, walking across the room, turning around, walking back to the chair, and sitting back down. This sequence of activities can be graded using a 1–5 rating scale (1 = normal, 2 = very slightly abnormal, 3 = mildly abnormal, 4 = moderately abnormal, and 5 = severely abnormal) *(30)* or a timed measurement of the same tasks *(31)*. This assessment may help to identify individuals with potential postural stability deficits predisposing them to falls. Recently, Studenski and colleagues have developed a simple maneuver called the "functional reach" test, which correlated with balance ability and may be a marker for general functional decline *(32,33)*. This test is performed using a leveled yardstick secured to a wall at the height of the acromion. The person being tested assumes a comfortable stance without shoes or socks, and stands so that his or her shoulders are perpendicular to the yardstick The individual makes a fist and extends the arm forward as far as possible without taking a step or losing balance. The total reach is measured along the yardstick and recorded. This yardstick reach correlated with an electronic measurement of the same maneuver ($r = 0.69$), and the test–retest intraclass correlation coefficient was 0.92. The functional reach maneuver also correlated with other physical performance measures, such as walking speed ($r = 0.71$), and various measures of balance, such as tandem walk (graded using an ordinal scale) ($r = 0.67$) and one-footed standing (measured as number of seconds able to maintain stance) ($r = 0.64$).

A more comprehensive performance-oriented assessment of balance has been used by Tinetti, and includes measures of sitting and standing balance, ability to withstand a nudge on the sternum, and ability to reach up, bend down, and extend the back and neck *(34)*. Each of these performances measures attempt to identify components of postural stability that might otherwise be untested by the standard physical examination, but that complement the standard physical assessment as outlined above. When deficits are identified using these assessments, an appropriate referral to physical therapy can be made. Physical therapists can also assess such patients, and design an individualized program for balance training, muscle strengthening, or safety education. Home visits by physical therapists can also be employed by the primary provider to ensure that the home environment is safe.

A complete medication history should focus specifically on vasodilators, diuretics, and psychoactive drugs, including antidepressants, antipsychotics, and benzodiazepines, because these agents have been associated with increased risk of falls. In any case where a medication is not deemed to be absolutely important, it should be eliminated.

3.1.2. PASSIVE PROTECTIVE SYSTEMS

Since falls to the side that impact on the hip are the primary determinant of hip fracture *(35)*, there is considerable interest in the design and evaluation of protective trochanteric padding devices. In early trials, padding devices were found to reduce hip fracture risk, but subject compliance was relatively low. Newer padding systems are designed to lower femoral impact force by shunting energy away from the femur and into the surrounding soft tissues. Laboratory methods of impact testing are available for comparing the ability of such devices to attenuate the forces of a fall on the trochanter. Using such laboratory tests, there are wide ranges of energy-reducing potential of the pads currently available (*see* Fig. 2). Not all pads attenuate the forces of a fall on the trochanter to levels that would be expected to reduce the risk of hip fracture. As optimal pad design evolves, it is expected

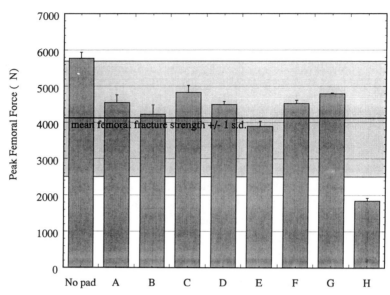

Fig. 2. Impact tests with a laboratory apparatus measuring force attenuation of eight energy-shunting pads compared with no pad. Bars show mean peak femoral force from five repeated measures, with error bars displaying 1 SD. Pad H is the pad currently being tested by the author in collaboration with Wilson C. Hayes.

that these devices may enjoy widespread use by elderly individuals who are at highest risk of fall-related fractures, such as nursing home residents. As with any therapeutic intervention, the hip pad would be expected to have the greatest protection among persons who are prone to fall to the side and who have very little soft tissue overlying the trochanter.

Related to protective trochanteric padding devices, another way to reduce the energy delivered to the hip during a fall is to design flooring materials that will absorb energy rather than deliver the energy of a fall directly to the trochanter. Toward this goal, such flooring materials are being tested with the goal of using them in high-risk environments, such as nursing homes.

3.2. Interventions that Reduce the Factor of Risk by Increasing the Force Required to Fracture

The intention here is to provide practical guidelines for the treatment of low bone density, specifically among older adults. No attempt will be made to provide an in-depth review of the use of these therapies in general, since they are covered in other chapters of this text. The approach to be described divides therapy into nutritional factors, antiresorptive drug therapy, and anabolic therapy.

3.2.1. NUTRITIONAL FACTORS

The major nutrients required for bone health are calcium and vitamin D. The role of trace minerals, such as magnesium, manganese, copper, and zinc, is somewhat uncertain, and the contribution of other dietary components, such as sodium, potassium, protein, vitamin K, and vitamin C, has not been adequately studied to be able to make general recommendations. Avoidance of excessive caffeine consumption may reduce bone loss and prevent fractures.

Although the bulk of evidence supports an important role for calcium intake in the health of adult bone, not all studies have been in agreement (36). Among randomized controlled clinical trials of calcium administration, however, almost all studies show that calcium slows or stops bone loss (36). Furthermore, calcium supplementation, an inexpensive, low-risk intervention, has been particularly successful among older women with very low calcium intakes (<500 mg/d). The recent NIH Consensus Conference on Optimal Calcium Intake recommended that "in women and men over 65 years of age, calcium intake of 1500 mg/day seems prudent" (37). To achieve a daily intake of 1500 mg/d among older persons may be difficult without resorting to the use of calcium supplements. Dietary intake of calcium is low in the US, because dairy product use declines with age. Constant reminders to limit fat intake can also constrain the consumption of dairy products. Many elderly persons may not recognize that low-fat dairy products provide adequate calcium. The role of calcium-fortified food products, including juices, fruit drinks, breads, and cereals, is not currently defined.

The calcium supplement most often recommended is calcium carbonate, because of its widespread availability, low price, and generally adequate absorption. Because some foods contain certain compounds that reduce calcium absorption (e.g., oxalates), the Consensus Conference recommended that calcium supplements be ingested between meals in doses not exceeding 500 mg. However, absorption of calcium carbonate is impaired in the absence of gastric acid when taken between meals and is actually enhanced when taken with foods. Alternatively, calcium citrate does not require gastric acid for optimal absorption and, thus, could be considered in older individuals with reduced gastric acid production.

Studies of vitamin D status among noninstitutionalized elderly performed in diverse populations estimate that the prevalence of vitamin D deficiency in the US among older individuals is between 30 and 50%. Compared with calcium, there is less agreement about the recommended daily allowance of vitamin D from dietary sources. However, a figure of 10 μg/d (400 IU) is widely accepted in the US. The data supporting this figure are limited, and the variable contribution of endogenous vitamin D_3 production in the skin must be factored into any recommendations of this kind. Furthermore, seasonal variations in 25-hydroxyvitamin D (25-OH-D) owing to sunlight exposure affect the measurements of plasma vitamin D. Among healthy elderly, the greatest vitamin D deficiency occurs among North Americans during the winter months. Several recent studies have been performed among institutionalized elderly, including nursing home residents, chronic hospital residents, home-bound community-dwellers, and hospital patients As measured by either dietary intake or 25-OH-D levels, institutionalized elderly persons have extremely poor vitamin D status.

Support for the use of vitamin D supplementation in the prevention of hip fractures has recently been highlighted by a large randomized, double-blind, placebo-controlled clinical trial of vitamin D_3 and calcium supplements to reduce the incidence of hip and nonvertebral fractures in elderly women living in French nursing homes. This 18-mo study of 3270 women demonstrated that the supplemented group enjoyed a significant reduction in the incidence of fractures without any unfavorable side effects, suggesting that the major effect of this regimen is to correct osteomalacia, a reversible disorder. The favorable effects of calcium and vitamin D_3 on fracture incidence, bone density, and biochemical markers in that study support the routine use of these supplements for elderly person in institutions, and probably for all elderly, although the optimal dose and formulation of vitamin D have not been established. From the available clinical trials of vitamin D supplementation, a dose of at least 10 μg (400 IU)/d should be given to all elderly persons *(38,39)*.

3.3. Resorptive Inhibitors

Virtually all of the drugs available for treatment of osteoporosis fall into the category of antiresorptive agents (*see* Chapters 13, 14, and 15), because they act to inhibit osteoclast activity. These include estrogen, calcitonin, and the bis-phosphonates.

3.3.1. ESTROGEN

The use of estrogen therapy by older women has been somewhat controversial. However, several studies of women age 70 and older have demonstrated protective effects on BMD *(40,41),* but suggest that these protective effects decline after cessation of therapy *(42,43),* so consideration must be given to the continuation of therapy for at least 10 yr. Furthermore, its cardiologic and urogenital effect may be particularly helpful in this age group compared to the potential carcinogenic effects on the uterus and breast. Compounds related to estrogen, such as tamoxifen, behave as estrogen agonist/antagonists and, thus, have potential for use in fracture prevention. New compounds with agonist effects on bone and lipids, and antagonist effects on breast and uterus are currently being tested in clinical trials. These agents could prove to be an important addition to the pharmacologic treatment of osteoporosis in the future.

Elderly women are usually reticent to take estrogens because of a reluctance to resume menses. These individuals should be informed that only about a half of elderly women who begin estrogen many years after menopause ever have menses. Either continuous estrogen/progesterone regimens or intermittent progesterone use can be offered as an option to women who object to having monthly cycles. Regarding the fear of breast cancer from estrogen therapy, older women should probably have less concern since their duration of use may be limited by their life expectancy, and it appears that longer durations of use are associated with the slight increase in the risk of breast cancer with estrogen use.

3.3.2. CALCITONIN

The use of salmon calcitonin by elderly individuals with osteoporosis has been limited by expense and need to administer the drug by injection. The recent approval in the US of a nasally administered preparation of salmon calcitonin offers an alternative to the injectable preparation. Studies outside the US have confirmed the ability of nasal calcitonin to slow or prevent bone loss.

The experience among elderly women involved in clinical trials of the nasally administered calcitonin has been favorable. The overall incidence of nasal side effects has been comparable between placebo and drug-treated women. Nasal irritation was reported in 12% of patients receiving nasal calcitonin vs 6.9% of placebo patients in clinical trials; other nasal symptoms were reported in 10.6% of patients vs 16% of placebo patients. In foreign marketing experience, no serious allergic-type reactions have been reported. The only potentially unique characteristic attributed to calcitonin that may have implications for elderly patients suffering from painful osteoporotic vertebral fractures is the analgesic effect that some physicians have observed with its use. This effect has not been confirmed in any large-scale trials.

3.3.3. BISPHOSPHONATES

The bisphosphonates, analogs of pyrophosphate in which the oxygen of the P—O—P bond is replaced by a carbon atom, resulting in a P—C—P bond, have a strong affinity for bone mineral despite their poor absorption. The most striking effect of the bisphosphonates is on the inhibition of bone resorption. Since the bone loss characteristic of osteoporosis and other bone diseases is the result of an imbalance between bone resorption and bone formation, inhibition of bone resorption is thus a rational approach to the prevention and treatment of osteoporosis.

The bisphosphonates represent a class of drug that may be particularly suited for the elderly person for a number of reasons. First, the drug is taken once a day by mouth. Second, there are few side effects. Finally, since elderly persons are most at risk of fractures, the therapeutic effect of these agents (fracture prevention) may be realized after only a relatively short duration of therapy compared to therapies initiated early after the menopause, which must be continued into old age to achieve fracture prevention. Thus, even thought the expense of daily therapy may be great, the benefits may also be great in this age group.

Despite these theoretical advantages in the elderly, the studies in this age group are limited. Etidronate, one of the bisphosponates currently available for oral use in the US, has not been tested in the elderly group. In the randomized clinical trial of this agent conducted in the US, the age requirement for entry was limited to women 75 yr and younger.

A new bisphosphonate, alendronate, recently approved by the Food and Drug Administration, has been tested in older persons. In an ongoing study of 359 women of age range 59–85 yr, alendronate led to statistically significant increases in BMD of the spine (4.6%) and hip (1.4%) after 1 yr of treatment. Ongoing studies involving women up to age 80 will provide information regarding the effects of this bis-phosphonate on fracture prevention.

3.4. Anabolic Therapy

Although there may be small anabolic effects of estrogen and alendronate, there has been little progress in the development of effective anabolic agents that can lead to new bone accretion beyond that created during normal remodeling.

3.4.1. FLUORIDE

Early trials of fluoride held promise that new bone formation could be stimulated. Unfortunately, at the doses and with the preparations used, the observed increase in bone density was not accompanied by increases in bone strength or by fracture reduction. However, a recent trial in women with existing osteoporosis (mean age 68 yr), using a sustained-release form of sodium fluoride, demonstrated a reduction in vertebral fractures without an increase in other fractures (44). This type of therapy would have particular appeal in the elderly population, since many persons with low bone density would benefit from new bone-forming therapy. Further studies are needed in older persons to be able to recommend the use of such preparations by this group.

4. FRACTURE REHABILITATION IN ELDERLY PERSONS

4.1. Hip Fracture

Following a hip fracture, most rehabilitation is performed at a rehabilitation facility, either at a special hospital, a unit in a long-term care facility, or at home. Since the length of stay for hospitalization of hip fracture has dropped to 5 d or less, elderly patients are discharged to the rehabilitation setting in a more unstable condition. This situation may require the primary care physician to become involved earlier than had traditionally been the case. Medical complications, including delirium, infection, and fluid overload, as well as anticoagulation management, become the domain of the primary care physician. The goals of rehabilitation are fairly standard, including relief of pain, maintaining the bony union in ideal position, maintenance of the normal range of motion of joints, prevention of muscle atrophy and weakness, restoration of function, and prevention of complications, such as malunion and prolongation of bed rest (45). Ensuring adequate nutritional support during the perioperative period may improve outcomes.

During the rehabilitation period, the occupational therapist trains the patient in dressing, bathing, and other activities of daily living. The physical therapist works with the patient to learn proper transfer techniques, exercises to strengthen various muscle groups, and the proper use of assistive devices. Activities and exercises begin at a low level and progress. The patient is started on breathing exercises, range of motion for the upper extremities, and isometric lower extremity exercises before working on transfers. The important decision to begin any degree of weight bearing depends on characteristics of the individual patient, such as weight, cognition, type and site of hip fracture, and type of operative procedure. For example, weight bearing can begin almost the day after the operation in the case of a cemented arthroplasty, whereas after nail and plate operations, it may take a number of weeks before weight bearing can be initiated.

When the patient returns to the care of the primary physician, all of the fracture prevention strategies outlined above are important to consider in the prevention of subsequent hip fractures, which are more common in individuals with a previous fracture.

4.2. Vertebral Fracture

For the subset of vertebral fractures that are symptomatic, the general approach is initial bedrest, analgesics, and local ice packs. The period of rest must be individualized for each patient, but may extend up to 3 wk. After the initial bedrest, hot packs and increasing activities as tolerated by the patient are started, including instructions in transfer activities, gait training, and activities of daily living. Flexion of the spine is generally avoided, since most of the fractures are of the anterior wedge variety. Extension exercise of the back muscles are extremely important. Referral to physical therapy to achieve these aims is appropriate.

5. SUMMARY

The problem of osteoporotic fractures in the elderly person is a complex one that involves both falling and underlying osteoporosis. Both factors need to be considered when assessing an individual's risk of fracture. In fact, special attention to fall prevention is particularly important in a person with low bone density, and attention to low bone density is particularly important in a person with a propensity to fall. Thus, pharmacologic therapy is not the only way to prevent fractures. Fall prevention may even be more important than maintaining bone density in the elderly patient. Even the best efforts at fall prevention will leave some individuals vulnerable for injurious falls. Newer developments in protective padding devices and energy-absorbing surfaces may provide additional approaches to fracture prevention.

REFERENCES

1. Buchner DM, Wagner EH. Preventing frail health. *Clin Geriatr Med* 1992; 8: 1–17.
2. Marottoli RA, Berkman LF, Leo-Summers L, et al. Predictors of mortality and institutionalization after hip fracture: the New Haven EPESE cohort. *Am J Pub Health* 1994; 84: 1807–1812.
3. Cooper C, Atkinson EJ, Jacobsen SJ, et al. Population-based study of survival after osteoporotic fractures. *Am J Epidemiol* 1993; 137: 1001–1005.
4. Thorngren KG, Ceder L, Svensson K. Predicting results of rehabilitation after hip fracture. *Clin Orthop Rel Res* 1993; 287: 76–81.
5. Ceder L, Thorngren KG, Wallden B. Prognostic indicators and early home rehabilitation in elderly patients with hip fractures. *Clin Orthol Rel Res* 1980; 152: 173–184.
6. Cobey JC, Cobey JH, Conant L. Indicators of recovery from fractures of the hip. *Clin Orthop Rel Res* 1976; 117: 258–262.
7. Marottoli RA, Berkman LF, Cooney LM. Decline in physical function following hip fracture. *J Am Geriatr Soc* 1992; 40: 861–866.
8. Mossey JM, Mutran E, Knott K, et al. Determinants of recovery 12 months after hip fracture: the importance of psychosocial factors. *Am J Pub Health* 1989; 79: 279–286.
9. Cummings SR, Phillips, SL, Wheat ME, et al. Recovery of fixation after hip fracture the role of social supports. *J Am Geriatr Soc* 1988; 36: 801–806.
10. Foster MR, Heppenstall B, Friedenberg ZB, et al. A prospective assessment of nutritional status and complications in patients with fractures of the hip. *J Orthopaedic Trauma* 1990; 4: 49–57.
11. Kennie DC, Reid J, Richardson IR, et al. Effectiveness of geriatric rehabilitative care after fractures of the proximal femur in elderly women: a randomised clinical trial. *Br Med J* 1988; 297: 1083–1086.
12. Reid J, Kennie DC. Geriatric rehabilitative care after fractures of the: proximal femur: one year follow up of a randomised clinical trial. *Br Med J* 1989; 299: 25, 26.
13. Tinetti ME, Speechley M, Ginter F. Risk factors for falls among elderly persons living in the community. *N Engl J Med* 1988; 319: 1701–1707.
14. Nevitt MC, Johnell O, Black DM, et al. Bone mineral density predicts non-spine fractures in very elderly women. *Osteo Int* 1994; 4: 325–331.
15. Campbell AJ, Borrie MJ, Spears GF. Risk factors for falls in a community-based prospective study of people 70 years and older. *J Gerontol* 1989; 44: M112–M117.
16. Province MA, Hadley EC, Hornbrook MC, et al. The effects of exercise on falls in elderly patients. *JAMA* 1995; 273: 1341–1347.
17. Hayes WC, Myers ER, Morris JN, Gerhart TN, Yett HS, Lipsitz LA. Impact near the hip dominates fracture risk in elderly nursing home residents who fall. *Calcif Tissue Int* 1993; 52: 192–199.
18. Nevitt MC, Cummings SR. Type of fall and risk of hip and wrist fractures: the study of osteoporotic fractures. *J Am Geriatr Soc* 1993; 41: 1226–1234.
19. Lauritzen JB, Petersen MM, Lund B. Effect of external hip protectors on hip fractures. *Lancet* 1993; 341: 11–13.
20. Hui, SL, Slemenda CW, Johnston CC. Baseline measurement of bone mass predicts fracture in white women. *Ann Intern Med* 1989; 111: 355–361.
21. Gardsell P, Johnell O, Nilsson BE. Predicting fractures in women by using forearm bone densitometry. *Calcif Tissue Int* 1989; 44: 235–242.
22. Cummings SR, Black DN, Nevitt MC, et al. Bone density at various sites for prediction of hip fractures. *Lancet* 1993; 341: 72–75.
23. Hui SL, Wiske PS, Norton JA, et al. A prospective study of change in bone mass with age in postmenopausal women. *J Chron Dis* 1982; 35: 715–725.
24. Hannan MT, Kiel DP, Mercier CE, Anderson JJ, Felson DT. Longitudinal bone mineral density (BMD) change in elderly men and women: the Framingham osteoporosis study. *J Bone Miner Res* 1994; 9(Suppl. 1): S130.
25. Cali CM, Kiel DP. Age-related bone loss in the "old" old: a longitudinal study of institutionalized elderly. *J Bone Miner Res* 1995; 10 (suppl. 1) S450.
26. Greenspan SL, Maitland LA, Myers ER, et al. Femoral bone loss progresses with age: a longitudinal study in women over age 65. *J Bone Miner Res* 1994; 9: 1959–1965.
27. Ensrud KE, Palermo L, Black DM, et al. Hip bone loss increases with advancing age: longitudinal results from the study of osteoporotic fractures. *J Bone Miner Res* 1994; 9(Suppl. 1): S153.
28. Jones G, Nguyen T, Sambrook P, et al. Progressive loss of bone in the femoral neck in elderly people: longitudinal findings from the Dubbo osteoporosis epidemiology study. *Br Med J* 1994; 309: 691–695.

29. Tobin JD, Fox KM, Cejku ML, et al. Bone density changes in normal men: a 4–19 year longitudinal study. *J Bone Miner Res* 1993; 8(Suppl. 1): S142.

30. Mathias S, Nayak USL, Isaacs B. Balance in elderly patients: the "Get-up and Go" test. *Arch Phys Med Rehabil* 1986; 67: 387–389.

31. Podsiadlo D, Richardson S. The timed "up and go": a test of basic functional mobility for frail elderly persons. *J Am Geriatr Soc* 1991; 39: 142–148.

32. Duncan PW, Weiner DK, Chandler J, Studenski S. Functional reach: a new clinical measure of balance. *J Gerontol* 1990; 45: M192–M197.

33. Weiner DK, Duncan PW, Chandler J, et al. Functional reach: a marker of physical frailty. *J Am Geriatr Soc* 1991; 40: 203–207.

34. Tinetti ME. Performance-oriented assessment of mobility problems in elderly patients *J Am Geriatr Soc* 1986; 34: 119–126.

34a. Robinovitch SN, Hayes WC, McMahon TA. Energy shunting hip padding system attenuates femoral impact force in a simulated fall. *Asne J Bio Eng* 1995; 117: 409–413.

35. Greenspan SL, Myers ER, Maitland LA, Resnick NM, Hayes WC. Fall severity and bone mineral density as risk factors for hip fracture in ambulatory elderly. *JAMA* 1994; 271: 128–133.

36. Heaney RP. Editorial: thinking straight about calcium. *N Engl J Med* 1993; 328 : 503–505.

37. NIH consensus development panel on optimal calcium intake. Optimal calcium intake. *JAMA* 1994; 272: 1942–1948.

38. Ooms ME, Roos JC, Bezemer PD, et al. Prevention of bone loss by vitamin D supplementation in elderly women: a randomized double-blind trial. *J Clin Endocrinol Metab* 1995; 80: 1052–1058.

39. Dawson-Hughes B, Harris SS, Krall EA, et al. Rates of bone loss in postmenopausal women randomly assigned to one of two dosages of vitamin D. *Am J Clin Nutr* 1995; 61: 1140–1145.

40. Lindsay R, Tohme JF. Estrogen treatment of patients with established postmenopausal osteoporosis. *Obstet Gynecol* 1990; 76: 290–295.

41. Quigley MET, Martin PL, Burneir AM, et al. Estrogen therapy arrests bone loss in elderly women. *Am J Obstet Gynecol* 1987; 156: 1516–1523.

42. Felson DT, Zhang Y, Hannan MT. The effect of postmenopausal estrogen therapy on bone density in elderly women. *N Engl J Med* 1994; 329: 1141–1146.

43. Cauley JA, Seeley DG, Ensrud K, et al. Estrogen replacement therapy and fractures in older women. *Ann Intern Med* 1995; 122: 9–16.

44. Pak CYC, Saknaee K, Piziak V, et al. Sow-release sodium fluoride in the management of postmenopausal osteoporosis. A randomized controlled trial. *Ann Intern Med* 1994; 120: 625–632.

45. Mehta AJ, Nastasi AE. Rehabilitation of fractures in the elderly. *Clin Geriatr Med* 1993; 9: 717–730.

20 Preventing and Treating Glucocorticoid Osteoporosis

Robert A. Adler, MD

CONTENTS

CASE STUDY

A 42-yr-old white female presents with severe upper thoracic back pain. Her history includes the fact that she has been on glucocorticoid therapy for Crohn's disease for more than 20 yr. She is premenopausal with regular periods and has no obvious risk factors for osteoporosis aside from her history of glucocorticoid therapy. Previous studies have not demonstrated any evidence of malabsorption. X-rays reveal three compression fractures of the thoracic spine (T_{8-11}). Lumbar spine bone density is 3 SD below the mean for a 35-yr-old woman (t-score = −3.0).

1. WHAT IS DIFFERENT ABOUT GLUCOCORTICOID OSTEOPOROSIS?

The classic patient with osteoporosis is a thin, white postmenopausal woman with loss of height, dowager's hump, or hip fracture. One important aspect of glucocorticoid osteoporosis is that the disorder can affect all sorts of people, including relatively young people, men, premenopausal women (such as the patient noted above), and blacks, all groups less susceptible to garden variety osteoporosis. The second clinical aspect of importance is that this bone loss can be quite severe over a relatively short period of time. Indeed, there is evidence that serum markers of bone formation are altered within hours

From: *Osteoporosis: Diagnostic and Therapeutic Principles*
Edited by: C. J. Rosen Humana Press Inc., Totowa, NJ

of the first pharmacologic dose of a glucocorticoid *(1)*. Finally, there are multiple mechanisms of glucocorticoid osteoporosis, which implies that one single treatment modality is unlikely to improve all parts of this problem. An understanding of the treatment and prevention of this disorder requires knowledge of the multifaceted pathophysiology of glucocorticoid osteoporosis.

2. PATHOGENESIS OF GLUCOCORTICOID OSTEOPOROSIS

2.1. Direct Effects on Osteoblast Function

What separates glucocorticoid osteoporosis from other forms is the profound and direct effect of glucocorticoids on osteoblast function. As stated above, within hours of a dose of prednisone, a serum marker of osteoblast activity, serum osteocalcin, is decreased *(1)*. The reader is directed to reviews of glucocorticoid osteoporosis *(2,3)* for details of this phenomenon, but the important point is that the glucocorticoid-induced decrease in osteoblast function is what separates this form of osteoporosis from the others. In garden variety osteoporosis, both bone resorption and formation may be increased, but the formation is less than the resorption. In glucocorticoid osteoporosis, formation is greatly decreased at a time of increased resorption. Thus, the osteoporosis affects all sorts of patients, is often severe, and happens soon after a high glucocorticoid state begins *(4)*.

2.2. Effects on Osteoclast Function

Through various mediators, such as cytokines and prostaglandins, glucocorticoids stimulate osteoclastic activity *(2)*. Thus, in the face of decreased bone formation, bone resorption is increased.

2.3. Effects in the Gut and Kidney

Glucocorticoids decrease the absorption of calcium in the gut by a mechanism that is not dependent on vitamin D *(5)*. However, some patients may also be vitamin D deficient *(6)*, leading to a further decrease in intestinal calcium absorption. Increased urinary loss of calcium is also found in patients with endogenous or exogenous Cushing's syndrome *(2,3)*.

2.4. Secondary Hyperparathyroidism

The decreased intestinal calcium absorption and increased urinary calcium excretion lead to an imperceptible decrease in the serum calcium level. However, this decrease is enough to increase serum levels of parathyroid hormone (PTH), which leads to loss of bone mineral and increase in urinary phosphate excretion *(7)*.

2.5. Catabolic Effects of Glucocorticoids

The generalized catabolic effects of glucocorticoids may lead to loss of protein—in the form of muscle and bone matrix. Muscle strength is positively correlated with bone mineral density (BMD) *(8)*, and inactivity leads to bone loss. Thus, the patient with the classic loss of muscle in Cushing's syndrome has another reason to have osteoporosis. Similarly, patients taking glucocorticoids (i.e., with exogenous Cushing's syndrome) also manifest muscle wasting. This muscle loss is additive to that associated with many of the inflammatory diseases for which glucocorticoids are prescribed.

2.6. Effects of Glucocorticoids on Sex Hormones

Women receiving glucocorticoids have adrenal suppression, leading to loss of adrenal androgen secretion. There is some evidence that the level of the adrenal androgen DHEA is positively correlated with BMD *(9)*. In addition, glucocorticoids (and many of the diseases for which they are prescribed) suppress the hypothalamic-pituitary–gonadal axis *(10)*. This leads to a functional hypogonadism, another contributor to bone loss.

2.7. Summary of Glucocorticoid Effects

It is, thus, easy to see why the osteoporosis of glucocorticoid excess is so severe and found in people thought not generally susceptible to osteoporosis. The amount of glucocorticoid excess need not be extreme. For example, there is some evidence *(11,12)* that patients with adrenal insufficiency receiving what we believe are replacement doses of glucocorticoids may be at increased risk for osteoporosis. Considering the frequency of glucocorticoid use for inflammatory diseases, the potential prevalence of osteoporosis is very high.

3. DIAGNOSIS OF GLUCOCORTICOID OSTEOPOROSIS

If the risk of this disorder is high and if bone formation is decreased soon after starting systemic glucocorticoid therapy, can the diagnosis be made from the clinical situation? A case can certainly be made that all patients taking pharmacologic doses of glucocorticoids for extended time periods will have a significant loss of bone mineral. The difficulty is determining how much glucocorticoid for how long will lead to clinically important bone loss.

3.1. Serum and Urine Markers of Bone Formation and Resorption

There are no serum or urine tests that will make this diagnosis of glucocorticoid osteoporosis. However, it is likely that serum markers of bone formation, such as osteocalcin or bone alkaline phosphatase, will be decreased by glucocorticoid therapy. Early in the course of the disorder, markers of bone resorption will likely be increased in these patients. A recent study *(13)* suggests that later in the course of glucocorticoid osteoporosis, there is evidence of both decreased bone formation and resorption, but the changes were small. However, there are no studies to demonstrate that prospective use of bone markers is helpful to determine which patients with glucocorticoids require therapy for borne loss. Some authorities *(6)* advocate measuring serum levels of 25-OH-D to determine if specific replacement is necessary. This step is supported by the recent study *(14)* demonstrating efficacy of calcitriol therapy for patients with glucocorticoid osteoporosis. However, measurements of circulating vitamin D metabolites in serum were not helpful in this study.

3.2. Measurement of BMD

The most widely accepted measure of bone mass is the BMD measurement by dual-energy X-ray densitometry. Patients with glucocorticoid-induced osteoporosis have decreased BMD in the spine and hip, and effective therapy will increase such measurements *(14)*. The question not answered by prospective studies is whether all patients who will need steroids require a BMD measurement at baseline. A strong case *(15)* can be made that for patients at highest risk, assessment of BMD is indicated: those patients who are likely to be on glucocorticoids for more than a few weeks and those patients who are at risk for other types of osteoporosis, such as postmenopausal women.

3.3. Measurement of Urinary Calcium Excretion

Some authorities *(6)* suggest that measurement of the 24-h urinary calcium excretion will show which patients are most vitamin D deficient and who would benefit from vitamin D replenishment. In addition, a baseline urinary calcium will be helpful in assessing the response to therapy. Unfortunately, in practice, 24-h urine collections are difficult to obtain. A reasonable substitute is a 2-h timed urine specimen. Sambrook et al. *(14)* measured a 2-h urine specimen for calcium and creatinine after their patients fasted overnight. The average ratio (in mg/mg) was about 0.09 ± 0.07 before treatment. Treatment with calcium, calcitriol, and calcitonin had little effect on urinary calcium/creatinine in the patients as a group. However, there may be patients who will need to have treatment adjusted (such as a decrease of oral calcium supplements or addition of hypocalciuric agents, such as hydrochlorothiazide) if the urinary calcium/creatinine ratio increases to >0.16. It would be reasonable to measure this ratio after a few months of therapy and again after 1 yr of therapy. In addition, measurement of serum calcium is important in patients receiving vitamin D and/or thiazide diuretics, because these agents may raise the serum calcium and/or unmask underlying primary hyperparathyroidism.

4. PREVENTION AND TREATMENT

4.1. Adjustment of Glucocorticoid Therapy

Prevention is almost always better than treatment, and alteration of glucocorticoid therapy to minimize systemic side effects is important in prevention. For example, shorter-acting glucocorticoids (prednisone rather than dexamethasone) should be used, so that there is not a constantly high level of glucocorticoids. If alternate-day therapy is possible, it should be used for the same reason. Topical or inhaled glucocorticoids should be used whenever possible to minimize systemic effects.

4.2. Other Preventive Maneuvers

Although the disorders for which patients receive glucocorticoids often compromise mobility, every opportunity should be used to maintain exercise and muscle mass. In addition, adequate calcium intake is necessary; at least 1 g of elemental calcium plus 400–800 U of vitamin D should be ingested by the patient each day. If the patient becomes hypercalciuric on this regimen (urinary calcium/creatinine > 0.16 mg/mg), then an agent such as a thiazide diuretic may be added. An alternative is amiloride. Low doses, such as 25 mg of hydrochlorothiazide, are often effective. Diuretics that decrease the urinary excretion of calcium may also raise the serum calcium. Thus, it is necessary to assess this when therapy is changed.

4.3. Other Medications

Several recent studies have suggested that it is possible to prevent glucocorticoid osteoporosis with a variety of medications. As mentioned previously, Sambrook et al. *(14)* treated patients with calcium (1000 mg of elemental calcium/d) and calcitriol (0.5–1.0 µg/d) with or without calcitonin (salmon calcitonin 400 IU/d intranasally) starting with the onset of glucocorticoid treatment. As measured by lumbar spine BMD, calcitriol was clearly better than calcium alone in preventing bone loss. There was some additional benefit of calcitonin as well, particularly in the second year of the study, during which the patients received no further treatment. The calcitonin used in this study was administered intranasally. A nasal spray preparation of calcitonin has recently been approved by the FDA and is now available in the US. Among patients taking calcium alone, hypercalcemia was rare, but about 25% of those patients also taking calcitriol or calcitriol plus calcitonin had hypercalcemia. Many of the patients had an increase in the urinary calcium/creatinine ratio during the first few months of treatment. By 12 mo, the ratio had decreased to normal. There were no urinary tract stones reported, nor was there a change in the serum creatinine. Nonetheless, this was a 2-yr study with therapy only in the first year. In patients with recent compression fracture of the spine, calcitonin has an analgesic effect (16) that is helpful in acute management. There are no long-term studies of the incidence of urolithiasis in patients taking calcium supplements and low-dose vitamin D for glucocorticoid osteoporosis, but in general, calcium supplements are safe (17).

In a recent study (18) from Australia, the osteoclast-inhibiting bis-phosphonate etidronate was given to postmenopausal women about to commence glucocorticoid therapy. They also received ergocalciferol and calcium, and were compared with patients treated with calcium alone. The most exciting aspect of this study was that the combination therapy resulted in an actual increase in BMD in the lumbar spine and femoral neck. Another etidronate study (19) appears to corroborate the findings. The newer bis-phosphonate, pamidronate, has also been reported (20) to be effective in preventing glucocorticoid osteoporosis. Other newer bis-phosphonates, such as alendronate and risedronate, that seem to be effective in postmenopausal osteoporosis (21,22) are also being tested for usefulness in glucocorticoid osteoporosis. It is hoped that they will also be efficacious without the potential side effects of etidronate (23). For the moment, bis-phosphonate therapy is instituted with etidronate 400 mg/d for 2 wk every 3 mo. It is important to note that all bis-phosphonates are poorly absorbed in the gastrointestinal tract. Thus, the drugs need to be taken on an empty stomach with water only. Other medications should not be administered at the same time. One possible mode of pamidronate administration is periodic iv infusion (30 mg every 3 mo; 24). This therapy is appealing for patients taking multiple oral medications.

4.4. Androgens and Estrogens

There is considerable debate about the use of estrogen replacement therapy in post-menopausal women. Although many authorities believe that the beneficial effects of estrogen replacement (decreased cardiac risk, decreased osteoporosis) outweigh the potential harm (small increased risk of breast cancer), only a small minority of women actually take estrogen after menopause. The postmenopausal patient with glucocorticoid osteoporosis is even more likely to benefit from hormone replacement therapy. In a recent study (25) of postmenopausal women, estrogen and etidronate had additive salutary effects on bone. Although this combination has not been studied in glucocorticoid osteoporosis, it makes intuitive sense that such double therapy would be helpful for the postmenopausal woman taking glucocorticoids. There is one caveat, however. Estrogens may cause a worsening of certain connective tissue diseases treated with glucocorticoids, such as systemic lupus erythematosus. Thus, it may not be possible to treat such patients with estrogen replacement, despite their very high risk.

In young men *(26)*, hypogonadism is clearly associated with low BMD, and testosterone replacement is effective in restoring bone mineral. Thus, a young man with glucocorticoid-induced hypogonadism would be a good candidate for testosterone replacement. Measurement of serum testosterone is indicated for younger men who will be on glucocorticoids for extended periods. The usual treatment of hypogonadism is testosterone esters in oil given as an im injection. Doses are 200–400 mg every 3–4 wk, although some men are treated every 2 wk. Newer modes of androgen replacement are becoming available. For example, a daily testosterone patch can be applied to the scrotum (or another preparation to the torso) to result in closer to physiologic replacement. In older men, the connection between hypogonadism and decreased bone mineral mass is less clear *(27,28)*. In addition, the use of testosterone replacement in older men has the potential side effect of stimulating growth of the prostate gland. Studies are in progress to determine if testosterone is a safe and effective treatment for older men. Until the results are known, men with glucocorticoid-induced hypogonadism or with glucocorticoid osteoporosis and hypogonadism owing to another cause should at least be considered for testosterone replacement. Perhaps a case can be made for a less than replacement dose to increase the serum testosterone into the normal range. In any event, careful surveillance of the prostate gland will be necessary in men so treated. There is also evidence *(29,30)* that medroxyprogesterone is effective for men with glucocorticoid osteoporosis, although the mechanism of this effect is unclear.

In women, another source of sex steroids is the adrenal gland. Specifically, adrenal androgens are responsible for pubic and axillary hair growth in females. Women with Addison's disease (primary adrenal insufficiency) are sometimes treated with small doses of androgens for improvement in general well-being and for libido. Women receiving glucocorticoid therapy are likely to lack adrenal androgens, and a case can be made for giving the women small doses of androgens. In one study *(9)* of postmenopausal osteoporosis (not owing to glucocorticoids), there was a strong relationship between the level of the adrenal androgen DHEA and the BMD. Thus, it will be necessary to study whether any androgen will help women with glucocorticoid osteoporosis, or whether DHEA or another specific steroid will be necessary for effective treatment. Although oral androgens are not used for testosterone replacement in men, oral nandrolone has been used safely as an anabolic steroid in frail elderly women *(31)*. As newer methods of androgen administration are developed, such as skin patches, low doses may be available for certain women with glucocorticoid osteoporosis.

ILLUSTRATIVE CASES

Case 1

The patient is a 65-yr-old man with a 10-yr history of biopsy-proven temporal arteritis and polymyalgia rheumatica. He has been on prednisone for most of the time and experiences stiffness, soreness, difficulty in walking, and pain in his legs and hips whenever his dose of prednisone is decreased below 15 mg/d. He has had a rib fracture after minimal trauma. Even on prednisone, his sedimentation rate is 40 mm/h. His rheumatologist ordered a BMD of the spine and hip. In lumbar vertebrae 1–4, his total BMD was 0.710 g/cm^2, which is about 3.5 SD from the mean of normal young men and about 2.7 SD from the mean of men his age. Similarly decreased BMD was found in his right hip. All of his measurements showed that he was at risk for fracture. His rheumatologist attempted to taper his prednisone dose by alternating 15 mg with 12.5 mg followed by 12.5 mg/d, and then 12.5 mg alternating with 10 mg/d. In addition, the patient was given calcium carbonate, 500 mg twice a day (approx 400 mg elemental calcium/d) and a multivitamin containing 400 IU of vitamin D. After 6 mo, the patient complained of lower back and chest pain. He was stiff, lacked energy, and felt depressed. His sedimentation rate was 28 mm/h. His prednisone was again increased to 15 mg/d, but later it was tapered slightly as sertraline was added for his depression. The patient was referred to the Metabolic Bone Disease Clinic. His testosterone level was found to be normal, and a 24-h urine collection for calcium was unsatisfactory. His calcium carbonate dose was increased, and he was started on etidronate 400 mg/d for 2 wk every 3 mo. He was instructed to take the last-mentioned on an empty stomach separately from his other medications. The patient seemed to feel better over the next several months, allowing gradual tapering of his prednisone (about 1 mg/mo) to 8 mg/d. Interestingly, his sedimentation rate fell to 10 mm/h. The patient returned for a BMD after two cycles of etidronate therapy. There was a 4% increase in the lumbar spine BMD measurement, but no significant change in the measurements of the hip.

COMMENTS

This patient had a demonstrable improvement in his lumbar spine BMD soon after starting cyclic therapy with etidronate, but actually his repeat BMD was done too soon. Although the precision of the dual-energy X-ray densitometers is excellent, waiting 1 yr before remeasuring BMD is best for most patients—unless there is clear clinical indication that the therapy is not working and must be changed. The patient also points out the difficulties in collecting 24-h urine samples. He will have a fasting 2-h urinary calcium-to-creatinine ratio determined instead. Finally, it is important to remember that the dose of various calcium preparations must be adjusted for the content of elemental calcium.

Case 2

A 44-yr-old woman with a long history of asthma was referred to the Metabolic Bone Disease Clinic because of low BMD noted on dual-energy X-ray densitometry. She had this measurement because she had been dependent on oral glucocorticoids for over 3 yr. Despite taking inhaled steroids and many other anti-asthma medications, the patient had multiple visits to the Emergency Department and multiple hospital admissions for exacerbations of her asthma. On prednisone she gained weight and became diabetic. After the low BMD was found, the patient was given 1 g of calcium carbonate three times a day (approx 1200 mg of elemental calcium/d) by her primary care physician. She was also given a multivitamin tablet containing 400 IU of vitamin D.

In the Metabolic Bone Disease Clinic, the patient had no symptoms of compression fractures or any other problems that could be ascribed to her glucocorticoid osteoporosis. At this time, she was taking 10 mg of prednisone each day. Review of her BMD measurements showed that her total lumbar spine BMD was 2.3 SD below the mean for young women and almost 2 SD below the mean for women her age. This number was below the so-called fracture threshold. The readings from her right hip were not as severe, with the total hip number about 1 SD below that of average young women. However, the reading at Ward's triangle was over 3 SD lower than a young women's average level. The patient was Cushingoid in appearance, and the lungs were clear to auscultation.

It was decided to continue the calcium and vitamin D treatment, and attempt to taper the prednisone. Over the next few months, there were many attempts at tapering, each one followed by an exacerbation of the asthma leading to a visit to the Emergency Department and one more hospital admission. Despite many adjustments in her anti-asthma treatment, the possibility that the patient will have to remain on prednisone indefinitely seems more likely. She was scheduled to measure the urinary calcium-to-creatinine ratio and then begin therapy with hydrochlorothiazide, 25 mg/d.

COMMENTS

The patient has reasonably normal menstrual periods, but she is approaching the age of menopause. She has a sister with breast cancer, and the patient is concerned about taking estrogen after menopause. What are the possible treatments for this woman, who also takes antihypertensive medications and medication for supraventricular tachycardia, in addition to her medications for asthma? This is important because if she is to take bis-phosphonates, she must take them on an empty stomach without other medications. She should be considered for calcitonin treatment, although her allergic history might concern us. She has allergic rhinitis, so the new preparation of nasal calcitonin is also less appealing. Tamoxifen, the agent used in patients with breast cancer, has some appeal because it has estrogen-like qualities in bone *(32)*, while having no stimulatory effect on mammary tissue. In the future, raloxifene, a related drug *(33)*, may be even better, because it appears to help bone without stimulating either mammary or uterine tissue. In the meantime, this patient might be a candidate for some sort of intermittent therapy, perhaps the iv injection of pamidronate, 30 mg, every 3 mo *(24)*. One might also consider a small dose of androgen to make up for lack of adrenal androgens. Nandrolone is appealing because other androgens can be aromatized to estrogens, causing possible breast stimulation. Thus, this is a difficult patient for whom perfect therapy is not yet available. Aggressive treatment of her asthma is important to keep her mobile and active. She should have reassessment of BMD after a trial of conservative therapy with calcium, vitamin D, and hydrochlorothiazide before adding another drug.

STRATEGIC OUTLINE FOR PREVENTION OR TREATMENT OF GLUCOCORTICOID OSTEOPOROSIS

History
1. Disorder requiring glucocorticoids
   a. Mode of administration
   b. Duration of administration
   c. Mobility of patient
2. Other medical problems
   a. Fracture history
   b. Other risk factors for osteoporosis
   c. General health and prognosis

Physical examination
1. Evidence of osteoporosis
   a. Evidence of fracture
   b. Kyphosis, loss of height
   c. Muscle strength, size

2. General physical findings
    a. Assessment of underlying disorder
    b. Other medical conditions

Laboratory
1. Serum calcium (and other screening tests; e.g., protein electrophoresis)
2. 2-h Fasting urinary calcium/creatinine measurement
3. Consider serum estradiol or testosterone
4. BMD of spine and hip
5. X-rays of appropriate areas

Plans—at start of glucocorticoid therapy
1. Minimize glucocorticoid dose
2. Use alternate-day therapy, topical steroids if possible
3. Prescribe exercise, physical therapy
4. Assure adequate calcium intake
5. Add supplemental calcium, up to 1 g calcium/d
6. Add multivitamin containing 400 IU vitamin D

Reassessment at 2–3 mo
1. Review glucocorticoid therapy; attempt to decrease or discontinue
2. Assess exercise
3. Assess calcium intake
4. Measure serum calcium, 2-h fasting urinary calcium
5. Add hydrochlorothiazide, if necessary

Reassessment at 6 mo
1. Review glucocorticoid therapy and minimize
2. Assess exercise and calcium intake
3. Repeat serum and urinary calcium measurements
4. Alter calcium/vitamin D/thiazide therapy, if necessary
5. If patient is to continue glucocorticoids, consider
    a. Cyclic etidronate, 400 mg/d for 2 wk/ 3 mo
    b. Nasal calcitonin, 400 U/d
6. Consider repeat BMD

Reassessment at 1 yr
1. Review glucocorticoid therapy and minimize
2. Review exercise and calcium intake
3. Repeat serum and urinary calcium/creatinine
4. Measure BMD in spine and hip
5. Alter calcium/vitamin D/thiazide therapy, if necessary
6. Alter further therapy if bone loss continues

Reassessment thereafter if glucocorticoids continue
1. Repeat annual assessment as above
2. Change therapy as needed
3. Consider newer drugs as they become available

REFERENCES

1. Godschalk MF, Downs RW. Effect of short-term glucocorticoids on serum osteocalcin in healthy young men. *J Bone Miner Res* 1988; 13: 113–115.
2. Adler RA, Rosen CJ. Glucocorticoids and osteoporosis. *Endocrinol Metab Clin North Am* 1994; 23: 641–654.

3. Lukert BP, Raisz LG. Glucocorticoid-induced osteoporosis: pathogenesis and management. *Ann Intern Med* 1990; 122: 352–364.

4. LoCascio V, Bonnucci E, Imbimbo B, Ballanti P, Taratarotti D, Galvanini G, Fuccella L, Adami S. Bone loss after glucocorticoid therapy. *Calcif Tissue Int* 1984; 36: 435–438.

5. Morris HA, Need AG, O'Loughlin PD, Horowitz M, Bridges A, Nordin BEC. Malabsorption of calcium in corticosteroid-induced osteoporosis. *Calcif Tissue Int* 1990; 46: 305–308.

6. Libanati CR, Baylink DJ. Prevention and treatment of glucocorticoid-induced osteoporosis. *Chest* 1992; 102: 1426–1435.

7. Suzuki Y, Ichikawa Y, Saito E, Homma M. Importance of increased urinary calcium excretion in the development of secondary hyperparathyroidism of patients under glucocorticoid therapy. *Metabolism* 1983; 32: 151–156.

8. Adler RA. Osteoporosis and exercise. *Curr Opinion Orthop* 1991; 2: 98–102.

9. Wild RA, Buchanan JR, Myers C, Demers LM. Declining adrenal androgens: an association with bone loss in aging women. *Proc Soc Exper Biol Med* 1987; 186: 355–360.

10. MacAdams MR, White RH, Chipps BE. Reduction of serum testosterone levels during chronic glucocorticoid therapy. *Ann Intern Med* 1986; 104: 648–651.

11. Zeilissen PMJ, Croughs RJM, van Rijk PP, Raymakers JA. Effect of glucocorticoid replacement therapy on bone mineral density in patients with Addison Disease. *Ann Intern Med* 1994; 12: 207–210.

12. Devogelaer JP, Crabbe J, De Deuxchaisnes CN. Bone mineral density in Addison's Disease: evidence for an effect of adrenal androgens on bone mass. *Br Med J* 1987; 294: 798–800.

13. Lukert BP, Higgins J. Markers of bone remodeling in patients taking glucocorticoids. *J Bone Miner Res* 1995; 10(Suppl. 1): S181, no. P211.

14. Sambrook P, Birmingham J, Kelly P, Kempler S, Nguyen T, Stat M, Pocock N, Eisman J. Prevention of corticosteroid osteoporosis. *N Engl J Med* 1993; 328: 1747–1752.

15. Johnston CC Jr, Slemenda CW, Melton LJ III. Clinical use of bone densitometry. *N Engl J Med* 1991; 324: 1105–1109.

16. Lyritis GP, Tsakalakos N, Magiasis B, Karachalios T, Yiatzides A, Tsekoura M. Analgesic effect of salmon calcitonin in osteoporotic vertebral fractures: a double-blind placebo-controlled clinical study. *Calcif Tissue Int* 1991; 49: 369–373.

17. Ringe JD. The risk of nephrolithiasis with oral calcium supplementation. *Calcif Tissue Int* 1991; 48: 69–73.

18. Diamond T, McGuigan L, Barbagallo S, Bryant C. Cyclical etidronate plus ergocalciferol prevents glucocorticoid-induced bone loss in postmenopausal women. *Am J Med* 1995; 98: 459–463.

19. Mulder H, Struys A. Intermittent cyclical etidronate in the prevention of corticosteroid-induced bone loss. *Br J Rheum* 1994; 33: 348–350.

20. Reid IR, Schooler BA, Stewart AW. Prevention of glucocorticoid-induced osteoporosis. *J Bone Miner Res* 1990; 5: 619–6:23.

21. Liberman UA, Weiss SR, Bröll J, Minne HW, Quan H, Bell NH, et al. Effect of oral alendronate on bone mineral density and the incidence of fractures in postmenopausal osteoporosis. *N Engl J Med* 1995; 333: 1437–1443.

22. Mortensen L, Bekker P, Ouweland Fvd, Horowitz Z, Rupich R, DiGennaro J, Axelrod D, Charles P, Johnston C. Prevention of early postmenopausal loss, by risedronate: a two year study. *J Bone Miner Res* 1995; 10(Suppl. 1): S140, no. 5.

23. Conference report. Consensus Development Conference: diagnosis, prophylaxis and treatment of osteoporosis. *Am J Med* 1993; 94: 646–650.

24. Gallacher SJ, Fenner JAK, Anderson K, Bryden FM, Banham SW, Logue FC, Cowan RA, Boyle IT. Intravenous pamidronate in the treatment of osteoporosis associated with corticosteroid dependent lung disease: an open pilot study. *Thorax* 1992; 47: 932–936.

25. Wimalawansa SJ. Combined therapy with estrogen and etidronate has an additive effect on bone mineral density in the hip and vertebrae: four-year randomized study. *Am J Med* 1995; 99: 36–42.

26. Greenspan SL, Oppenheim DS, Klibanski A. Importance of gonadal steroids to bone mass in men with hyperprolactinemic hypogonadism. *Ann Intern Med* 1989; 110: 526–531.

27. Orwoll ES, Klein RF. Osteoporosis in men. *Endocr Rev* 1995; 16: 87–116.

28. Stanley HL, Schmitt BP, Poses RM, Deiss WP. Does hypogonadism contribute to the occurrence of a minimal trauma hip fracture in elderly men? *J Am Geriatr Soc* 1991; 39: 766–771.

29. Grecu EO, Simmons R, Baylink DJ, Haloran BP, Spencer ME. Effects of medroxyprogesterone acetate on some parameters of calcium metabolism in patients with glucocorticoid-induced osteoporosis. *Bone Miner* 1991; 13: 153–161.

30. Grecu EO, Weinshelbaum A, Simmons R. Effective therapy of glucocorticoid-induced osteoporosis with medroxyprogesterone acetate. *Calcif Tissue Int* 1990; 46: 294–299.

31. Sloan JP, Wing P, Dian L, Meneilly GS. A pilot study of anabolic steroids in elderly patients with hip fractures. *J Am Geriatr Soc* 1992; 40: 1105–1111.

32. Fornander T, Rutqvist LE, Wilking N, Carlstrom K, Schoultz B. Oestrogenic effects of adjuvant tamoxifen in postmenopausal breast cancer. *Eur J Cancer* 1993; 29A: 497–500.

33. Wang Q, Hassager C, Wang S, Heegaard AM, Riis BJ, Christiansen C. Raloxifene prevents bone loss in lumbar spine and femur in aged ovariectomized rats. *J Bone Miner Res* 1995; 10(Suppl. 1): S249, no. S392.

21

Therapy for Osteoporosis in Men

Eric S. Orwoll, MD and Robert F. Klein, MD

CASE STUDY

A 63-yr-old man experienced acute, severe back pain while digging in the garden. He was seen in the Emergency Department, and found to have a new anterior compression fracture of T-11. Although his back pain had been somewhat relieved by analgesics, he was still, 3 wk later, in some pain and unable to be active. He had suffered a fracture of his humerus 2 yr before during a fall on an icy sidewalk.

His past history was notable for a 40 pack-year history of tobacco abuse, and the routine consumption of 2 alcoholic drinks/d. He had little dietary calcium intake and worked at a sedentary job with few physical activities. An examination showed a slightly overweight man in some distress because of back pain. There was mild lower thoracic tenderness, but no gibbous deformity or frank kyphosis. Secondary sexual characteristics were normal, but the testes were somewhat small with a soft consistency.

The patient's major concerns were "This is supposed to happen in old women—why am I having these fractures?" "What can I do to prevent any more in the future?"

Despite the tremendous personal and public health impact of osteoporosis in men, its therapy is virtually unexplored. There have been no randomized trials of fracture prevention in men. Although a limited numbers of observational trials are available (primarily of the effects of dietary calcium intake), there is large variability in the reported results. As a result, the degree to which fracture risk can be reduced in men by any therapy cannot be confidently assessed. Similarly, the incidence of adverse effects resulting from thera-

From: *Osteoporosis: Diagnostic and Therapeutic Principles*
Edited by: C. J. Rosen Humana Press Inc., Totowa, NJ

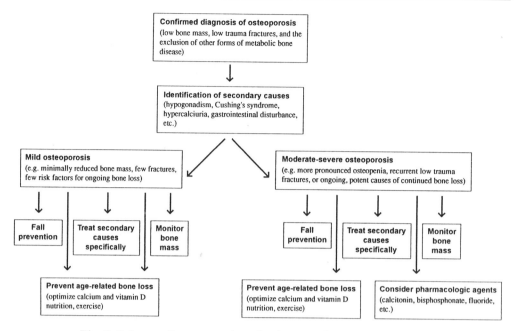

Fig. 1. Schema of an approach to the therapy of osteoporosis in men.

pies in men has not been reported. Finally, there have been no adequate assessments of either the functional benefit to patients, or of the economic benefit to be expected, by any therapy of osteoporosis in men. In general, therefore, it is very difficult to assess the likelihood of success of any therapeutic approach in male subjects. Expectedly, there are no approved pharmacological therapies for osteoporosis in men in the US. For all these reasons, the strength of recommendations developed for the therapeutic approach to osteoporosis prevention and therapy in men must be considered weak. Any recommendations are based on very limited data in men and extrapolations from a much more comprehensive experience in women.

As in women, the most important proximate causes of osteoporotic fracture in men are trauma (most commonly falls) and a reduction in skeletal mechanical strength *(1)*. The prevention of falls and the optimization of skeletal health both must be considered essential in the clinical management of patients. The general approach to the therapy of osteoporosis in men is described below and summarized in Fig. 1.

1. PREVENTION OF FALLS

In addition to bone mass, the risk of falling has been identified as a major determinant of fracture in women. In men, there are few prospective data that directly relate fall propensity to subsequent fractures, but a variety of factors indirectly related to risk of falling are associated with fracture. For instance, Nguyen et al. found that men who had experienced a nontraumatic fracture exhibit more body sway and lower grip strength (as well as lower bone density) than nonfracture controls *(1)*. Similarly, in a study of men with hip fractures *(2)*, a number of factors associated with falls were found to be more prevalent than in controls. These included neurological disease, confusion, "ambulatory problems," and alcohol use. As in women, the use of several classes of psychotropic drugs is associated with hip fracture risk in men *(3,4)*. Finally, men with hip fracture are of lower weight, have lower fat and lean body mass, and more commonly live alone than control subjects *(5)*. These differences suggest a body habitus and lifestyle more conducive to falls and injury, as well as the possibility of other interacting risk factors (nutritional deficiencies, comorbidities).

In all patients with an increased risk of falls and fracture, an assessment of contributing factors is important. Several studies have documented the success of nutritional and exercise interventions in increasing strength and mobility in the elderly of both sexes *(6,7)*, and optimizing physical capacity should be an important goal. An active approach to physical conditioning is described in Chapter 16.

2. PREVENTION AND THERAPY OF BONE LOSS

2.1. Categories of Osteopenia in Men

There are several broad categories of osteoporotic disorders in men that reflect basic pathophysiologic processes. It is useful to consider them independently to establish clearly the rational for specific preventative and therapeutic approaches. In many individual patients, the causation of osteoporosis will be multifactorial, and when designing therapy simultaneous consideration must be given to the contributions of each etiologic component.

2.1.1. AGE-RELATED OSTEOPOROSIS

Bone loss that occurs with aging is an important feature of osteoporosis in men. In some, age-related bone loss may alone suffice to cause nontraumatic fractures, but even when other causes of bone loss are present (i.e., hypogonadism, alcoholism), the loss of bone that universally accompanies aging unquestionably contributes to the propensity for fractures.

Aging in normal men is associated with detectable appendicular and substantial axial bone loss. The cause of this loss in unknown, but has been speculated to be related to a number of factors. Histomorphometric techniques demonstrate a reduction in bone formation (mean wall thickness) in both sexes *(8–13)* that probably contributes to the decline. An additional age-related increase in bone resorption in men is not apparent using these methods *(9,12)*, but may be subtly present as well. The mechanisms responsible for these changes in cellular activity are undoubtedly complex and are currently too unclear to use to base therapeutic decisions on. In addition to these putative influences, several other processes probably contribute to the pathophysiology of bone loss with aging and deserve consideration when recommending therapy. These include nutritional calcium deficiency, inactivity, and loss of gonadal function.

2.1.2. IDIOPATHIC OSTEOPENIA

Osteoporosis in men has been termed idiopathic if no known cause of bone disease can be identified on clinical and laboratory grounds. Although at least one identifiable cause of bone loss is found in the majority of men with osteoporosis, many patients have bone disease of unknown etiology *(14–17)*. The age of men with idiopathic osteoporosis varies widely with an average in midlife. This age range overlaps that of "senile" osteoporosis, and differentiation of idiopathic and senile osteoporosis is somewhat arbitrary. Riggs and Melton *(18)* defined senile (or Type II) osteoporosis as occurring in either sex after the age of 70, but this definition obviously does not exclude the potential for pathophysiological overlap between older and younger patients.

The character of idiopathic osteoporosis in men is relatively indistinct. After major secondary contributors to bone loss have been eliminated, more detailed biochemical and histomorphometric analyses of men with idiopathic disease fail to reveal consistent features *(16,17,19–21)*. Osteoblastic dysfunction may contribute to osteoporosis in men *(20–22)*, but does not seem to be a consistent finding *(15,19)*. Nordin et al. have suggested that accelerated resorption may also be a primary mediator *(23)*, but others have not found evidence of such *(17)*. Undoubtedly, the cause of osteopenia in these patients is heterogeneous. Currently, the therapies available for these patients must be considered generic.

2.1.3. Secondary Osteopenias

Metabolic bone disease in men has been traditionally considered to be more commonly related to "secondary" causes *(14,16,18,20,24)*, and many men with osteoporosis will have medical conditions, drugs, or lifestyles that contribute to the etiology of bone loss. Often these exist in concert with aging. The nature of the bone loss in each of these conditions is distinct and often complex. Each should be carefully considered and, if present, approached with specific therapeutic choices based on its pathophysiology.

3. PREVENTION OF AGE-RELATED BONE LOSS IN MEN

Although previously considered clinically insignificant, it is now clear that the rate of age-related bone loss in men is important *(25)*, and fractures in older men are an important public health issue. Nevertheless, there is very little information available concerning the prevention and treatment of the problem. It is unclear when bone loss begins in the course of aging in men. Some have suggested that a fall in bone mass is detectable only after the age of 50 yr *(26–29)*, whereas others indicate a fairly linear decrease in cortical and trabecular bone mass during adulthood *(26–28,30–34)*. In any man in whom osteoporosis has developed or is considered a clinically important possibility, efforts should be made to prevent this component of bone loss. Reasonable guidelines can be developed on the basis of current pathophysiologic models and from experience in women, but these approaches lack validation. Efforts to prevent age-related bone loss are the foundation on which a successful treatment plan is based, and should always be a part of the prevention and therapy of osteoporosis, regardless of the other etiologies of bone disease that may be present in addition.

3.1. Exercise

Mechanical force exerts major effects on bone mass, and is probably one of the fundamental variables responsible for the sexual dimorphism in bone mass and structure. In cross-sectional studies, bone mass is greater in physically active men *(35–41)*, an effect that can be demonstrated at both the regional (i.e., the particular anatomic region affected) and systemic levels. Activity and muscle strength and lean body mass in men also correlate with bone density both regionally and systemically *(35,36,42,43)*. Furthermore, muscle strength is related to bone bending stiffness in men, an index of strength independent of mass, suggesting that mechanical force has effects not only on bone mass, but also on quality *(44)*. The character of senile bone loss closely mimics that of chronic disuse *(45)*, but this tentative conclusion requires confirmation in longitudinal studies.

Longitudinal studies tend to corroborate the effect of mechanical force on skeletal character in men *(46)*, but are very few in number. Importantly, exercise has been strongly related to a reduction in hip fracture rates in men *(47,48)*, an effect that may also relate to a reduced risk of falls. Unfortunately, the fairly consistent finding of positive correlations between exercise history and/or strength and bone mass in cross-sectional studies has not been confirmed in longitudinal investigations.

In sum, the available data strongly suggest a powerful effect of weight and mechanical force on the male skeleton. In view of the clear decline in physical activity and muscle strength with aging *(49,50)*, senile bone loss in men may, in part, relate to a diminution of the trophic effects of mechanical force on skeletal tissues.

There have been few controlled, longitudinal, or comparison trials of exercise in men. Nevertheless, activity is probably beneficial in several ways. Reductions in strength and coordination contribute to fracture via an increased risk of falling *(51)*. In addition, inactivity is associated with bone loss, and exercise may increase or maintain bone mass. Specific exercise prescriptions to accomplish these goals have not been confirmed in men or women, although it is clear that strength can be dramatically increased and risk of falls reduced in the elderly with achievable levels of exercise *(51)*. That fracture rates have been reported to be lower in elderly men who exercise modestly buttresses this contention *(48)*, but those findings have been difficult to verify. In one large longitudinal study by Greendale et al., activity was associated with a higher bone mineral density (BMD) in older men, but no reduction in fracture rates *(52)*.

In view of the lack of adequate data, a specific exercise prescription is difficult to generate with currently available information. At present, general guidelines include the use of weight-bearing exercise to the extent it can be safely undertaken, and the avoidance of situations that might materially increase the risk of trauma and fracture *(53)*. Conditioning and muscle strengthening probably have benefits (fall protection) beyond those associated with bone mass.

3.2. Calcium and Vitamin D Nutrition

Riggs and Melton *(18)* have suggested that senile (Type II) osteoporosis in men and women is owing, at least in part, to alterations in calcium economy. Aging in men has been associated with biochemical changes that suggest physiological stress on bone and mineral metabolism. Calcium absorption declines with aging in men as in women, particularly after the age of 60. Also, there is evidence of increased parathyroid hormone (PTH) levels *(54,55)*, reduced 25-hydroxyvitamin D (25-OH-D) levels *(56)*, and (in some studies) subnormal 1,25-dihydroxyvitamin D (1,25-[OH]$_2$-D) levels *(57–60)*. In the Baltimore Longitudinal Study of Aging *(61)*, lower radial bone density in men was related to higher PTH levels and lower 25-OH-D concentrations. In sum, these data suggest both that optimal levels of calcium intake may change with age and that inadequate calcium nutrition can have an adverse effect on skeletal mass.

Several reports have linked dietary calcium intake to levels of bone density in men, but the evidence is not yet conclusive *(62,63)*. Most results suggest that calcium intake may play a role in the determination of axial, but not (or to a lesser extent) of appendicular bone mass *(26,64,65)*. However, in the only published controlled trial of calcium supplementation in adult men, no beneficial effects were found on the rate of bone mineral loss from either spinal or radial sites *(27)*, despite the fact that urine calcium excretion increased and PTH levels were suppressed. Osteocalcin levels were not altered. The results of this trial are somewhat muted by the relatively large dietary calcium intake of the subjects before supplementation began (>1100 mg/d), and supplementation in a less calcium-replete population may prove to be more effective. There have been no studies of the relationship between calcium intake and skeletal structure (e.g., cortical thickness, trabecular architecture, remodeling rates, material properties).

A variety of studies have examined the relationship between dietary calcium intake and hip fracture in men, with inconsistent results. Significant associations between calcium intake and fracture rates have been reported in small case-controlled trials (66,67). Similarly, in several longitudinal observational trials (including the NHANES I followup study [35], the Rancho Bernardo study [68], and a study of eight communities in Britain [47]), hip fracture risk in men was strongly suggested to be related to dietary calcium intake, although the relationships did not reach statistical significance. However, two other very large studies (1,48) found no relationship between calcium intake and hip fracture risk in men. Looker et al. (35) have pointed out the pitfalls inherent in these trials, including low power, difficulties in estimating calcium intake and the effects of confounding variables, and so forth, and they apply to studies involving both sexes. In general, these evaluations of the relationship between calcium nutrition and hip fracture in men suggest a beneficial effect, but remain inconclusive. Moreover, there have been no attempts to examine the effects of calcium intake on other fractures, in particular, vertebral fractures. Although incomplete, the data are probably consistent with a limited role for dietary calcium insufficiency in the determination of the rate of bone loss and fractures in men.

The amount necessary to maintain calcium balance in men is unclear. Calcium balance studies are available in young men and have been recently reviewed by Nordin (69). From these limited data, it would appear that calcium balance is maintained in the average individual at an intake of about 500 mg. However, the range of intakes required for the maintenance of calcium balance is wide, and an intake of 900 mg/d was required to ensure balance in 90% of subjects studied. This individual variability may be amplified by the influence of other dietary constituents that strongly influence calcium economy (e.g., protein, fiber, and so on) (70–72). Although US men achieve a mean dietary calcium intake considerably greater than that of women (~800 vs ~500 mg/d in the 1978 NHANES survey), these data still indicate that about one-half of men ingest less than the recommended daily allowance (800 mg), and many ingest much less. The bioavailability of calcium supplements does not appear to be different in men and women (73).

The level of calcium intake, however, that should be recommended is unclear. Only one prospective study has addressed this issue, and no benefit from calcium supplements was observed in an already well-nourished population (dietary calcium intake >800 mg/d) (27). Based on suggestive, but not definitive data, a recent NIH Consensus Development Conference recommended a calcium intake of 1000 mg/d in young men and 1500 mg/d in those over 65 yr. A concern regarding dietary calcium supplementation has been the possible precipitation of calcium stone disease in susceptible individuals. Recent data, though, suggest dietary calcium intake is actually negatively correlated with the risk of nephrolithiasis in men (74), potentially by increasing gastrointestinal oxalate binding.

Optimal vitamin D intake in men is also a matter of some debate. Whereas the relationship between vitamin D intake and bone health is extensively studied in women, there are few data on men. On the basis of data extrapolated from studies in women, it would seem appropriate to use vitamin D supplements in a patient with osteoporosis, or in whom osteoporosis prevention is an important issue, if necessary to maintain adequate 25-OH-D levels (>30 ng/mL). Even in normal men 25-OH-D levels may be <20 ng/mL *(75)*, but small vitamin D supplements (1000 IU/d) were sufficient to ensure adequate 25-OH-D availability *(75)*. In men with impaired baseline vitamin D nutrition (poor nutrition, inadequate sun exposure), impaired absorption, or increased metabolism, higher amounts of supplementation (25,000–50,000/wk or more) are frequently required to maintain adequate levels. In all these situations, serum 25-OH-D levels should be useful as an index of adequate (and not excessive) supplemental doses.

4. PHARMACOLOGICAL APPROACHES TO THE THERAPY OF AGE-RELATED AND IDIOPATHIC OSTEOPOROSIS

In men with moderate-severe osteopenia, those who are at high risk for bone loss because of coexisting and unremediable conditions, or those who have been demonstrated to have sustained bone loss, measures designed merely to prevent further age-related bone loss may be insufficient. In these situations, additional pharmacological therapies should be considered.

4.1. Calcitonin

There has been one trial of calcitonin therapy in a small group of men with idiopathic osteoporosis *(76)* in which total body calcium tended to increase during a 24-mo treatment interval (100 IU calcitonin/d with a calcium and vitamin D supplement). However, the change was not significantly different than that observed in the control groups (receiving calcium plus vitamin D supplements, or vitamin D alone), and there were no changes in radial bone mass. Men have been included in several other trials of calcitonin therapy, but the effects in men are not separable from those in the women subjects *(77,78)*.

Although there are few data in men, theoretically, calcitonin should be effective in reducing osteoclastic activity in men and, hence, reducing the risk of continuing bone loss. This may be particularly true if there is evidence of increased bone resorption (via histomorphometric analysis of bone or increases in biochemical indices of resorption). Doses and treatment schedules have not been developed in men, but an initial approach using 100 IU sc every other day, or 200 IU intranasally, may be reasonable. Dose adjustments should be based on longitudinal studies of biochemical markers of bone remodeling and bone mass. The appropriate duration of treatment should be individualized, taking into account the response to therapy and the ongoing medical condition. For instance, a patient whose general medical condition improves in parallel with calcitonin therapy, allowing the discontinuation of medications with adverse skeletal effects and an increase in activity levels, thus may be at less risk of bone resorption and continued bone loss, setting the stage for discontinuation of calcitonin.

4.2. Bisphosphonates

There have been no trials of any bisphosphonates performed exclusively in men. Male patients with osteoporosis have been included in mixed patient populations, and have seemed to experience beneficial effects on calcium balance and lumbar spine bone density during treatment with pamidronate *(79)*. Similarly, men have been included (in fact, the majority of subjects were male) in a trial of the effects of pamidronate on glucocorticoid-induced bone loss, in which therapy had a beneficial effect on metacarpal cortical area and vertebral bone density *(80)*. Although specific data are lacking, there is no theoretical reason bisphosphonates would not be effective in reducing osteoclastic work in men as in women *(81)*. Recently, potent forms of bisphosphonates have been developed (e.g., alendronate, residronate). No treatment information is currently available in men using these newer compounds, but an initial dose of 10 mg/d of alendronate may be appropriate, given the data developed in women.

4.3. Thiazide Diuretics

There is evidence to support a beneficial effect of thiazide administration on BMD *(82)*, rates of bone mineral loss *(83)*, and hip fracture risk *(84)* in men. These effects were quite robust. For instance, the use of thiazides reduced calcaneal BMD loss rates by 49% compared to controls *(83)*, and the relative risk of hip fracture was halved by an exposure to thiazides for more than 6 yr *(84)*. Other diuretics did not seem to impart the same positive effects. The source of the benefit is unclear. Although it has been postulated to stem from the hypocalciuric effects of thiazides *(85)*, there are also data to suggest a direct effect of thiazides on bone cells *(86)*. In patients requiring diuretic therapy for other indications, thiazides should be used preferentially if there is concern for bone loss.

4.4. PTH

PTH administration to osteoporotic subjects has been shown to increase trabecular bone formation and bone volume in concert with an increase in calcium balance *(87–89)*. Slovik et al. reported that in a small group of men with idiopathic osteoporosis, combined PTH and 1,25-OH$_2$D administration increased trabecular (spinal) bone mass and improved intestinal calcium absorption *(88)*. Although the role of PTH administration in the treatment of osteoporosis, either alone or in concert with other agents *(89)*, remains unclear, the potential appears similar in men and women.

4.5. Growth Hormone

Growth hormone may have anabolic actions on the skeleton in the elderly *(90,91)* and in subjects with osteoporosis, but the available data are inconclusive *(34)*. Low levels of IGF-I have been reported to be present in men with idiopathic osteoporosis *(92)*, and in a study of healthy men over 60 yr of age with low IGF-I levels, Rudman et al. *(93)* found that in addition to positive effects on lean mass, fat mass, and skin thickness, vertebral BMD was increased slightly (1.6%) by the administration of growth hormone for 6 mo. Radial and proximal femoral density was unaffected. In either sex, growth hormone therapy may thus be of potential, but as of yet unproven, usefulness *(94)*.

4.6. Fluoride

The use of fluoride in the therapy of osteoporosis remains controversial. Although consistent and sometimes dramatic increases in BMD can be achieved with supplemental fluoride, the biomechanical competence of fluoride-treated bone is uncertain *(95)*. In one large, controlled trial of fluoride therapy for postmenopausal osteoporosis, BMD was increased, but fracture rate was not reduced, and the incidence of skeletal (stress fractures) and nonskeletal (primarily GI) adverse effects was high *(96)*. Epidemiological studies of the effects of water-borne fluoride suggest that an increased exposure to fluoride may actually increase fracture risk *(97)*. Nevertheless, there remains an active interest in refining the form of administration and dose of fluoride in the hope of taking better

advantage of its anabolic properties. In fact, recent evaluations of a cyclically administered slow-release form of fluoride demonstrated an increase in BMD and a reduction in
fracture rates in older women *(98,99)*. As with many of the other therapies discussed,
there have been no specific trials of fluoride administration in men. In some studies,
osteoporotic men have been included in the treatment groups *(100–109)*, but it is difficult
to ascertain whether responses were in any way sex-specific.

5. THERAPEUTIC APPROACHES
TO SECONDARY CAUSES OF OSTEOPOROSIS

5.1. Hypogonadism

5.1.1. AGE-RELATED CHANGES IN GONADAL FUNCTION

Aging in men is associated with changes in the hypothalamic–pituitary–gonadal axis
that result in notable declines in total and free testosterone levels *(110,111)*. These changes
have given rise to considerable speculation regarding whether several of the concomi-
tants of aging are the result, at least in part, of the decline in testosterone levels. For
instance, the well-documented declines in muscle strength and bone mass with aging
have been suggested to be potential sequelae *(112)*. Indeed, there are several lines of
evidence firmly linking androgen action to skeletal mass in men *(113)*, and there have
been several attempts to link bone mass to testosterone levels. Kelly et al. *(63)* found that
free testosterone levels correlated with ultradistal bone density (but not with a variety of
other densitometric measurement sites) in a group of men aged 21–79 even after the
effects of age were considered. Similarly, in a study of randomly selected older men in
England, androgen levels were found to correlate (although weakly) with proximal femoral BMD *(114)*. However, these findings have not been corroborated by other investigators *(115–117)*. In an attempt to test the hypothesis that relative androgen deficiency has
a skeletal impact in older men, Tenover et al. reported in a small study (13 men) that
parenteral testosterone supplementation reduced urinary hydroxyproline excretion *(118)*.
Clarke et al. have suggested that changes in testosterone are not as important as the
skeletal effects of age-related declines in adrenal androgens *(119)*. The study of this and
similar issues is made particularly difficult by the inability to assess adequately the long-
term, integrated level of sex steroid action on bone with cross-sectional or relatively
short-term study designs. Obviously, the issue of the importance of gonadal insufficiency
in the genesis of senile bone loss in men remains unresolved. Currently, the use of
androgenic compounds in men without frank hypogonadism—for instance, the older
man with low normal testosterone levels—remains highly speculative. Not only are there
no studies supporting a beneficial effect in these patients (e.g., on bone mass or fracture
rates), but there should be serious concern regarding potential toxicity. Parenteral testosterone administration is associated with reductions in HDL cholesterol levels *(120)*,
and orally administered androgens have dramatically adverse effects on lipid concentrations *(121)*. In case reports, testosterone replacement therapy has been associated with
prostatic disease *(122)*, an issue that needs more clarification.

5.1.2. ESTABLISHED HYPOGONADISM

The effectiveness of androgen replacement therapy in hypogonadal men is unclear.
One experience with a small number of hypogonadal adolescents suggested an improvement in bone mass that was lacking in untreated subjects *(123)*. There have also been

several reports of small increases in BMD with androgen replacement in hypogonadal adult men *(124–127)*. The reversal of hyperprolactinemia and the subsequent achievement of eugonadism in men with pituitary adenomas also lead to an improvement in vertebral bone mass *(128)*. However, the effect of variables, such as time since onset of gonadal disease and age, on the likelihood of a positive response is not well defined. In general, the response of BMD to androgen replacement has been modest. The histomorphometric response to androgen replacement is unknown, but a single case report suggested that an impairment in bone formation was improved *(129)*. All these reports suggest that at least in the short term, androgen replacement therapy may have beneficial effects on bone mass. However, it is not certain that all men respond, or whether other factors (e.g., age, duration of hypogonadism) influence the success of treatment.

The role of estrogen action in the male skeleton is controversial, but replacement studies in castrated animals *(130)*, as well as binding studies in human osteoblastic cell lines *(131)*, indicate that testosterone and dihydrotestosterone are equally active in bone. Nevertheless, essentially all evaluations of the effectiveness of androgen replacement therapy in hypogonadal men have examined the use of parenteral testosterone *(123,124,126,127,129)* or the response to the restoration of endogenous testicular function after treatment of reversible causes of hypogonadism (hyperprolactinemia) *(128)*. However, the most appropriate route of androgen administration and the specific androgen to be used have also not been examined. For instance, transdermal testosterone therapy is now available for treatment of hypogonadism *(128,132–134)* and the use of transdermal dihydrotestosterone has been explored *(135)*, but neither have been examined in the treatment or prevention of bone loss. The minimal effective dose of androgen is also unknown. Moreover, all studies that suggest a beneficial effect of androgen therapy are of short duration (1–5 yr), and whether there is a sustained increase in bone mass with therapy or whether bone mass ever reaches eugonadal levels is uncertain. In patients with Klinefelter's syndrome (in which the basic disease process is not known to affect bone directly), there is evidence that bone mass does not recover after therapy is begun *(136)* or is capable of recovery (or osteopenia is prevented) only if therapy is begun early after the onset of puberty *(137)*. Of great importance, the potential risks of androgen replacement therapy, particularly in the elderly, are uncertain in relation to the possible skeletal benefits to be gained *(112)*. Nevertheless, the concern of bone loss and fractures should represent one of the indications for androgen therapy of gonadal failure.

There is essentially no experience with other pharmacological approaches in the therapy of hypogonadal bone disease in men. The character of hypogonadal bone loss in men suggests it is similar to that in women (an early phase of resorption followed by lower turnover), so approaches that have been effective in the postmenopausal period (bisphosphonates, calcitonin) may be useful in men as well. In a study of the early hypogonadal period in men, Stepan and Lachman *(138)* found that calcitonin therapy reduced biochemical evidence of increased resorption, but measures of bone mass were not assessed.

5.2. Glucocorticoid Excess

The current clinical management of glucocorticoid-induced osteoporosis is based on limited data, not only with regard to the efficacy of preventative and therapeutic regimens, but also in terms of our limited understanding of the pathophysiology of the disease. Various therapies—including calcium, vitamin D, calcitonin, bisphosphonates, sex steroids, and fluoride, have been examined, but usually in open studies of limited subjects measuring effects on bone mass, rather than large-scale investigations evaluating fracture risk.

Certainly, management of patients receiving long-term glucocorticoid therapy should include minimally effective doses, at all times; discontinuation of the drug, when practical; and topical administration, if possible. Although alternate-day glucocorticoid dosing preserves normal function of the hypothalamic–pituitary–adrenal axis, there is little evidence that such a regimen offers any advantage in terms of preventing bone loss *(139,140)*.

Calcium supplements diminish indices of bone resorption *(141)*, and thiazide diuretics combined with reduced dietary sodium intake improve gastrointestinal absorption of calcium and attenuate urinary calcium losses *(142,143)*. Pharmacologic doses of vitamin D have been widely used to treat glucocorticoid-induced osteoporosis in the past. Such therapy is not justified on the basis of vitamin D deficiency *(144)* and has not consistently shown therapeutic benefit *(145–150)*. However, in some studies that included male patients, vitamin D therapy appeared beneficial. For instance, Sambrook et al. *(150)* demonstrated a preservation of lumbar spine (but not femoral or radial) BMD with calcium and calcitriol therapy. In this study, the addition of nasal calcitonin to calcium and calcitriol therapy had no additional benefit. Vitamin D toxicity can accompany therapy with pharmacological doses of vitamin D *(145,147,148,150,151)* and limits the vitamin D dose utilized. Supplementation with lower doses (800–1000 IU/d) is certainly safe. Because long-term glucocorticoid therapy reduces serum testosterone levels and administration of testosterone to hypogonadal men has been shown to improve bone mass, such therapy may be helpful, but has not been adequately evaluated. Sodium fluoride stimulates replication and function of osteoblasts and, as such, might be particularly useful in overcoming the primary inhibitory effects of glucocorticoids on the osteoblast. Several open and uncontrolled studies have revealed variable responses to treatment. One study of only 6 mo duration found no effect on the rate of glucocorticoid-induced bone loss *(149)*, whereas another study examining long-term fluoride therapy demonstrated marked histologic improvement in indices of bone formation and trabecular mass *(152)*. Agents that inhibit bone resorption, such as calcitonin and bis-phosphonates, have also been shown to be of therapeutic benefit *(80,150,153–156)*. However, the efficacy of these agents appears to be greatest when administered in a preventative fashion from the time of initial exposure to glucocorticoids *(150,153)*.

5.3. Alcoholism

Osteoporosis should be suspected in every chronic alcohol abuser, and patients with "idiopathic" osteoporosis should be routinely and thoroughly questioned about drinking habits. Once the diagnosis of alcohol-induced bone disease has been established, a number of measures are recommended. Aggressive medical and psychiatric treatment should be pursued in the hopes of interrupting the cycle of chronic alcohol ingestion and thereby diminish the risk of further skeletal deterioration. A careful dietary history should be followed by an adequate well-balanced diet rich in calcium-containing products. Evidence that calcium supplementation will improve the bone disease of alcoholics has not been reported, but it is reasonable to minimize other potential risk factors for bone loss if possible. Adequate vitamin D nutrition and physical exercise should be encouraged. Tobacco use and excessive consumption of phosphate-binding antacids should be discouraged.

Presumably, the cessation of alcohol intake will stop further progression of bone loss, but data are scant. Studies on alcohol abstainers have demonstrated a rapid recovery of osteoblast function (as assessed histomorphometrically and by biochemical parameters of bone remodeling) within as little as 2 wk after cessation of drinking, but no significant differences in bone mineral content (BMC) were observed between abstainers and actively drinking men *(138,157–160)*. The relatively short period of abstinence, however, makes these results inconclusive. Recently, Peris and colleagues reported slight gains in both trabecular (2.9%) and cortical (2.8%) bone mass in alcoholics after 2 yr of abstinence *(161)*. No significant changes in hormonal parameters were observed in the study participants, lending further support to the hypothesis that alcohol directly inhibits bone formation by the osteoblast.

Thus, the challenge in alcohol-induced bone disease is to stimulate bone formation. Most of the drugs currently used to treat other forms of osteoporosis work primarily by inhibiting osteoclastic bone resorption. Such agents as fluoride, PTH, or growth hormone may stimulate bone formation, but such regimens remain investigational and no therapeutic trials in alcoholic men have been reported. The toxic effects of alcohol and fluoride on the gastrointestinal tract may likely preclude its use in the individual who continues to drink.

5.4. Tobacco

The ideal approach to osteoporosis associated with tobacco use is smoking cessation. Whether cessation leads to reduced rates of bone loss or to a gain in bone mass is unknown. In the studies by Slemenda et al. *(64),* there was apparently a protective effect of heavy physical activity on the bone loss induced by smoking. Other interventions (nutritional supplements, antiresorptive drugs) might potentially reduce the incidence of low bone mass in men who did not abstain, although these possibilities are untested.

5.5. Gastrointestinal Disorders

The therapeutic approach to low bone mass in men (as in women) with gastrectomy or small bowel disease should be based on an understanding of gastrointestinal function and mineral metabolism. Vitamin D insufficiency should be treated with replacement doses sufficient to restore adequate serum 25-OH-D levels. In some patients with severe malabsorption, this may require large doses of vitamin D, parenteral vitamin D administration, or stimulation of endogenous dermal vitamin D synthesis with UV irradiation *(162)*. Dietary calcium intake should be supplemented when necessary, but the amounts needed to achieve adequate calcium balance vary greatly. PTH levels and rates of urinary calcium excretion may help to gage the severity of dietary calcium deficiency and the adequacy of replacement doses. With this therapy for classic hypovitaminosis D, improvement in bone mass should be expected, but the bone deficit existing before therapy is, to a large extent, not fully reversible *(163)*. In patients with low bone mass who show either histomorphometric evidence of a mineralization defect or low-turnover osteoporosis in the absence of vitamin D insufficiency, there is no therapy yet shown to be effective in restoring bone mass. Many patients with low bone mass and mineralization defects with normal vitamin D levels fail to improve with calcium/vitamin D replacement therapy *(164)*.

5.6. Hypercalciuria

Attempts to treat low bone mass associated with idiopathic hypercalciuria are not yet reported. Since the most likely cause of defects in bone remodeling result from the mineral abnormalities induced by the renal calcium disturbance, it seems prudent to prevent hypercalciuria. In those with either renal or absorptive hypercalciuria, thiazide diuretics would be appropriate (and their use is associated with positive effects on bone density in other settings).

REFERENCES

1. Nguyen T, Sambrook P, Kelly P, Jones G, Lord SJ. Prediction of osteoporotic fractures by postural instability and bone density. *BMJ* 1993; 307: 1111–1115.
2. Grisso JA, Chiu GY, Maislin G, Steinmann WC, Portale J. Risk factors for hip fractures in men: a preliminary study. *J Bone Miner Res* 1991; 6: 865–868.
3. Ray WA, Griffin MR, Schaffner W, Baugh DK, Melton LJ III. Psychotropic drug use and the risk of hip fracture. *N Engl J Med* 1987; 316: 363–370.
4. Ray WA, Griffin MR, Downey W. Benzodiazepines of long and short elimination half-life and the risk of hip fracture. *JAMA* 1989; 262: 3303–3307.
5. Karlsson MK, Johnell O, Nilsson BE, Sernbo I, Obrant KJ. Bone mineral mass in hip fracture patients. *Bone* 1993; 14: 161–165.
6. Fiatarone MA, O'Neill E, Ryan ND, Clements KM, Solares GR, Nelson ME, Roberts SB, Keyhayias JJ, Lipsitz LA, Evans WJ. Exercise training and nutritional supplementation for physical frailty in very elderly people. *N Engl J Med* 1994; 330: 1769–1775.
7. Tinetti ME, Baker DI, McAvay G, Claus EB, Garrett P, Gottschalk M, Koch ML, Trainor K, Horwitz RI. A multifactorial intervention to reduce the risk of galling among elderly people living in the community. *N Engl J Med* 1994; 331: 821–827.
8. Aaron JE, Makins NB, Sagreiya K. The microanatomy of trabecular bone loss in normal aging men and women. *Clin Orthop Related Res* 1987; 215: 260–271.
9. Eriksen EF. Normal and pathological remodeling of human trabecular bone: three dimensional reconstruction of the remodeling sequence in normals and in metabolic bone disease. *Endocr Rev* 1986; 7: 379–408.
10. Eriksen EF, Mosekilde L, Melsen F. Trabecular bone resorption depth decreases with age: differences between normal males and females. *Bone* 1985; 6: 141–146.
11. Croucher PI, Mellish RWE, Vedi S, Garrahan NJ, Compston JE. The relationship between resorption depth and mean interstitial bone thickness: age-related changes in man. *Calcif Tissue Int* 1989; 45: 15–19.
12. Melsen F, Melsen B, Mosekilde L, Bergmann S. Histomorphometric analysis of normal bone from the iliac crest. *Acta Pathol Microbiol Scand* 1986; 86: 70–81.
13. Kragstrup J, Melsen F, Mosekilde L. Thickness of bone formed at remodeling sites in normal human iliac trabecular bone: variations with age and sex. *Metab Bone Dis and Related Res* 1983; 5: 17–21.
14. Seeman E, Melton LJ III. Risk factors for spinal osteoporosis in men. *Am J Med* 1983; 75: 977–983.
15. Parfitt AM, Duncan H. Metabolic bone disease affecting the spine. In: Rothman R, ed. *The Spine,* 2nd ed. Philadelphia, PA: Saunders, 1982; pp. 775–905.
16. Resch H, Pietschmann P, Woloszczuk W, Krexner E, Bernecker P, Willvonseder R. Bone mass and biochemical parameters of bone metabolism in men with spinal osteoporosis. *Eur J Clin Invest* 1992; 22: 542–545.
17. Kelepouris N, Harper KD, Gannon F, Kaplan FS, Haddad JG. Severe osteoporosis in men. *Ann Int Med* 1995; 123: 452–460.
18. Riggs BL, Melton LJ. Medical progress: involutional osteoporosis. *N Engl J Med* 1986; 314: 1676–1686.
19. Francis RM, Peacock M, Marshall DH, Horsman A, Aaron JE. Spinal osteoporosis in men. *Bone Miner* 1989; 5: 347–357.
20. DeVernejoul MC, Bielakoff J, Herve M. Evidence for defective osteoblastic function. A role for alcohol and tobacco consumption in osteoporosis in middle-aged men. *Clin Orthop* 1983; 179: 107–115.
21. Hills E, Dunstan CR, Wong SYP, Evans RA. Bone histology in young adult osteoporosis. *J Clin Pathol* 1989; 42: 391–397.

22. Marie PJ, de Vernejoul MC, Donnes D, Hott M. Decreased DNA synthesis by culture osteoblastic cells in eugonadal osteoporotic men with defective bone formation. *J Clin Invest* 1991; 88: 1167–1172.

23. Nordin BEC, Aaron J, Speed R, Francis RM, Makins N. Bone formation and resorption as the determinants of trabecular bone volume in normal and osteoporotic men. *Scott Med J* 1984; 29: 171–175.

24. Jackson JA, Kleerekoper M. Osteoporosis in men: diagnosis, pathophysiology, and prevention. *Medicine* 1990; 69: 137–152.

25. Jones G, Nguyen T, Sambrook P, Kelly PJ, Eisman JA. Progressive loss of bone in the femoral neck in elderly people: longitudinal findings from the Dubbo osteoporosis epidemiology study. *Br Med J* 1994; 309: 691–695.

26. Garn SM, Sullivan TV, Decker SA, Larkin FA, Hawthorne VM. Continuing bone expansion and increasing bone loss over a two-decade period in men and women from a total community sample. *Am J Human Biol* 1992; 4: 57–67.

27. Orwoll ES, Oviatt SK, McClung MR, Deftos LJ, Sexton G. The rate of bone mineral loss in normal men and the effects of calcium and cholecalciferol supplementation. *Ann Int Med* 1990; 112: 29–34.

28. Mazess RB, Barden HS, Drinka PJ, Bauwens SF, Orwoll ES, Bell NH. Influence of age and body weight on spine and femur bone mineral density in U.S. white men. *J Bone Miner Res* 1990; 5: 645–652.

29. Tobin JD, Fox KM, Cejku ML. Bone density changes in normal men: a 4-19 year longitudinal study. *J Bone Miner Res* 1993; 8: 102.

30. Gotfredsen A, Hadberg A, Nilas L, Christiansen C. Total body bone mineral in healthy adults. *J Lab Clin Med* 1987; 110: 362–368.

31. Hannan MT, Felson DT, Anderson JJ. Bone mineral density in elderly men and women: results from the Framingham osteoporosis study. *J Bone Miner Res* 1992; 7: 547–553.

32. Davis JW, Ross PD, Vogel JM, Wasnich RD. Age-related changes in bone mass among Japanese-American men. *Bone Miner* 1991; 15: 227–236.

33. Meier DE, Orwoll ES, Jones JM. Marked disparity between trabecular and cortical bone loss with age in healthy men: measurement by vertebral computed tomography and radioal photon absorptiometry. *Ann Intern Med* 1984; 101: 605–612.

34. Mann T, Oviatt SK, Wilson D, Nelson D, Orwoll ES. Vertebral deformity in men. *J Bone Miner Res* 1992; 7(11): 1259–1265.

35. Looker AC, Harris TB, Madans JH, Sempos CT. Dietary calcium and hip fracture risk: the NHANES I epidemiologic follow-up study. *Osteoporosis Int* 1993; 3: 177–184.

36. Snow-Harter C, Whalen R, Myburgh K, Arnaud S, Marcus R. Bone mineral density, muscle strength, and recreational exercise in men. *J Bone Miner Res* 1992; 7: 1291–1296.

37. Colletti LA, Edwards J, Bordon L, Shary J, Bell NH. The effects of muscle-building exercise on bone mineral density of the radius, spine and hip in young men. *Calcif Tissue Int* 1989; 45: 12–14.

38. Block JE, Genant HK, Black D. Greater vertebral bone mineral mass in exercising young men. *West J Med* 1986; 145: 39–42.

39. Block JE, Friedlander AL, Brooks GA, Steiger P, Stubbs HA, Genant HK. Determinants of bone density among athletes engaged in weight-bearing and non-weight-bearing activity. *J Appl Physiol* 1989; 67: 1100–1105.

40. Jones HH, Priest JD, Hayes WC, Tichenor CC, Nagel DA. Humeral hypertrophy in response to exercise. *J Bone Jt Surg* 1977; 59–A: 204–208.

41. Orwoll ES, Ferar J, Oviatt SK, McClung MR, Huntington K. The relationship of swimming exercise to bone mass in men and women. *Arch Int Med* 1989; 149: 2197–2200.

42. Need AG, Durbridge TC, Nordin BE. Anabolic steroids in postmenopausal osteoporosis. *Wien Med Wochenschr* 1993; 143: 392–395.

43. Bevier WC, Wiswell RA, Pyka G, Kozak KC, Newhall KM, Marcus R. Relationship of body composition, muscle strength, and aerobic capacity to bone mineral density in older men and women. *J Bone Miner Res* 1989; 4: 421–432.

44. Myburgh KH, Zhou L-J, Steele CR, Arnaud S, Marcus R. In vivo assessment of forearm bone mass and ulnar bending stiffness in healthy men. *J Bone Miner Res* 1992; 7: 1345–1350.

45. Frost HM. The role of changes in mechanical usage set points in the pathogenesis of osteoporosis. *J Bone Miner Res* 1992; 7: 253–261.

46. Williams JA, Wagner J, Wasnich R, Heilbrun L. The effect of long-distance running upon appendicular bone mineral content. *Med Sci Sports Exerc* 1984; 16: 223–227.

47. Wickham CAC, Walsh K, Cooper C, Barker DJP, Margetts BM, Morris J, Bruce SA. Dietary calcium, physical activity, and risk of hip fracture: a prospective study. *BMJ* 1989; 299: 889–892.

48. Paganini-Hill A, Chao A, Ross RK, Henderson BE. Exercise and other factors in the prevention of hip fracture: the Leisure World study. *Epidemiology* 1991; 2: 16–25.

49. Larsson L, Sjodin B, Karlsson J. Histochemical and biochemical changes in human skeletal muscle with age in sedentary males, age 22-65 years. *Acta Physiol Scand* 1978; 103: 31–39.

50. Aniansson A, Gustaffson E. Physical training in elderly men with special reference to quadriceps muscle strength and morphology. *Clin Physiol* 1981; 1: 89–98.

51. Rubenstein LZ, Josephson KR. Causes and prevention of falls in elderly people. In: Vellas B, Toupet M, Rubenstein L, Albarede JL, Christen Y, eds. *Falls, Balance and Gait Disorders in the Elderly*. Paris: Elsevier, 1992, pp. 21–36.

52. Greendale GA, Barrett CE, Edelstein S, Ingles S, Haile R. Lifetime leisure exercise and osteoporosis. *Am J Epidemiol* 1995; 141: 951–959.

53. American College of Medicine. ACSM position stand on osteoporosis and exercise. *Med Sci Sports Exerc* 1995; 27: i–vii.

54. Young G, Marcus R, Minkoff JR, Kim LY, Segre GV. Age-related rise in parathyroid hormone in man: the use of intact and midmolecule antisera to distinguish hormone secretion from retention. *J Bone Miner Res* 1987; 2: 367–374.

55. Endres DB, Morgan CH, Garry PJ, Omdahl JL. Age-related changes in serum immunoreactive parathyroid hormone and its biological action in healthy men and women. *J Clin Endocrinol Metab* 1987; 65: 724–731.

56. Orwoll ES, Meier DE. Alterations in calcium, vitamin D, and parathyroid hormone physiology in normal men with aging: relationship to the development of senile osteopenia. *J Clin Endocrinol Metab* 1986; 63: 1262–1269.

57. Slovik DM, Adams JS, Neer RM, Holick MF, Potts JR. Deficient production of 1,25-dihydroxyvitamin D in elderly osteoporotic patients. *N Engl J Med* 1981; 305: 372.

58. Manolagas SC, Culler FL, Howard JE. The cytoreceptor assay for 1,25-dihydroxyvitamin D in elderly osteoporotic patients. *J Clin Endocrinol Metab* 1983; 56: 751–760.

59. Epstein S, Bryce G, Hinman JW. The influence of age of bone mineral regulating hormones. *Bone* 1986; 7: 421–425.

60. Halloran BP, Portale AA, Lonergan ET, Morris RCJ. Production and metabolic clearance of 1,25-dihydroxyvitamin D in men: effect of advancing age. *J Clin Endocrinol Metab* 1990; 70: 318–323.

61. Sherman SS, Tobin JD, Hollis BW, Gundberg CM, Roy TA, Plato CC. Biochemical parameters associated with low bone density in healthy men and women. *J Bone Miner Res* 1992; 7: 1123–1130.

62. Kroger H, Laitinen K. Bone mineral density measured by dual-energy x-ray absorptiometry in normal men. *Eur J Clin Invest* 1992; 22: 454–460.

63. Kelly PJ, Pocock NA, Sambrook PN, Eisman JA. Dietary calcium, sex hormones, and bone mineral density in men. *Br Med J* 1990; 300: 1361–1364.

64. Slemenda CW, Christian JC, Reed T, Reister TK, Williams CJ, Johnston CCJ. Long-term bone loss in men: effects of genetic and environmental factors. *Ann Intern Med* 1992; 117: 286–291.

65. Matkovic V, Kostial K, Simonovic I, Buzina R, Brodarec A, Nordin BEC. Bone status and fracture rates in two regions of Yugoslavia. *Am J Clin Nutr* 1979; 32: 540–549.

66. Lau E, Donnan S, Barker DJP, Cooper C. Physical activity and calcium intake in fracture of the proximal femur in Hong Kong. *BMJ* 1988; 297: 1441–1443.

67. Cooper C, Barker DJ, Wickham C. Physical activity, muscle strength, and calcium intake in fracture of the proximal femur in Britain. *BMJ* 1988; 297(6661): 1443–1446.

68. Holbrook TL, Barrett-Connor E, Wingard DL. Dietary calcium and risk of hip fracture: 14-year prospective population study. *Lancet* 1988; II: 1046–1049.

69. Nordin BEC, Marshall PH. Dietary requirements for calcium. In: Nordin BEC, ed. *Calcium in Human Biology*. New York: Springer-Verlag, 1988, pp. 447–471.

70. O'Brien KO, Allen LH, Quatromoni P, Siu-Caldera M-L, Vieira NE, Perez A, HOlick MF, Yergey AL. High fiber diets slow bone turnover in young men but have no effect on efficiency of intestinal calcium absorption. *J Nutr* 1993; 123: 2122–2128.

71. Orwoll ES. The effects of dietary protein insufficiency and excess on skeletal health. *Bone* 1992; 13: 343–350.

72. Heaney RP. Nutritional factors in bone health in elderly subjects: methodological and contextual problems. *Am J Clin Nutr* 1989; 50: 1182–1189.

73. Miller JZ, Smith DL, Flora L, Slemenda C, Jiang X, Johnston CCJ. Calcium absorption from calcium carbonate and a new form of calcium (CCM) in healthy male and female adolescents. *Am J Clin Nutr* 1988; 48: 1291–1294.

74. Curhan GC, Willett WC, Rimm EB, Stampfer MJ. A prospective study of dietary calcium and other nutrients and the risk of symptomatic kidney stones. *N Engl J Med* 1993; 328: 833–838.

75. Orwoll ES, Weigel RM, Oviatt SK, McClung MR, Deftos LJ. Calcium and cholecalciferol: effects of small supplements in normal men. *Am J Clin Nutr* 1988; 48: 127–130.

76. Agrawal R, Wallach S, Cohn S, Tessier M, Verch R, Hussain M, Zanzi I. Calcitonin treatment of osteoporosis. In: Pecile A, ed. *Chemistry, Physiology, Pharmacology, and Clinical Aspects.* Exerpta Medica, Amsterdam, 1981; p. 237–246.

77. Burckhardt P, Burnand B. The effect of treatment with calcitonin on vertebral fracture rate in osteoporosis. *Osteoporosis Int* 1993; 3: 24–30.

78. McDermott MT, Kidd GS. The role of calcitonin in the development and treatment of osteoporosis. *Endocr Rev* 1987; 8: 377–390.

79. Valkema R, Vismans F-JFE, Papapoulos SE, Pauwels EKJ, Bijvoet OLM. Maintained improvement in calcium balance and bone mineral content in patients with osteoporosis treated with the bisphosphonate APD. *Bone Miner* 1989; 5: 183–192.

80. Reid IR, Alexander CJ, King AR, Ibbertson HK. Prevention of steroid-induced osteoporosis with (3-amino-1-hydroxypropylidene)-1, 1-bisphosphonate(APD). *Lancet* 1988; January 23: 143–146.

81. Papapoulos SE, Landman JO, Bijvoet OLM, Lowik CWGM, Valkema R, Pauwels EKJ, Vermeij P. The use of bisphosphonates in the treatment of osteoporosis. *Bone* 1992; 13: S41–S49.

82. Morton DJ, Barrett-Connor EL, Edelstein SL. Thiazides and bone mineral density in elderly men and women. *J Bone Miner* 1993; 8: S265.

83. Wasnich R, Davis J, Ross P, Vogel J. Effect of thiazide on rates of bone mineral loss: a longitudinal study. *Br Med J* 1990; 301: 1303–1305.

84. Ray WA, Griffin MR, Downey W, Melton LJI. Long-term use of thiazide diuretics and risk of hip fracture. *Lancet* 1989; I: 687–690.

85. Costanza LS, Weiner IM. On the hypocalciuric action of chlorothiazide. *J Clin Invest* 1974; 54: 628–637.

86. Song X, Wergedal JE. Hydrochlorothiazide stimulates proliferation of human osteoblasts in vitro. *J Bone Miner Res* 1993; 8: S362.

87. Reeve J, Neunier PJ, Parsons JA, Bernat M, Bijvoet OLM, Courpron P, Edouard C, Klenerman L, Neer RM, Renier JC, Slovik D, Vismans FJFE, Potts JRJ. Anabolic effect of human parathyroid hormone fragment on trabecular bone in involutional osteoporosis: a multicentre trial. *Br Med J* 1980; June 7: 1340–1344.

88. Slovik DM, Rosenthal DI, Doppelt SH, Potts JRJ, Daly MA, Campbell JA, Neer RM. Restoration of spinal bone in osteoporotic men by treatment with human parathyroid hormone (1-34) and 1,25-dihydroxyvitamin D. *J Bone Miner Res* 1986; 1: 377–381.

89. Reeve J, Bradbeer JN, Arlot M, Davies UM, Green JR, Hampton L, Edouard C, Hesp R, Hulme P, Ashby JP, Zanelli JM, Meunier PJ. hPTH 1-34 treatment of osteoporosis with added hormone replacement therapy: biochemical, kinetic and histological responses. *Osteoporosis Int* 1991; 1: 162–170.

90. Marcus R, Butterfield G, Holloway L, Gilliland L, Baylink DJ, Hintz RL, Sherman BM. Effects of short term administration of recombinant human growth hormone to elderly people. *J Clin Endocrinol Metab* 1990; 70: 519–527.

91. Mann DR, Rudman CG, Akinbami MA, Gould KG. Preservation of bone mass in hypogonadal female monkeys with recombinant human growth hormone administration. *J Clin Endocrinol Metab* 1992; 74: 1263–1269.

92. Ljunghall S, Johansson AG, Burman P, Kampe O, Lindh E, Karlsson FA. Low plasma levels of insulin-like growth factor 1 (IGF-1) in male patients with idiopathic osteoporosis. *J Intern Med* 1992; 232: 59–64.

93. Rudman D, Feller AG, Hoskote S, Nagraj S, Gergans GA, Lalitha PY, Goldberg AF, Schlenker RA, Cohn L, Rudman IW, Mattson DE. Effects of human growth hormone in men over 60 years old. *N Engl J Med* 1990; 323: 1–6.

94. Marcus R, Holloway L, Butterfield G. Clinical uses of growth hormone in older people. *J Reprod Fertil Suppl* 1993; 46: 115–118.

95. Heaney RP, Baylink DJ, Johnston CJ, Melton LJI, Meunier PJ, Murray TM, Nagant de Deuxchaisnes C. Fluoride therapy for the vertebral crush fracture syndrome. *Ann Int Med* 1989; 111(8): 678–680.

96. Riggs BL, Hodgson SF, O'Fallon WM, Chao EYS, Wahner HW, Muhs JM, Cedel SL, Melton LJI. Effect of fluoride treatment on the fracture rate in postmenopausal women with osteoporosis. *N Engl J Med* 1990; 322: 802–809.

97. Danielson C, Lyon JL, Egger M, Goodenough GK. Hip fractures and fluoridation in Utah's elderly population. *JAMA* 1992; 268(6): 746–748.

98. Pak YC, Sakhaee K, Adams-Huet B, Piziak V, Peterson RD, Poindexter JR. Treatment of postmenopausal osteoporosis with slow-release sodium fluoride. *Ann Int Med* 1995; 123: 401–408.

99. Pak CYC, Sakhaee K, Piziak V, Peterson RD, Breslau NA, Boyd P, Poindexter JR, Herzog J, Heard-Sakhaee A, Haynes S, Adams-Huet B, Reisch JS. Slow-release sodium fluoride in the management of postmenopausal osteoporosis: a randomized controlled trial. *Ann Int Med* 1994; 120: 625–632.

100. Mamelle M, Meunier PJ, Dusan R, Guillaume M, Martin JL, Gaucher A, Prost A, Zeigler G. Risk-benefit ratio of sodium fluoride treatment in primary vertebral osteoporosis. *Lancet* 1988; II: 361–365.

101. Pak CYC, Sakhaee K, Zerwekh JE, Parcel C, Peterson R, Johnson K. Safe and effective treatment of osteoporosis with intermittent slow release sodium fluoride: augmentation of vertebral bone mass and inhibition of fractures. *J Clin Endocrinol Metab* 1989; 68: 150–159.

102. Schulz EE, Engstrom H, Sauser DD, Baylink DJ. Osteoporosis: radiographic detection of fluoride-induced extra-axial bone formation. *Radiology* 1986; 159: 457–462.

103. Farley SMG, Wergedal JE, Smith LC, Lundy MW, Farley JR, Baylink DJ. Fluoride therapy for osteoporosis: characterization of the skeletal response by serial measurements of serum alkaline phosphatase activity. *Metabolism* 1987; 36(3): 211–218.

104. El-Khoury GY, Moore TE, Albright JP, Huang HK, Martin RK. Sodium fluoride treatment of osteoporosis: radiologic findings. *AJR* 1982; 139: 39–43.

105. Jowsey J, Riggs BL, Kelly PJ, Hoffman DL. Effect of combined therapy with sodium fluoride, vitamin D and calcium in osteoporosis. *Am J Med* 1972; 53: 43–49.

106. Meunier PJ, Galus K, Briancon D, Edouard C, Charhon SA. Treatment of idiopathic osteoporosis with sodium fluoride. Frances and Anthony D'Anna Memorial Symposium, Detroit, MI, 1983.

107. Inkovaara J, Heikinheimo R, Jarvinen K, Kasurinen U, Hanhijarvi H, IIsalo E. Prophylactic fluoride treatment and aged bones. *Br Med J* 1975; 3: 73–74.

108. Riggs BL, Hodgson SF, Hoffman DL, Kelly PJ, Johnson KA, Taves D. Treatment of primary osteoporosis with fluoride and calcium. *JAMA* 1980; 243(5): 446–449.

109. Zerwekh JE, Antich PP, Sakhaee K, Gonzales J, Gottschalk F, Pak CYC. Assessment by reflection ultrasound method of the effect of intermittent slow-release sodium fluoride-calcium citrate therapy on material strength of bone. *J Bone Miner Res* 1991; 6(3): 239–244.

110. Vermeulen A. Clinical review 24: androgens in the aging male. *J Clin Endocrinol Metab* 1991; 73: 221–223.

111. Vermeulen A, Kaufman JM. Editorial: role of the hypothalamo-pituitary function in the hypoandrogenism of healthy aging. *J Clin Endocrinol Metab* 1992; 75: 704–706.

112. Bardin CW, Swerdloff RS, Santen RJ. Special article-androgens: risk and benefits. *J Clin Endocrinol Metab* 1991; 73: 4–17.

113. Orwoll ES, Klein RF. Osteoporosis in men. *Endocr Rev* 1995; 16: 87–116.

114. Murphy S, Khaw KT, Cassidy A, Compston JE. Sex hormones and bone mineral density in elderly men. *Bone Miner* 1992; 20: 133–140.

115. Johansson AG, Forslund A, Hambraeus L. Growth-hormone-dependent insulin-like growth factor binding protein is a major determinant of bone mineral density in healthy men. *J Bone Miner Res* 1994; 9: 915–921.

116. Drinka PJ, Olson J, Bauwens S, Voeks S, Carlson I, Wilson M. Lack of association between free testosterone and bone density separate from age in elderly males. *Calcif Tissue Int* 1993; 52: 67–69.

117. Meier DE, Orwoll ES, Keenan EJ, Fagerstrom RM. Marked decline in trabecular bone mineral content in healthy men with age: lack of association with sex steroid levels. *JAGS* 1987; 35: 189–197.

118. Tenover JS. Effects of testosterone supplementation in the aging male. *J Clin Endocrinol Metab* 1992; 75: 1092–1098.

119. Clarke BL, Ebeling PR, Jones JD. Increased bone turnover with aging in men is not due to testosterone deficiency (abstract). Endocrine Society Program & Abstracts, Las Vegas, NV, 1993.

120. Bagatell CJ, Knopp RH, Vale WW, Rivier JE, Bremner WJ. Physiologic testosterone levels in normal men suppress high-density lipoprotein cholesterol levels. *Ann Int Med* 1992; 116: 967–973.

121. Thompson PD, Cullinane EM, Sady SP, Chenevert C, Saritelli AL, Sady MA. Contrasting effects of testosterone and stanozolol on serum lipoprotein levels. *JAMA* 1989; 261: 1165–1168.

122. Jackson JA, Waxman J, Spiekerman M. Prostatic complications of testosterone replacement therapy. *Arch Intern Med* 1989; 149: 2365–2366.

123. Arisaka O, Arisaka M. Effect of testosterone on radial bone mineral density in adolescent male hypogonadism. *Acta Paediatr Scand* 1991; 80: 378–380.

124. Diamond T, Stiel D, Posen S. Effects of testosterone and venesection on spinal and peripheral bone mineral in six hypogonadal men with hemochromatosis. *J Bone Miner Res* 1991; 6: 39–43.

125. Isaia G, Mussetta M, Pecchio F, Sciolla A, Di Stefano M, Molinatti GM. Effect of testosterone on bone in hypogonadal males. *Maturitas* 1992; 15: 47–51.

126. Devogelaer JP, De Cooman S, de Deuxchaisnes CN. Low bone mass in hypogonadal males. Effect of testosterone substitution therapy, a densitometric study. *Maturitas* 1992; 15: 17–23.

127. Finkelstein JS, Klibanski A, Neer RM, Doppelt SH, Rosenthal DI, Segre GV, Crowley WFJ. Increases in bone density during treatment of men with idiopathic hypogonadotropic hypogonadism. *J Clin Endocrinol Metab* 1989; 69: 776–783.

128. Greenspan SL, Oppenheim DS, Klibanski A. Importance of gonadal steroids to bone mass in men with hyperprolactinemic hypogonadism. *Ann Int Med* 1989; 110: 526–531.

129. Baran DT, Bergfeld MA, Teitelbaum SL, Avioli LV. Effect of testosterone therapy on bone formation in an osteoporotic hypogonadal male. *Calcif Tissue Res* 1978; 26: 103–106.

130. Turner RT, Wakley GK, Hannon KS. Differential effects of androgens on cortical bone histomorphometry in gonadectomized male and female rats. *J Orthopaed Res* 1990; 8: 612–617.

131. Orwoll ES, Stribrska L, Ramsay EE, Keenan E. Androgen receptors in osteoblast-like cell lines. *Calcif Tissue Int* 1991; 49: 182–187.

132. Findlay JC, Place V, Snyder PJ. Treatment of primary hypogonadism in men by the transdermal administration of testosterone. *J Clin Endocrinol Metab* 1989; 68: 369–373.

133. Findlay JC, Place VA, Snyder PJ. Transdermal delivery of testosterone. *J Clin Endocrinol Metab* 1987; 64: 266–268.

134. Ahmed SR, Boucher AE, Manni A, Santen RJ, Bartholomew M, Demers LM. Transdermal testosterone therapy in the treatment of male hypogonadism. *J Clin Endocrinol Metab*' 1988; 66: 546–551.

135. Vermeulen A, Deslypere JP. Long-term transdermal dihydrotestosterone therapy: effects on pituitary gonadal axis and plasma lipoproteins. *Maturitas* 1985; 7: 182–287.

136. Wong FHW, Pun KK, Wang C. Loss of bone mass in patient with Klinefelter's syndrome despite sufficient testosterone replacement. *Osteoporosis Int* 1993; 7: 281–287.

137. Kubler A, Schulz G, Cordes U, Beyer J, Krause U. The influence of testosterone substitution on bone mineral density in patients with Klinefelter's syndrome. *Exp Clin Endocrinol* 1992; 100: 129–132.

138. Stepan JJ, Lachman M. Castrated men with bone loss: effect of calcitonin treatment on biochemical indices of bone remodeling. *J Clin Endocrinol Metab* 1989; 69: 523–527.

139. Nordborg E, Hansson T, Jonson R. Glucocorticosteroid-induced osteoporosis in giant-cell arteritis (GCA). *Scand J Rheum* 1990; 85: 7.

140. Gluck OS, Murphy WA, Hahn TJ. Bone loss in adults receiving alternate day glucocorticoid therapy: a comparison with daily therapy. *Arthritis Rheum* 1985; 24: 833–838.

141. Reid IR, Ibbertson HK. Calcium supplements in the prevention of steroid-induced osteoporosis. *Am J Clin Nutr* 1986; 44: 287–290.

142. Adams JS, Wahl TO, Luker BP. Effects of hydrochlorothiaize and dietary sodium restriction on calcium metabolism in corticosteroid treated patients. *Metabolism* 1981; 30: 217–221.

143. Suzuki Y, Ichikawa Y, Saito E. Importance of increased urinary calcium excretion in the development of secondary hyperparathyroidism of patients under glucocorticoid therapy. *Metabolism* 1983; 151–156.

144. Bikle DD, Halloran B, Fong L. Elevated 1,25-dihydroxyvitamin D levels in patients with chronic obstructive pulmonary disease treated with prednisone. *J Clin Endocrinol Metab* 1993; 76: 456–461.

145. Condon JR, Nassim JR, Dent CE. Possible prevention and treatment of steroid-induced osteoporosis. *Postgrad Med J* 1978; 54: 249–252.

146. Braun JJ, Birkenhager-Frenkel DH, Reitveld AH. Influence of 1a-(OH)D3 administration on bone mineral metabolism in patients on chronic glucocorticoid treatment: a double-blind controlled study. *Clin Endocrinol (Oxf)* 1983; 19: 265–273.

147. Dykman TR, Haralson KM, Gluck OS. Effect of oral 1,25-dihydroxyvitamin D and calcium on glucocorticoid-induced osteopenia in patients with rheumatic disease. *Arthritis Rheum* 1984; 27: 1336–1341.

148. Bijlsma JW, Raymakers JA, Mosch C. Effect of oral calcium and vitamin D on glucocorticoid-induced osteopenia. *Clin Exp Rheumatol* 1988; 6: 113–119.

149. Rickers H, Deding A, Christiansen C. Mineral loss in cortical and trabecular bone during high-dose prednisone treatment. *Calcif Tissue Int* 1984; 36: 269–273.

150. Sambrook P, Birmingahm J, Kelly P. Prevention of corticosteroid osteoporosis—a comparison of calcium, calcitriol and calcitonin. *NEJM* 1993; 328: 1747–1752.

151. Schwartzman MS, Frank WA. Vitamin D toxicity complicating the treatment of senile, postmenopausal. *Am J Med* 1987; 82: 224–230.

152. Meunier PJ, Birancon D, Chavassieux P. Treatment with fluoride: bone histomorphometric findings. In: Christiansen C, Johansen JS, Riis BJ, eds. *Osteoporosis*. Copenhagen, Denmark: Osteopress, 1987; pp. 824–828.

153. Montemurro L, Schiraldi G, Fraioli P, Tosi G, Riboldi A, Rizzato G. Prevention of corticosteroid-induced osteoporosis with salmon calcitonin in sarcoid patients. *Calcif Tissue Int* 1991; 49: 71–76.

154. Luengo M, Picado C, Del Rio L. Treatment of steroid-induced osteoporosis with calcitonin in corticosteroid-dependent asthma. *Am Rev Respir Dis* 1990; 142: 104–107.

155. Nishioka T, Kurayama H, Yasuda T. Nasal administration of salmon calcitonin for prevention of glucocorticoid-induced osteoporosis in children with nephrosis. *J Pediatr* 1991; 118: 703–707.

156. Reid JR, Heap SW, King AR. Two-year followup of bisphosphonate (APD) treatment in steroid osteoporosis. *Lancet* 1988; ii: 1144.

157. Feitelberg S, Epstein S, Ismail F. Deranged bone mineral metabolism in chronic alcoholism. *Metabolism* 1987; 36: 322–326.

158. Diamond T, Stiel D, Lunzer M, Wilkinson M, Posen S. Ethanol reduced bone formation and may cause osteoporosis. *Am J Med* 1989; 86: 282–288.

159. Laitinen K, Lamberg-Allardt C, Tunninen R. Bone mineral density and abstention-induced changes in bone and mineral metabolism in noncirrhotic male alcoholics. *Am J Med* 1992; 93: 642–650.

160. Jaouhari J, Schiele F, Pirollet P. Concentration and hydroxyapatite binding capacity of plasma osteocalcin in chronic alcoholic men: effect of a three-week withdrawal therapy. *Bone Miner* 1993; 21: 171–178.

161. Peris P, Pares A, Guanabens N, Delrio L, Pons F, Deosaba MJM, Monegal A, Caballeria J, Rodes J, Munozgomez J. Bone mass improves in alcoholics after 2 years of abstinence. *J Bone Miner Res* 1994; 9: 1607–1612.

162. Jung RT, Davie M, Hunter JO. Ultraviolet light: an effective treatment of osteomalacia in malabsorption. *Br Med J* 1978; i: 1668–1669.

163. Parfitt AM, Rao DS, Stanciu J, Villanueva AR, Kleerekoper M, Frame B. Irreversible bone loss in osteomalacia—comparison of radial photon absorptiometry with iliac bone histomorphometry during treatment. *J Clin Invest* 1985; 76: 2403–2412.

164. McKenna MJ, Freaney R, Casey OM, Towers RP, Muldowney FP. Osteomalacia and osteoporosis: evaluation of a diagnostic index. *J Clin Pathol* 1983; 36: 245–252.

22 Bone Mass in Renal Disease

Paul D. Miller, MD

CONTENTS

INTRODUCTION
CASE REPORTS
CONCLUSION
REFERENCES

1. INTRODUCTION

Renal metabolic bone disease is a heterogenous group of bone disorders, some delineated as distinct entities, each of which has distinct pathophysiological mechanisms, and other, often interlinked mechanisms, which are incompletely understood (Table 1).

Most types of renal osteodystrophy have been studied by bone histomorphometry and/ or biochemical assessment *(1)*. It is often difficult to discriminate which type of renal osteodystrophy is present in individual patients using biochemical tests alone. Overlap exists in biochemical testing as a means of diagnosing a specific type of renal bone disease, even though mean values for groups are generally diagnostic and specific *(2,3)*. However, because of such overlap, the most objective method for diagnosing the current form of renal metabolic bone disease is quantitative bone histomorphometry *(4)*. The examination of bone histology in patients with end-stage renal disease (ESRD) can also assist in making therapeutic intervention decisions. For example, it would be a mistake to perform a parathyroidectomy in an ESRD patient who had an abundant aluminum burden in bone. It would also be a mistake to perform a parathyroidectomy in an ESRD patient presenting with hypercalcemia caused by adynamic bone disease. Experienced, skilled nephrologists, however, often make such diagnostic and therapeutic decisions in ESRD patients without quantitative bone histomorphometry because the bone biopsy procedure is invasive, expensive, and not readily accepted by all patients. It would be ideal if additional noninvasive methods were available to enhance the specificity of the diagnosis of the various forms of renal bone disease.

Bone mass measurement data is scarce in these heterogeneous disorders. There are presently only cross-sectional studies, which are not well controlled, most of which were performed prior to the development of DXA, SXA, and QCT technology. There may be a relationship between the duration of ESRD and/or hemodialysis and bone mineral content *(5)*. In some patients, bone mass increases following parathyroidectomy

From: *Osteoporosis: Diagnostic and Therapeutic Principles*
Edited by: C. J. Rosen Humana Press Inc., Totowa, NJ

Table 1
Metabolic Bone Diseases Associated with Renal Disease

1. Osteitis Fibrosa Cystica
2. Osteomalacia
   a. Vitamin D related
   b. Non-vitamin D related
      i. Chronic metabolic acidosis
      ii. Aluminum accumulation
   c. Phosphate depletion
3. Adynamic Bone Disease
4. Mixed Uremic Osteodystrophy
5. Amyloid Bone Disease
6. Osteoporosis

Table 2
Anticipated Bone Mass Measurement Results in Renal Osteodystrophy

	Cancellous Bone	Cortical Bone
Hyperparathyroidism	Normal	Decreased
Aluminum	Normal to high	Normal
Adynamic	Normal to high	Increased
Osteomalacia	Low, normal	Low, normal
Osteoporosis	Decreased	Decreased

(6). However, longitudinal data, utilizing newer bone mass measurement techniques, which control for gonadal status, types of ESRD, and prior drug exposure, are lacking.

One could anticipate the results of bone mass measurement in subjects with recognized classifications of renal bone disease (Table 2).

2. CASE REPORTS

However, to emphasize the difficulties of accurately diagnosing renal bone disease by bone mass measurements, three representative cases are presented.

2.1. Case 1

B.S., a 56-yr-old Caucasian male with ESRD received maintenance hemodialysis for 6 yr. (Table 3). His ESRD was a result of obstructive uropathy. He developed sustained hypercalcemia (10.8–11.8 mg/dL), rising bone alkaline phosphatase (466 IU), elevated intact PTH (six times normal), and sustained three vertebral compression fractures and a nontraumatic hip fracture. His bone mineral density was 0.682 g/cm^2 (–4.1 T-score) and his DFO challenge test was negative. Bone histomorphometry is shown.

2.2. Case 2

T.Q., a 34-yr-old Caucasian female was treated with chronic peritoneal dialysis for 6 yr (Table 4). Her ESRD was a result of hereditary interstitial nephritis. She too developed sustained hypercalcemia (10.9–12.5 mg/dL), and elevated intact PTH (four times normal). Her bone mineral density was 1.243 g/cm^2 (+1.54 T-score) at the AP spine and 1.036 g/cm^2 (+1.36 T-score) at the femoral neck. Bone histomorphometry is shown.

Table 3
Bone Biopsy of Patient B. S.

		Normal
OS/BS, %	100.0	4–18
OTh, μ	17.5	6–12
MS/BS, %	75.5	1–17
MLT, d	31.8	15–50
Oc N/B Ar	35.2	0–2
Aluminum: Positive		
Diagnosis: Aluminum deposition		

Table 4
Bone Biopsy of Patient T. Q.

		Normal
OV/BV, %	3.4	0–6.0
OS/BS, %	21.5	4–18
MS/BS, %	3.0	1–17
MAR, μ/d	.730	.4–.7
Mlt, d	111.0	15–50
Oc N/B Ar	.5	0–2
Aluminum	14.2	0
Diagnosis: Aluminum deposition, low bone formation, low bone resorption.		

Table 5
Bone Biopsy of Patient S. B.

		Normal
OV/BV, %	9.39	0–6.0
OS/BS, %	53.2	4–18
MS/BS, %	47.5	1–17
MAR, μp/d	.859	0.2–0.5
Mlt, d	11.6	15–50
Oc N/B Ar	1.17	0–2
Aluminum: Negative		
Diagnosis: Osteitis fibrosa, osteopenia.		

2.3. Case 3

S.B., a 60-yr-old Caucasian female receiving maintenance hemodialysis for 16 yr also developed sustained hypercalcemia (mean 11.8 mg/dL), elevated PTH (10 times normal), rising bone alkaline phosphatase, and vertebral compression fractures (Table 5). She had bone histomorphometry diagnostic of hyperparathyroidism. Her bone mineral density was 0.783 g/cm^2 (3.58 T-score) at the AP spine and 0.803 g/cm^2 (–1.47 T-score) at the femoral neck. She underwent a subtotal parathyroidectomy and her alkaline phosphatase fell from 688 to 210 IU/ serum calcium normalized, PTH declined but remained elevated (two times normal), and bone mineral density remained low (0.724 g/cm^2 at the AP spine and 0.814 g/cm^2 at the femoral neck).

CONCLUSION

These cases highlight the complexities of renal bone disease, the diagnostic problems of biochemical testing, and the lack of cross-sectional and longitudinal data correlating the types of bone histology with biochemical tests and bone mass measurements.

A prospective, systematic study of all the forms of renal bone disease examined at baseline and longitudinally using bone histomorphometry, biochemical markers, and bone mass measurements is needed. This is the only way to competently determine if bone mass measurements can be used to diagnose the form of renal osteodystrophy, and, to determine it the changes in bone histology that often occur longitudinally in renal bone disease can be monitored by bone mass technology.

Perhaps the greatest contribution bone mass measurement can provide in renal osteo-dystrophy is the identification of low bone mass (particularly osteoporosis) in these patients. This would alert the nephrologist that osteoporosis is prevalent in patients with ESRD, which might, in turn, lead to increased attention to the disorders that might cause osteoporosis in patients living longer with ESRD.

REFERENCES

1. Malluche HH, Faugere M-C. Renal bone disease 1990: An unmet challenge for the nephrologist. *Kidney Int* 1990; 38: 193–211.
2. Pei Y, Hercz G, Greenwood C, et al. Risk factors for renal osteodystrophy. *J Bone Miner Res* 1995; 10: 149–156.
3. Hutchison A, Whitehouse RW, Boulton HF, et al. Correlation of bone histology with parathyroid hormone, Vitamin D and radiology in end-stage renal disease. *Kidney Int* 1993; 44: 1071–1077.
4. Malluche HH, Monier-Faugere M-C. The role of bone biopsy in the management of patients with renal osteodystrophy. *J Am Soc Nephrol* 1994; 41: 1631–1642.
5. Gabay C, Rvedin P, Slosman D, et al. Bone mineral density in patient with end-stage renal disease. *Am J Nephrol* 1993 13: 115–123.
6. Copley JB, Hui SL, Leapman S, Slemenda CW, Johnston CC. Longitudinal study of bone mass in end-stage renal disease patients: Effects of parathyroidectomy for renal osteodystrophy. *J Bone Miner Res* 1993; 8: 415–422.

23 Prevention of Osteoporosis
Making Sense of the Published Evidence

Peter S. Millard, MD, PhD

CONTENTS

1. INTRODUCTION

In this chapter, we will discuss the complexities of applying osteoporosis research findings to clinical practice, review the evidence for some specific preventive interventions, and suggest an algorithm that primary care providers can use to help make decisions about screening for osteoporosis and the prevention of fractures.

2. BASIC PRINCIPLES TO USE IN ASSESSING THE EVIDENCE

2.1. The Burden of Proof Is High for Preventive Interventions

No medical intervention benefits everyone, and almost every intervention has unwanted effects in some people. When patients are ill, they are generally willing to assume a small risk if the likelihood of benefit is substantial. The burden of proof, however, is greater when caregivers recommend interventions for healthy people, especially when the benefits are likely to be delayed for a long time, or the intervention is expensive, unpleasant to take, or adversely affects other body systems. The intervention, on the whole, may improve the quality or duration of life, but some patients may be unwilling to risk adverse effects, especially if they may be life-threatening. It is essential that primary care providers communicate honestly with their patients about the risks, as well as the benefits, of prevention and that each patient's personal preferences be taken into account.

From: *Osteoporosis: Diagnostic and Therapeutic Principles*
Edited by: C. J. Rosen Humana Press Inc., Totowa, NJ

2.2. Limitations of the Existing Evidence

Those evaluating the evidence for the prevention of osteoporotic fractures should keep in mind that clinical studies of osteoporosis began relatively recently, and clinical studies have not progressed to the point that they have in areas such as cardiovascular disease prevention *(1)*. This has important implications for providers, because many of the published studies are cross-sectional or case-control designs, which are generally more susceptible to bias ("getting the wrong answer") than are longitudinal studies (which are often called "cohort" or "follow-up" studies). Even fewer long-term experimental studies (randomized controlled trials) have been published. Providers should generally not change clinical practice based on cross-sectional or case-control studies, and they may need specific training in methodological issues to adequately interpret these studies.

Cross-sectional studies, in which the presence of disease and the "risk factor" (often referred to as the "exposure") are determined at the same time, often suffer from problems in determining the direction of causality. For example, a recent study showed that women with existing osteopenia had less muscle strength compared to women with normal bone mineral density (BMD) *(2)*. Readers might assume that the lack of exercise resulted in osteopenia, but the direction of causality is ambiguous. Case-control studies are also difficult to interpret because they are susceptible to bias in the selection of appropriate controls ("selection bias") and in recall by patients who have already experienced the disease of interest ("recall bias"). Several recent case-control studies have shown that women who have suffered fractures ("cases") are less likely to have taken hormone replacement therapy (HRT) compared to women without fractures ("controls"), but it is difficult to interpret from these studies whether or not there is a causal relationship between lack of hormone use and subsequent fractures.

Ideally, studies should be longitudinal and the follow-up period should have been sufficiently long for all important outcomes to have occurred *(3)*. Longitudinal studies are generally less prone to bias than cross-sectional and case-control studies, because we can be more certain that information collected at baseline (before the outcome of interest has occurred) is accurate. Longitudinal studies, however, may also suffer from bias as a result of incomparability between the "exposed" and "unexposed" groups. Statistical adjustments are frequently performed when the unexposed group differs from the exposed group in age, social class, smoking, menopausal status, and a host of other potential "confounders," but this is not always reassuring. For example, women who take estrogen replacement therapy (ERT) tend to eat healthier diets, to exercise more, to be more compliant, and have more contacts with medical providers than women who do not take ERT; these factors may be responsible for some of the apparent benefits of estrogen replacement therapy *(4)*. Randomized controlled trials, on the other hand, largely alleviate the effects of "hidden" or "partially controlled" confounders, because randomization makes it likely that treatment and control groups will have nearly identical characteristics (except for the assigned treatment).

In summary, primary care providers should generally have the most confidence in the results of randomized controlled trials, slightly less confidence in the results of cohort (longitudinal) studies, and should be skeptical of the results of case-control studies *(5)*.

2.3. Individual vs Community-Based Approaches

Primary care providers have a unique responsibility to their patients and to the community at large to consider seriously where best to focus their efforts toward prevention.

We generally use "risk stratification" in practice; i.e., we select patients for preventive advice and interventions based on identified risk factors. On the other hand, community-based efforts (for example, efforts to reduce smoking, to improve diet, and to exercise) seem less attractive because they are not patient centered, but they may ultimately have a greater impact on the health of the community *(6)*. In the case of fracture prevention, medical intervention based on individual risk factors for osteoporosis is satisfying because we are attempting to treat those who are most likely to benefit, but our ability to predict those at risk is limited. Community-based interventions may, on the other hand, shift the entire distribution of bone density (or other risk factors for fractures) and may prevent fractures in individuals thought to be at "low risk." Our efforts as primary care providers, then, need to be divided between the (traditional) individual-centered role, and the more fundamental role we play in our communities.

3. THE EVIDENCE REGARDING PREVENTION OF OSTEOPOROTIC FRACTURES

3.1. Exercise

When we evaluate the evidence for exercise, it is important to keep in mind that our objective is to prevent disability and death from fractures, and maximizing bone density is only one way to prevent fractures. The importance of conditioning to increase muscle strength, coordination, and balance, combined with environmental measures to prevent falls, may be as important in preventing hip and wrist fractures as the effect of exercise on strengthening bone *(7)*.

Longitudinal studies have generally supported the role of aerobic and strength training in preserving bone density *(8–12)*, but two studies indicated that aerobic exercise had little effect on bone density *(13,14)*. A recent longitudinal study showed that postmenopausal women who were on their feet for at least 4 h/day had a 42% lower risk of hip fracture after 4 yr, compared to women with lesser activity levels *(15)*.

The only two published randomized trials have shown substantial benefits of strength training in postmenopausal women *(16,17)*. Nelson randomized 40 postmenopausal women to either high-intensity strength training 2 d weekly for 1 yr, or their usual level of physical activity. Muscle mass, muscle strength, and dynamic balance increased in the trained subjects and declined in the controls after 1 yr. Femoral neck and lumbar spine bone mineral density each increased by 1% in the trained subjects and decreased by 2.5% and 1.8%, respectively, in the controls *(17)*. Although this study was too small to draw conclusions about the effect of strength training on falls, reduced muscle mass and strength have been shown in previous prospective studies to be risk factors for falls in elderly persons *(18,19)*.

Unfortunately, existing studies on exercise and osteoporosis tend to have small sample sizes and have short follow-up periods, which means that the end points in which we are most interested-namely, fractures-, are unlikely to occur in a sufficient number of women for us to draw conclusions about the benefits of the intervention. For example, two women in the control group of Nelson's study fell and broke their wrists, but the small sample size does not allow us to conclude whether or not this was a chance occurrence. This means that we need to depend on surrogate end points, such as changes in BMD. While bone density is an important predictor of fractures *(15,20)*, other factors (such as the propensity to fall) will be ignored if we simply rely on bone density as the end point.

4. HORMONE REPLACEMENT THERAPY

Few areas of medicine provide more complex decision making for primary care physicians than the issue of using hormone replacement therapy (HRT) for primary prevention in asymptomatic postmenopausal women. At the same time, the decision about whom to recommend for HRT illustrates many issues common to other preventive and therapeutic interventions: the necessity of relying on data from observational studies and the lack of long-term randomized trials; the need to attempt to extrapolate the findings of studies conducted using an earlier therapy (in this case estrogen monotherapy) to current therapy (estrogen with progestins); the necessity of balancing therapeutic effects against some potentially serious adverse effects and how therapy may affect longevity and quality of life; the need for patients to consistently take a long-term treatment for gains that, in the aggregate, may be positive but are not guaranteed for any individual; and an appreciation of the importance of assessing the values that individuals place on different outcomes.

4.1. Estrogen Replacement Therapy

4.1.1. ERT AND OSTEOPOROSIS

Much information is still missing about the risks and benefits of ERT, but far more data is available than on combined HRT. A wealth of observational studies and several randomized trials have shown that ERT reduces the rate of bone loss in postmenopausal women; longitudinal studies also suggest that postmenopausal women who take ERT have a reduced likelihood of sustaining hip fractures (21). The best data that we have from longitudinal studies suggest that the benefits of estrogen replacement therapy are greatest if started shortly after the menopause and decline rapidly after stopping, so ERT should be started soon after the menopause and continued indefinitely (22–24). The fact that the median age of hip fracture among postmenopausal women in the US is 80 yr means that many years of ERT will need to be taken to be effective in reducing fracture.

4.1.2. OTHER EFFECTS OF ERT

ERT has effects on uterine bleeding, sexual function, and serum lipoproteins; it increases the incidence of endometrial carcinoma, but reduces the incidence of coronary heart disease. Because coronary heart disease is the leading cause of death among postmenopausal women, the effects of ERT on coronary heart disease weigh heavily in risk–benefit analyses of ERT use (25).

Unfortunately, part of the beneficial effects of ERT may result from the fact that women who take estrogens may lead healthier lifestyles than women who do not (4), and the lack of randomized studies, in which women are followed-up for many years and all important outcomes are assessed, will not be remedied soon (26).

4.1.3. ERT AND BREAST CANCER

The apparent increase in the incidence of breast cancer among women who take exogenous estrogens remains controversial (27). Overall, the risk of breast cancer appears to become substantial after 5 yr of estrogen use and to increase with increasing duration of use (28). A quantitative analysis of previous studies suggests that 10 yr of ERT is associated with a 20% increase in breast cancer incidence and breast cancer mortality (29).

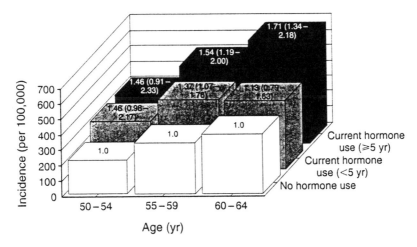

Fig. 1. Incidence and relative risk of breast cancer according to age and the duration of current postmenopausal hormone therapy. Relative risks and 95% confidence intervals are shown at the top of the bars; relative risks are expressed in comparison with the risk among women in each age group who never received hormone therapy. Data have been adjusted for age at menopause, type of menopause, and family history of breast cancer in a proportional hazards analysis. Reprinted from ref. *28* with permission.

4.2. Combination Hormone Replacement Therapy

Much less information is available concerning the risks and benefits of combination HRT. The addition of progestins prevents endometrial proliferative changes associated with ERT *(30),* and a recent randomized trial showed that combination HRT has similar protective effects on cardiovascular risk factors *(31).* Again, we should feel somewhat uncomfortable with the reliance on lipoproteins and fibrinogen measurements as surrogate markers for coronary disease risk, but long-term randomized trials with "hard" end points (myocardial infarction, death) have not yet been conducted *(26).*

The Nurses' Health Study is an ongoing study of over 100,000 nurses who have been followed regularly, almost without dropouts, since 1976, and it represents the best data yet available on the risk of breast cancer following long-term combined HRT *(28).* Current HRT users 55–59 yr of age who had used HRT for 5 yr or longer had a 54% greater incidence of breast cancer, compared to women who had never taken postmenopausal hormones. Figure 1 shows the graded increases in breast cancer incidence with age and with duration of hormone use -results, which are internally consistent and consistent with the bulk of other data. Women who had previously stopped taking HRT were not at increased risk for breast cancer, compared to women who had never taken hormone replacement.

5. BONE MINERAL DENSITY:
AN ADEQUATE PREDICTOR OF FRACTURES?

Routine radiographs frequently show spinal fractures and demineralization, but are insensitive to early changes of osteoporosis and poor tests of bone mineral density at other sites. More accurate tests have been developed, which are stronger predictors of future fractures in asymptomatic patients. Photon absorptiometry (single photon absorptio-

Table 1
Major Clinical Risk Factors for Hip Fracture (relative risk > 1.5)

Risk factor	Compared to	Relative risk	Ref.
White race	Black race	2	39
H/o maternal hip fracture	No history	2	15
H/o corticosteroid use	No history	—	
H/o stroke	No history	3.1	40
Current use of anticonvulsant drugs	No use	2.8	15
Inability to rise from a chair without using arms	Ability to rise from a chair without use of arms	2.1	15
Use of aids in walking	No use of aids	5.6	40
Previous hyperthyroidism	No h/o hyperthyroidism	1.8	15
On feet ≤ 4 h/d	On feet > 4 h/d	1.7	15
Current use of long-acting benzodiazepines	No current use	1.6	15
Resting pulse > 80 bpm	Resting pulse ≤ 80 bpm	1.8	15
Weight loss since age 25	No change in weight since age 25	2.2	15
Low body mass index	Normal body mass index	—	40,41
Consumption ≥ 7 alcoholic drinks/wk	≤ 1 alcoholic drink/wk	4.6	40

metry, dual photon absorptiometry, and dual energy X-ray absorptiometry [DEXA]) measures the transmission of photons through bone and is currently the most commonly used method to measure BMD. DEXA can provide precise measurements of total body calcium and can be used to measure BMD at all sites of osteoporotic fracture (32). Bone mineral density for each site is compared to the mean BMD for healthy 35-yr-olds, matched for sex, and expressed as T scores (or standard deviations from the mean). T scores of <–1 (i.e., 1 SD below the mean) are considered abnormal.

Longitudinal studies have shown that the results of densitometry correlate closely with the risk of fractures at multiple sites (15,20,33). Cummings showed that a T score of –1 in femoral neck bone density increased the age-adjusted risk of hip fracture by 2.6 times, and that women in the lowest quartile for bone density had an 8.5-fold greater risk of hip fracture than those in the highest quartile. Bone density of the calcaneus was nearly as good a predictor of future hip fracture as femoral neck bone density (20). Combining densitometry results with clinical risk factors for falling (e.g., a history of previous falls, benzodiazepine use, inability to rise from a chair without using the arms, and use of an aid in walking—see Table 1) sharpens our ability to predict fractures even further.

6. RISK STRATIFICATION—
THE NEED FOR A PREVENTIVE ALGORITHM

The approach taken by the US Preventive Services Task Force in its Guide to Clinical Preventive Services is important because it is based on a rigorous evaluation of the existing evidence and not on "expert opinion," which can sometimes be misleading (34).

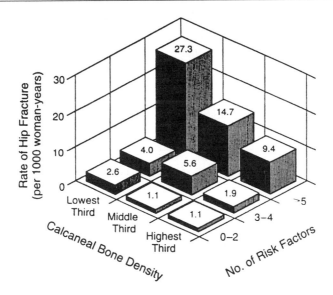

Fig. 2. Annual risk of hip fracture according to the number of risk factors and the age-specific calcaneal bone density. The risk factors are as follows: Age ≥ 80; maternal history of hip fracture; any fracture (except hip fracture) since the age of 50; fair, poor, or very poor health; previous hyperthyroidism; anticonvulsant therapy; current weight less than at the age of 25; height at the age of 25 ≥ 168 cm; caffeine intake more than the equivalent of two cups of coffee per day; on feet ≤ 4 h a day; no walking for exercise; inability to rise from chair without using arms; lowest quartile (standard deviation > 2.44) of depth perception; lowest quartile (≤ .70 U) of contrast sensitivity; and pulse rate > 80 per minute. Reprinted from ref. *15* with permission.

However, the Guide primarily makes recommendations concerning preventive interventions in low-risk populations, and, in practice, we often find that a surprisingly large proportion of our patients have risk factors, which makes them better candidates for screening tests and interventions than the general population. For example, low-risk individuals with hypercholesterolemia may receive little benefit from cholesterol-lowering therapy *(35,36)*, but high-risk individuals may benefit greatly *(37)*, because they are far more likely to experience death from myocardial infarction, and are probably no more likely to suffer adverse effects from treatment.

In practice, we often use risk stratification to determine who is most likely to benefit from a screening test or treatment. If we can successfully predict groups at high risk for developing an adverse outcome, we can focus our efforts on those individuals. Cummings' longitudinal study of over 9000 postmenopausal women, who were followed for an average of 4 yr, suggests that risk stratification is a viable strategy for predicting which women are at highest risk for hip fracture *(15)*. Figure 2 from Cummings' study shows how clinical risk factors and bone densitometry findings can be used to predict hip fracture. The low risk of subsequent hip fracture among the women with few clinical risk factors (regardless of bone densitometry results) suggests that densitometry should be reserved for women with pre-existing clinical risk factors. Women with the lowest calcaneal BMD and five or more clinical risk factors were 25 times more likely to fracture their hip, compared to women with the highest BMD and fewer than three clinical risk factors.

Table 2
A Summary of the Evidence Concerning Three Interventions
to Prevent Osteoporotic Fractures Among Unselected, Asymptomatic Postmenopausal Women

Intervention	Quality of evidence[a]	Strength of recommendations[b]
Physical exercise	I	A
Calcium (1.2 gm) and cholecalciferol (800 IU)	I	A
Combined HRT	II	B

[a]Quality of evidence: I, evidence from at least one properly-designed and conducted randomized controlled trial; II, evidence obtained from well-designed and conducted longitudinal studies without randomization; III, evidence from case-control studies.

[b]Strength of recommendations: A, there is good evidence to support the recommendation that the condition or treatment be specifically considered in a periodic health examination; B, there is fair evidence to support the recommendation that the condition or treatment be specifically considered in a periodic health examination; C, there is poor evidence regarding the inclusion of the condition or treatment in a periodic health examination.

7. WHAT DO OTHERS SAY?

There is currently insufficient information to model risks and benefits of HRT, but two decision analyses have been published on the risks and benefits of ERT for asymptomatic postmenopausal women (25,30). The assumptions for both studies were based on observational data and both may have underestimated the risks of breast cancer from long-term ERT. Grady concluded that ERT should be recommended for all women who have had a hysterectomy or are at high risk for coronary heart disease (30). Gorsky concluded that ERT would improve overall life expectancy and quality of life, and that all asymptomatic women should receive ERT, primarily because of expected large reductions in death from coronary heart disease (25). This conclusion was strengthened by a recent longitudinal study, which suggested that ERT use is associated with reduced mortality, primarily because of large reductions in death from cardiovascular disease (38).

The US Preventive Services Task Force, on the other hand, currently recommends counseling for all women with regard to dietary calcium and vitamin D intake, exercise, smoking cessation, and preventive measures to reduce the risk of falls and fall-related injuries. The current Guide to Clinical Preventive Services recommends bone densitometry measurements in those perimenopausal women who are at increased risk for osteoporosis and in whom HRT would otherwise not be advised, and recommends counseling for all perimenopausal women concerning the risks and benefits of hormone replacement therapy (34). Our own evidence-based recommendations are found in Table 2.

8. AN ALGORITHM FOR EVALUATION
AND PREVENTIVE INTERVENTIONS FOR OSTEOPOROSIS
IN ASYMPTOMATIC PERIMENOPAUSAL WOMEN

We follow with an algorithm for assessing asymptomatic postmenopausal women and treating those at high risk for osteoporotic fractures (Fig. 3). For simplicity, we have rated clinical risk factors as "major" or "minor" (Tables 1 and 3) and have speci-

2 major risk factors or 4 minor risk factors? (See tables 1 and 2)

Yes   No   Routine preventive advice*

Perform densitometry

BMD < 1 SD below that of standard (35 year old, matched for sex)?

Yes   No   Routine preventive advice*

Perform urinary N-telopeptide assay, serum PTH,
serum calcium, TSH

Urinary N-telopeptide increased?

Yes   No   Normal rate of bone resorption
                                                   Advise Ca with vit D, exercise,
                                                   consider HRT

Elevated rate of bone resorption

Start HRT if no contraindications, Ca with vit D, strengthening exercise program

---

Remeasure urinary N-telopeptide after 3 months

Urinary N-telopeptide still increased?

Yes   No   Densitometry after 3 additional months
                                                   (6 months after baseline)

Add calcitonin, bisphosphonates, or increase estrogen
dose

Densitometry after 3 additional months (6 months after baseline)

*Routine preventive advice = regular exercise, calcium and vitamin D supplementation,
assess for likelihood of falls

Fig. 3. An algorithm for the suggested workup and treatment of osteoporosis in postmenopausal
women.

fied the number of risk factors needed before we recommend densitometry, but it should
be kept in mind that these numbers are somewhat arbitrary and that the greater the
number of clinical risk factors present, the greater should be one's conviction that densitometry is indicated.

Table 3
Minor Clinical Risk Factors for Hip Fracture (relative risk 1.2–1.5)

Risk factor	Compared to	Relative risk	Ref.
Any fracture since age 50	No fracture since age 50	1.5	15
Current caffeine intake (per 190 mg increment)	No caffeine intake	1.3	15
Not walking for exercise	Walking for exercise	1.4	15
Current smoking	No current smoking	1.4	15
Fall in the previous year	No fall in previous year	1.4	15
Natural menopause before age 45	Menopause at or after age of 45	1.3	15
Past smoking	Never smoked	1.3	15
No alcohol use	Alcohol use	—	42

REFERENCES

1. Jacobs HS, Loeffler FE. Postmenopausal hormone replacement therapy. *BMJ* 1992; 305: 1403–1408.
2. Bauer DC, Browner WS, Cauley JA, et al. Factors associated with appendicular bone mass in older women. The Study of Osteoporotic Fractures Research Group. *Ann Intern Med* 1993; 118: 657–665.
3. Rothman KJ. *Modern Epidemiology*. Boston: Little, Brown and Company, 1986.
4. Barrett-Connor E. Postmenopausal estrogen and prevention bias. *Ann Intern Med* 1991; 115: 455,456.
5. Guyatt GH, Sackett DL, Cook DJ. Users' guides to the medical literature. II. How to use an article about therapy or prevention. A. Are the results valid? *JAMA* 1993; 270: 2598–2601.
6. Rose G. *The Strategy of Preventive Medicine*. New York: Oxford University Press, 1994.
7. Cooper C, Barker DJP. Risk factors for hip fracture. *N Engl J Med* 1995; 332: 815,816.
8. Chow R, Harrison JE, Notarius C. Effect of two randomised exercise programmes on bone mass of healthy postmenopausal women. *BMJ* 1987; 295: 1441–1444.
9. Dalsky GP, Stocke KS, Ehsani AA, Slatopolsky E, Lee WC, Birge SJ. Weight-bearing exercise training and lumbar bone mineral content in postmenopausal women. *Ann Intern Med* 1988; 108: 824–828.
10. Zylstra S, Hopkins A, Erk M, Hreshchyshyn MA, Anbar M. Effect of physical activity on lumbar spine and femoral neck bone densities. *Int J Sports Med* 1989; 10: 181–186.
11. Nelson M, Fisher E, Dilmanian F, Dallal G, Evans WJ. A 1-y walking program and increased dietary calcium in postmenopausal women: effects on bone. *Am J Clin Nutr* 1991; 53: 1304–1311.
12. Krall EA, Dawson-Hughes B. Walking is related to bone density and rates of bone loss. *Am J Med* 1994; 96: 20–26.
13. Cavanaugh DJ, Cann CE. Brisk walking does not stop bone loss in postmenopausal women. *Bone* 1988; 9: 201–204.
14. Prince RL, Smith M, Dick IM, et al. Prevention of postmenopausal osteoporosis: a comparative study of exercise, calcium supplementation, and hormone-replacement therapy. *N Engl J Med* 1991; 325: 1189–1195.
15. Cummings SR, Nevitt MC, Browner WS, et al. Risk factors for hip fractures in white women. *N Engl J Med* 1995; 332: 767–773.
16. Notelovitz M, Martin D, Tesar R, et al. Estrogen therapy and variable-resistance weight training increase bone mineral in surgically menopausal women. *J Bone Miner Res* 1991; 6: 583–590.
17. Nelson ME, Fiatrone MA, Morganti CM, Trice I, Greenberg RA, Evans WJ. Effects of high-intensity strength training on multiple risk factors for osteoporotic fractures. *JAMA* 1994; 272: 1909–1914.
18. Nevitt MC, Cummings SR, Kidd S, Black D. Risk factors for recurrent nonsyncopal falls: a prospective study. *JAMA* 1989; 261: 2663–2668.
19. Tinetti ME, Baker DI, McAvay G, et al. A multifactorial intervention to reduce the risk of falling among elderly people living in the community. *N Engl J Med* 1994; 331: 821–827.
20. Cummings SR, Black DM, Nevitt MC, et al. Bone density at various sites for prediction of hip fractures. The study of osteoporotic fractures research group. *Lancet* 1993; 341: 72–75.
21. Gordon M, Huang J. Monograph series on aging-related diseases: VI. Osteoporosis. *Chron Dis Canada* 1995; 16: 1–23.

22. Ettinger B, Grady D. The waning effect of postmenopausal estrogen therapy on osteoporosis. *N Engl J Med* 1993; 329: 1192,1193.

23. Felson DT, Zhang Y, Hannan MT, Kiel DP, Wilson PWF, Anderson JJ. The effect of postmenopausal estrogen therapy on bone density in elderly women. *N Engl J Med* 1993; 329: 1141–1146.

24. Cauley JA, Seeley DG, Ensrud K, Ettinger B, Black D, Cummings SR. Estrogen replacement therapy and fractures in older women. Study of osteoporotic fractures research group. *Ann Int Med* 1995; 122: 9–16.

25. Gorsky RD, Koplan JP, Peterson HB, Thacker SB. Relative risks and benefits of long-term estrogen replacement therapy: a decision analysis. *Obstet Gynecol* 1994; 83: 161–166.

26. Healy B. PEPI in perspective: good answers spawn pressing questions. *JAMA* 1995; 273: 240,241.

27. Adami HO, Persson I. Hormone replacement and breast cancer: a remaining controversy? *JAMA* 1995; 274: 178,179.

28. Colditz GA, Hankinson SE, Hunter DJ, et al. The use of estrogens and progestins and the risk of breast cancer in postmenopausal women. *N Engl J Med* 1995; 332: 1589–1593.

29. Steinberg KK, Thacker SB, Smith SJ, et al. A meta-analysis of the effect of estrogen replacement therapy on the risk of breast cancer. *JAMA* 1991; 265: 1985–1990.

30. Grady D, Rubin SM, Petitti DB, et al. Hormone therapy to prevent disease and prolong life in postmenopausal women. *Ann Int Med* 1992; 117: 1016–1037.

31. The Writing Group for the PEPI Trial. Effects of estrogen or estrogen/progestin regimens on heart disease risk factors in postmenopausal women. *JAMA* 1995; 273: 199–208.

32. Sartoris DJ, Resnicj D. Dual-energy radiographic absorptiometry for bone densitometry. Current status and perspective. *Am J Roentgenol* 1989; 152: 241.

33. Hui SL, Slemenda CW, Melton LJ. Baseline measurement of bone mass predicts fracture in white women. *Ann Int Med* 1989; 111: 355–361.

34. U.S. Preventive Services Task Force. *Guide to Clinical Preventive Services,* 2nd ed. Baltimore: Williams & Wilkins, 1996.

35. Muldoon MF, Manuck SB, Matthews KA. Lowering cholesterol concentrations and mortality: a quantitative review of primary prevention trials. *BMJ* 1990; 301: 309–314.

36. Brett AS. Treating hypercholesterolemia: how should practicing physicians interpret the published data for patients? *N Engl J Med* 1989; 321: 676–680.

37. Scandinavian Simvastatin Survival Study Group. Randomized trial of cholesterol lowering in 4444 patients with coronary heart disease: the Scandinavian Simvastatin Survival Study. *Lancet* 1994; 344: 1383–1389.

38. Ettinger B, Friedman GD, Bush T, Quesenberry CP. Reduced mortality associated with long-term postmenopausal estrogen therapy. *Obstet Gynecol* 1996; 87: 6–12.

39. Farmer ME, White LR, Brody JA, et al. Race and sex differences in hip fracture incidence. *Am J Public Health* 1984; 74: 1374–1380.

40. Grisso JA, Kelsey JL, Strom BL, et al. Risk factors for hip fracture in black women. *N Engl J Med* 1994; 330: 1555–1559.

41. Paganini-Hill A, Chao A, Ross RK, et al. Exercise and other factors in the prevention of hip fracture: the leisure world study. *Epidemiology* 1991; 2: 16–25.

42. Holbrook TL, Barrett-Connor E. A prospective study of alcohol consumption and bone mineral density. *BMJ* 1993; 306: 1506–1509.

Appendix 1: Glossary

Alendronate: A third generation bisphosphonate with an amino-terminal substitution on a methyl group off the carbon atom of the P-C-P skeleton; brand name is Fosomax®; approved by the FDA and released for the treatment of osteoporosis on October 15, 1995; single daily dose of 10 mg p.o.q AM 1 h prebreakfast.

Alleles: One of two or more alternative forms of a gene that occupy corresponding loci on homologous chromosomes; for example, there are several *alleles* in the vitamin D receptor gene.

Anterior wedge: A type of fracture where the anterior portion of the vertebral spine is collapsed in a wedge-shaped appearance.

Anti-estrogen: A class of estrogen derivatives that act via the estrogen receptor in a manner that simulate or oppose classic estrogen-like activity; an example of a first generation anti-estrogen is tamoxifen, which blocks estrogen activity on neoplastic breast tissue, but has agonistic properties to estrogen in bone and uterus; second and third generation anti-estrogens (estrogen agonist) are currently in phase II and III studies; these agents also act on estrogen responsive tissues, such as breast and uterus, as well as systemically (blood vessels, bone, elsewhere), but may have differential effects.

Anti-resorptive therapy: Agents that block bone resorption, thereby permitting bone formation to match or transiently exceed resorption. Examples include: estrogens, calcitonin, bisphosphonates.

Ashed bone: The weight of bone after it is ashed in a special oven at high temperature. Ash weight should correspond to actual bone density.

Biochemical markers: A general term that refers to laboratory tests that indirectly measure bone turnover. These markers can be reflective of bone formation (e.g., osteocalcin) or bone resorption (e.g., collagen crosslinks).

Bisphosphonates: The general class of compounds related to the pyrophosphates in which the oxygen middle atom is replaced by a carbon atom to form a P-C-P skeleton. This structure is very avid for calcium and this class of compounds hones into calcium-rich sites, such as bone. There are three generations of bisphosphonates that bind to hydroxyapatite and are potent inhibitors of bone resorption.

Bone mineral density (BMD): The mineral content of bone divided by its volume; by CT measurements this value is reported in mg/mm^3; by DXA (or other methods) it is reported in g/cm^2, which is representative of apparent bone density not strictly true volumetric density; BMD is reported for most areas of the body as spine BMD, hip BMD, total body BMD, wrist BMD, and so on.

Bone remodeling: The physiologic process whereby bone is resorbed and then reformed. This process provides a constant calcium source to the body and keeps the skeleton elastic enough to serve its structural functions. In general, there is no net change in bone mass with physiologic remodeling (resorption = formation), in contrast to modeling where scalloping of bone and addition of new bone is often a characteristic of the growing skeleton.

287

Calcitriol: This is the chemical name for 1,25 dihydroxyvitamin D_3.

Collagen crosslinks: The amino acid links between the three strands of collagen, which are added during the last stage of skeletal maturation; these crosslinks (pyridinoline and deoxypyridinoline) are removed during active bone resorption and are excreted unmetabolized into the urine. These chains and their associated peptides (from the collagen end of the molecule) can be measured by RIA or ELISA and reflect the degree of bone resorption.

Cytokines: Peptides produced by immune cells that act in autocrine, paracrine, or even endocrine fashion to affect cell activity; examples of cytokines include: the interleukin family, tumor necrosis factor, leukemia inhibitory factor, the interferons, colony-stimulating factors, and others. In bone, cytokines may be critical for activation of bone resorption and mediating tumor-induced osteolysis.

Dual-photon absorptiometry: An older method for measuring bone density using a radioactive source (Gd^{154}). It produces two sources of photons to determine bone density; this application has been surpassed by more efficient and less costly DXA machines where X-rays can generate photons necessary to measure bone density.

DXA: Dual energy X-ray absorptiometry (also referred to as DEXA); it uses a conventional X-ray tube to measure density; probably the most precise and accurate tool for measuring BMD currently available.

Ergocalciferol: Vitamin D_2 derived from the radiation of ergosterol, a yeast sterol (in contrast to cholecalciferol, which is derived from radiation of provitamin D_3).

Etidronate: Also called didronel®, a first generation bisphosphonate used in the treatment of Paget's disease and osteoporosis. For osteoporosis, treatment has been cyclical: 2 wk on, 3 mo off; has more capacity to inhibit mineralization than second and third generation agents; usual dose is 400 mg on an empty stomach for 2 wk q 3 mo; several studies have shown improvement in BMD (spine and hip) with some fracture efficacy.

HRT: Hormone replacement therapy, usually implying estrogen + progesterone.

Kyphosis: An abnormal condition of the vertebral column characterized by increased convexity in the curvature of the thoracic spine as viewed from the side. Kyphosis is often associated with osteoporotic thoracic compression fractures although uncommonly it can be caused by tuberculosis or rickets.

Meta-analysis: An analytic method of combining data from published studies to enhance (or reduce) the power of a particular effect; meta-analysis has been used to determine relative risks for particular situations, such as the relative risk of breast cancer with current or past use of estrogen; or the relative risk of coronary artery disease in postmenopausal women; the strengths of meta-analysis are the number of subjects and the diversity from where they are pooled.

N-telopeptide: The N (amino)-terminal end of the Type I collagen fibril is attached to the pyridinoline crosslink. During bone resorption, the N-terminal end (as well as the carboxy terminal, C-terminal) are released from the remaining part of the collagen helix, which is attached to the crosslink. This peptide can be measured in urine and is considered a marker of bone resorption. (The brand name for the marker is NTx or Osteomark®.)

Osteocalcin: the most abundant noncollagen protein in bone; it is synthesized by the osteoblast and is a late differentiation marker of that cell. Osteocalcin synthesis is regulated by several different factors including 1,25 dihydroxyvitamin D_3. The precise function of osteocalcin is unknown. Serum levels of osteocalcin can be used to indirectly determine bone turnover. The assay has high sensitivity and osteocalcin is relatively specific for bone.

However, recent data suggest osteocalcin in serum reflects the degree of bone resorption as well as bone formation (owing to release of stored osteocalcin within the bone matrix).

Osteoblast: The bone cell that is responsible for bone formation. This cell type is derived from mesenchymal stem cells, which can then differentiate into adipocytes or stromal cells. Stromal cells eventually can become osteoblasts through several differentiation steps. The osteoblast can produce collagen products and participates in the mineralization process as well as orchestrating the osteoclast.

Osteoclast: The bone cell responsible for bone resorption. This cell type is derived from a moncyte–macrophage precursor, and under the influence of 1,25 dihydroxyvitamin D_3, certain colony-stimulating factors, and interleukins can differentiate into a mature osteoclast able to secrete protons and resorb bone.

Osteogenesis imperfecta (OI): A genetic disorder involving defective development of the connective tissue. It is inherited as an autosomal dominant trait and is characterized by abnormally brittle and fragile bones that are easily fractured by the slightest trauma. It can be present in one of several different phenotypes (a pure form, a mixed form, or a late onset type) and is associated with translucent skin, hyperextensibility of ligaments, hypoplasia of teeth, epistaxis, easy bruisability, blue sclerae, and hearing loss. Various mutations in Type I collagen are responsible for the abnormalities associated with this condition.

Osteomalacia: Strictly defined as an abnormal condition of the lamellar bone characterized by a loss of calcification of the matrix resulting in softening of the bone, accompanied by weakness, fracture, pain, anorexia, and weight loss. In contrast to osteoporosis (reduction in bone mass) actual BMD is usually normal or only slightly reduced. The problem is a defect in mineralization leading to accumulation of unmineralized osteoid tissue. Although vitamin D deficiency (acquired or inherited) is the most frequent cause of osteomalacia, other conditions are associated with osteomalacia including various genetic disorders. Osteomalacia can co-exist with osteoporosis, especially in elders with vitamin D deficiency.

Osteopenia: Early definition was a reduction in bone mass noted by X-ray; now osteopenia has been considered as a reduction in bone mass measured by any instrument (densitometry, X-ray, radiogrammetry, and so on). The WHO has classified osteopenia as a BMD more than 1 SD below young normal (t-score < -1.0).

Osteopetrosis: An inherited disorder characterized by a generalized increase in bone density almost always related to a defect in bone resorption. In its most severe form, it is inherited as an autosomal recessive disease with almost complete obliteration of the marrow cavity resulting in anemia and marked deformities. The defect in this disorder occurs at the level of the osteoclast.

Peak bone mass: The time when bone acquisition is complete and bone mass is at its optimal point, probably somewhere between 15–25 yr of age.

Pyrophosphates: Naturally occurring compounds with a P-O-P structure. This class of compounds are substrates for pyrophosphatases also found in nature and especially in the skeleton. Pyrophosphates have a strong chemical affinity for calcium.

QCT: Quantitative CT measurements of true bone density (mineral/volume) usually performed in the spine or wrist.

Radiogrammetry: The measurement of dimensions of bone using skeletal radiographs; an example includes the metacarpal index, which is the cortical width divided by total width.

Radiographic absorptiometry (RA): Digitalization of high resolution X-rays with computerization to measure bone density. Currently two hand films are obtained by any X-ray machine and sent to an outside laboratory for digitalization. Accuracy and precision are reported to be excellent. Fracture prediction may be as good as DXA or QCT.

RFLP (restriction fragment length polymorphism): Allelic variation in a given gene owing to normal variations in human DNA that can be recognized by the variation in restriction enzyme patterns. RFLPs for certain alleles have provided insight into the importance of certain relationships between genetic variability and bone density. For example, RFLPs for the VDR gene have been shown to account for some of the variability in bone density among large groups of Caucasians.

RLFP (remaining lifetime fracture probability): This is a value based on meta-analysis and available data, which attempts to relate age, life span, and BMD to predict potential future fracture (*see* Chapter 7 by Wasnich).

Singh Index: A qualititative radiograph indicator of trabecular patterns in the hip.

Single photon absorptiometry (SPA): Use of a single radiation source to determine bone density in wrist; in older machines the source was either I^{125} or americium-241.

***t*-scores:** Units of standard deviation from the mean for bone mineral density compared to healthy 35-yr-old individuals presumably at peak bone mass. A *t*-score value (−5 to +5) is reported on most if not all densitometers at the time of bone density acquisition. A *t*-score of −1.0 is considered the upper limit for osteopenia or lower limit of normal (*see also* Z-score).

Tamoxifen: First generation anti-estrogen widely used to treat breast cancer at various stages; exhibits significant bone-sparing properties; several studies have shown that this drug can prevent bone resorption and lead to a mild increase in BMD among postmenopausal women. Its effect on the uterus is still being determined, although there are several documented cases of endometrial hyperplasia and tumor with continued use of the drug. Tamoxifen is the prototype of the newer anti-estrogens, which may have a greater effect on bone than breast or endometrium.

Type I collagen: the predominant protein within the organic matrix. Type I collagen is tightly bound by collagen crosslinks.

Z-scores: Units of standard deviation from the mean represented by age-, sex-, and height-matched controls. Z-scores tend to be higher than *t*-scores and underestimate the true extent of osteoporosis, since aging itself is associated with a significant reduction in BMD. It is possible to have a low *t*-score and still have a normal Z-score if the person being measured is old. Furthermore, a normal Z-score does not protect the individual from a future hip fracture. For example, an 80-yr-old woman has a BMD of 0.809 g/cm^2, which could translate into a normal Z score for her age but a *t*-score of −2.0. Use of the Z-score has diminished in recent years.

Appendix 2: Costs of Diagnostic Tests and Treatments for Osteoporosis

I. Diagnostic Tests

A. Biochemical Markers—Serum	*Cost*
Osteocalcin	$100–120
Serum irnmunoelectrophoresis	$70
PTH (intact)	$120–150
Calcium (total)	$20
Calcium (ionized)	$75
Alkaline phosphatase (total)	$20 (part of SMA)
Alkaline phosphatase isoenzymes	$67
25 hydroxyvitamin D (250HD)	$150–200
1,25 dihydroxyvitamin D (1,25D)	$195
TSH(second to third generation)	$35–70

B. Biochemical Markers—Urine	
24 h urinary calcium	$20–25
24 h urinary creatinine	$10
24 h collagen crosslinks (total HPLC)	$140
2 h Pyrilinks (free pyridinolines-Metra Biosystems)	N/A
2 h N-telopeptide (N-Tx; Ostex)	$85–110
Urine immunoelectrophoresis	$70

C. Bone Biopsy	
With tetracylcine labeling (total)	$300–800
Interpretation only (no procedure costs)	$200–280

D. Bone Density **	
DXA-1 site	$100–150
DXA-2 sites	$150–300
DXA-3 sites	$200+
Ultrasound of heel	Not available or approved
RA (hands)	$100–150
CT spine bone density	$150–250
pQCT (wrist)	$130–200
SXA	$100–200

*Costs are high/low for reference laboratories (average three reference labs).

**Reimbursed by Medicare in 41 states at different levels; costs of bone density varies according to location, machine, and ownership.

N/A = price not available.

II. Treatment Costs***

Drug	Cost (per 100 unless otherwise stated)
Alendronate (Fosomax®)	$150–200
Calcitonin	
nasal	$28/bottle [2cc] = 14 doses (200 IU/d)
parenteral (Calcimar® and Miacalcin®)	$33–50/bottle [400 IU/bottle]
Estrogen (Premarin®)	$38–43/100
Estrogen + progesterone	
(Provera®—5 mg)	
continuous (PEMPRO®)	$20.70/42 tablets
Estrogen + progesterone	
(Provera®—5 mg)	
cyclic(PEMPHASEX)	$22.32/28 days
Progesterone (10 mg for 14 days)	
Progesterone (Provera®—10 mg)	$12.50
Estrogen (Estraderm®—0.05 mg)	$23.00/28 days
Etidronate (Didronel®)—400 mg tablet	$300–423
Rocaltriol® (0.25 µg)	$39/28 days
Calcium Carbonate (Tums®—500 mg)	$3.50/150 pills
Calcium Carbonate (Oscal®—500 mg)	$9.15/150 pills
Multivitamins (with 400 U vitamin D/d)	$3–10/100

***These are low/high costs from two pharmacies (a discount and a family pharmacy—December 1, 1995 in Bangor, ME); generics are not included.

INDEX

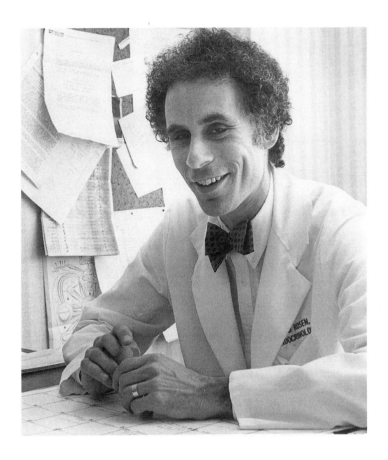

Dr. Clifford J. Rosen is currently Chief of Medicine at St. Joseph Hospital in Bangor, Maine. He is also an Associate Clinical Professor of Medicine at Boston University School of Medicine and Research Professor of Nutrition at the University of Maine. Besides being a practicing endocrinologist, Dr. Rosen is actively collaborating with The Jackson Laboratory in a major effort to map the genes responsible for determination of bone mass. He also conducts an active research program in Bangor, which has focused on the physiology of insulin-like growth factors and their role in skeletal diseases. Dr. Rosen is the author of more than 50 peer-reviewed publications and more than 100 abstracts. He is a member of the Scientific Advisory Board for the National Osteoporosis Foundation, the Public Affairs Committee of the American Society of Bone and Mineral Research, and a former officer of the Society of Clinical Densitometry. Dr. Rosen was recently nominated to Who's Who in Science and Engineering and is well known around the world for his lectures on osteoporosis and metabolic bone diseases.